RESEARCH PROJECT

A Guide to Success

Third Edition

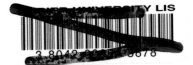

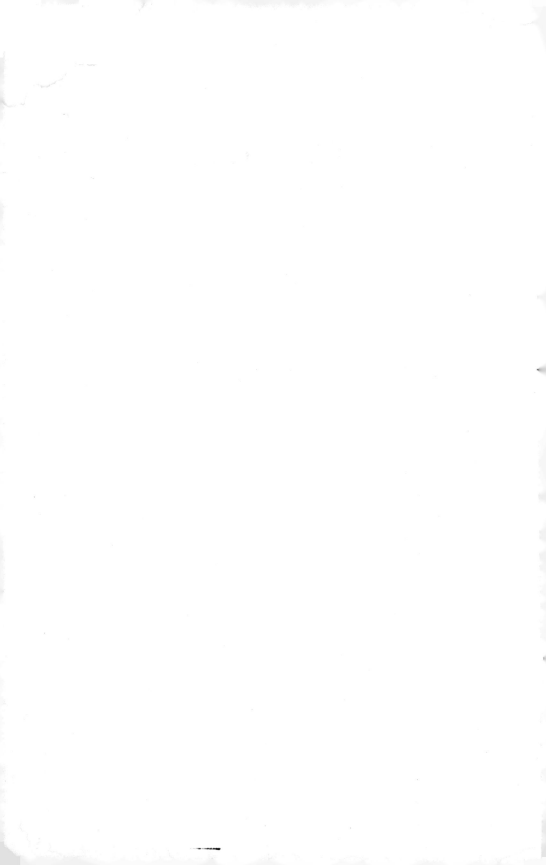

RESEARCH PROPOSALS
A Guide to Success

Third Edition

THOMAS E. OGDEN, M.D., PhD.
Professor Emeritus of Physiology and Biophysics
Keck School of Medicine
University of Southern California
Director of Research Development
Doheny Eye Institute
Los Angeles, California

Israel A. Goldberg, PhD.
President
Health Research Associates
Rockville, Maryland

This book is printed on acid-free paper. ∞

Copyright © 2002, 1995, 1991, Elsevier Science (USA).

Academic Press
An Elsevier Science Imprint
525 B Street, Suite 1900, San Diego, California 92101-4495, USA
http://www.academicpress.com

Academic Press
84 Theobalds Road, London WC1X 8RR, UK
http://www.academicpress.com

Library of Congress Catalog Card Number: 2002100888

International Standard Book Number: 0-12-524733-8

PRINTED IN THE UNITED STATES OF AMERICA
02   03   04   05   06   07   MM   9   8   7   6   5   4   3   2   1

Contents

v

Part Two: Advanced Grantmanship

Appendix

Preface to the First Edition

I learned about the fine art of research proposal preparation the hard way! I submitted a proposal that scored so poorly in priority that it was not funded. This came as a shock after 10 years of uninterrupted funding and a 5-year grant that started in 1967. Unbeknownst to me, the "Golden Years" of the 1960's had come to an end. During those years, funds for research exceeded the needs of the available workers and virtually every approved proposal was funded. A concerted program to interest young scientists in entering the life sciences was underway and very successful by the early 1970's. In the Nixon years, growth of NIH (National Institutes of Health) funding slowed, while the numbers of qualified life scientists burgeoned. There was no longer enough money to support every approved proposal and the process of peer review was taken much more seriously by the reviewers.

Since I had been previously funded, I was granted a site visit. The visiting team was headed by a most remarkable woman, Dr. Marie Jakus, an electron microscopist turned career NIH professional and executive secretary of the Vision Study Section. She made abundantly clear the shortcomings of my 5-page proposal! The visit successfully supplied the omitted information and my proposal was eventually funded. It must have been obvious to Marie that, although my science was credible, I needed exposure to grantsmanship. At any rate, shortly after the visit she invited me to join her study section. This was the beginning of my education in proposal preparation.

Marie was a severe, 90-pound taskmaster and ran her section with an iron, albeit benevolent, hand. She retired from the service before my 4 years as a member of her section were completed so I never received the honor she bestowed on her members at the end of their terms. She was fond of calling her graduation ceremony a "kiss-off " as she bussed them on the cheek! She was an activist and took a special interest in many of the researchers she encountered. This was certainly much to my benefit and I remember her with great fondness.

I received my graduate training in grantsmanship during 4 years as the chairman of BNSB, a special study section for the review of fellowship proposals in the field of vision, and then as grantsman for a rapidly growing eye institute. The experience at this private eye institute included clinical research proposals and institutional grants for core facilities, training, construction, renovation and instrumentation.

During the past 10 years a number of young investigators have been added to our faculty. Each was well trained and had shown evidence to suggest a bright future in science. None of them had been prepared by their training to write a research proposal and I found myself tutoring each in succession in the basics of proposal preparation. They have been successful but still benefit from inhouse review, a process which we have used to great advantage, but which I find peculiarly lacking in most departments and institutions. This is a surprising state-of-affairs since the institution derives great benefit from the success of its faculty in obtaining funds.

This book is an attempt to pass along a precious gift from Marie Jakus. It is a philosophy of support, probably somewhat paternalistic, for the efforts of scientists to gain research funding. It is based on the premise that those who are successful in the system have a responsibility to those, particularly the young ones, who are not. There is nothing controversial here since the principles of good grantsmanship are as universal as are those of good fellowship.

In a way, this book is a symptom of the times, of a growing malaise within the life-sciences research industry. Technology is progressing rapidly in sophistication and expense, and with it research budgets are escalating. Federal support for research in the life-sciences, however, has failed to keep pace with the demand. In part this is the direct result of a decision made several years ago to lengthen the duration of grants. The motivation for the decision was good: improvement of funding stability for the better investigators and reduction of paperwork. The result has been a disaster for biomedical research. In the past few years the average length of the individual research grant has increased from 3 to 4 years. Since funds are committed for the duration of the award, this has effectively reduced the funds available for new and competing awards by about 25%, and the overall award rate (the percent of approved proposals that are actually funded) of the NIH has fallen from 51.6% in 1979 to 35.3% in 1989, a 32% decrease!

Congress has been generous in maintaining funding levels against the inroads of inflation. In constant dollars, average awards for R01 grants (including indirect costs) rose from \$92,200 in 1979 to \$101,600 in 1989, an increase of 100% in excess of inflation. Congress has not provided additional funds to compensate for the longer duration of grants. Thus there is chronic starvation for research funds throughout academia. Graduate programs are languishing in many institutions for need of superior students or are filled with foreign students of marginal background. Employment opportunities in life-sciences research are so limited that one cannot in good conscience encourage students to enter the field. Those committed to such careers must accept the necessity of being selfsupporting.

Sources of support are severely limited. The only major source of funds for non-directed research in the life-sciences is the National Institutes of Health. The National Science Foundation (NSF) and the military provide some funds for life-sciences research, and private foundations also contribute. But the NIH is the primary source, at once easier and more difficult to master than the others. Easier because the peer review system used by the NIH is more predictable; more difficult because many more proposals are considered by the NIH, comparisons between proposals are more direct and the competition is probably greater. With assignment of priority scores differing by only 0. 1 point, funding may be dependent on differences in average scores as small as 0.01 point.

The focus of this book is the NIH system. Other sources of support are considered, but in less depth. The bottom line of the NIH review system is the priority score: 1.0 to 5.0, with 1.0 being best. NIH Institutes fund research according to availability of funds and priority rank of individual proposals within the group. It is unlikely that proposals with very poor priority scores can be improved sufficiently through good grantsmanship to be fundable. Such proposals are usually scientifically flawed. There is a mid-range of proposals, however, with good scores by any standard but that fall outside the funding cut-off range. Without exception, the priority scores of these proposals can be improved by better proposal preparation. This is true because no research proposal is perfect; proposals are written against a submission deadline, and although they represent the best efforts of the investigator given a host of conflicting time demands, there is always excess verbiage that can be trimmed and organization that can be tightened. Time management and commitment to the attainment of established goals are the basis of good grantsmanship. These are areas in which virtually everyone can stand some improvement.

This book is organized into three sections. Part I, Basic Grantsmanship

(Chapters 1-15), includes the R01 or individual research grant of the National Institutes of Health, National Science Foundation, private foundation, and military grants for research. Part II, Advanced Grantsmanship (Chapters 16-25), includes other NIH grant mechanisms. Part III is kind of an after thought. It contains some advice for young scientists at the brink of their first university appointment. Part I is directed to novice and unsuccessful applicants. Part II is directed to experienced investigators who may be applying for an institutional grant such as a Core Center, Training, or Construction Grant for the first time. The Appendix contains support material pertinent to a variety of grant mechanisms, and a fairly lengthy description of the categorical programs of each of the NIH institutes.

Some of the ideas expressed in this manual may seem a bit heretical or even cynical. I believe in the great value to society of scientific research, and I know how great are the personal rewards to the successful researcher. But I have also seen far too much scientific talent directed into other endeavors because of lack of funds. Without funds, there can be no research. The ideas expressed in this book are practical and, when used appropriately, will result in better proposals and a greater likelihood of funding. This is the end that justifies the means. There is a good deal of repetition in this book. It is intentional. The things that are repeated are presented in different settings, and, I think, bear repeating. Also, I expect each chapter to stand on its own. If a chapter is reread in the process of writing a section of a proposal, it should have all the salient points in it, hence the repetition.

I've tried to imagine how a new investigator would use this material. If you are preparing for an R01 proposal, I think the way to start is to read right through Chapters 1-15. You will see that I advise starting a proposal by writing down the Specific Aims page. Refer back to this chapter as this is done. When the Specific Aims are under control, proceed to the section on Experimental Design, rereading this chapter as the protocol is developed. You will probably want to do the Methods section next, then the Background and Significance section. The Experimental Design and the Background and Significance sections should follow the presentation and logic of the Specific Aims exactly. I suggest doing the Preliminary Data section after the other sections to facilitate incorporation of last minute findings and, hopefully, submitted manuscripts. When this section is finished, compare it with the Methods section and eliminate any repetitions. Finally complete the listing of Literature Cited, Biographical Sketch, and Budget. The last part I usually prepare is the Budget Justification. Base this justification on the Experimental Design section, and if you are tight for pages, consider moving some of the experimental design verbiage to the Budget Justification, as a table of procedures. These ideas are expanded in Chapter 4.

T. E. Ogden

= Preface to the Second Edition =

The principles of good grantsmanship do not change. Bureaucracies and bureaucrats do change. The NIH R01 grant situation has changed dramatically during the past 5 years. This second edition reflects those changes. It is difficult for an "outsider" (outside the Beltway) to keep current with NIH affairs. Because I am convinced that familiarity with the inner workings of the NIH is essential for successful grantsmanship, I have persuaded Israel Goldberg to co-author this edition. He was an NIH senior administrator for 13 years and for the past 8 years has established a grants consulting business. He has maintained many friendships and contacts within the NIH bureaucracy and is largely responsible for the accuracy of the latest NIH data presented herein.

Although we have made some minor changes in the chapters, and added current data, the basic grantsmanship section of the book is largely unchanged. A new chapter on Small Business Innovation Research (SBIR) grants has been added to the section on Advanced Grantsmanship.

The major changes in the grants process that have taken place are: (a) In 1993 only 11.5% of new proposals and 38.4% of competing renewals were funded on the initial submission. Second and third revisions were common and the overall award rate was 21.8%. Most of the proposals seen by any Study Section now are revised, and the necessity of planning for revision has taken on new importance; (b) The NIH now allows 25 pages of Research Plan, but the NSF has reduced the allowable pages to 15 and suggests reduction in descriptions of methods; (c) Study Sections are requested to consider the overall cost of a project in deciding its relative merit; (d) Proposals that previously would have been disapproved are classified as "not recommended for further consideration"; (e) Under a recent trial innovation, proposals that are considered by the primary reviewers to lack sufficient merit to be in the top half of their group are no longer presented to the entire IRG (triage), and are not assigned a priority score.

The dire consequences of our current climate of severe competition for funds are now apparent as a drastic reduction in the numbers of proposals submitted by young investigators. In 1985, 3,826 proposals (20% of the total) were submitted by investigators age 36 years or less. In 1993 this cohort submitted only 2,177 proposals (10% of the total). In 1985 1,308 of these young investigators were funded, but in 1993 only 527 were funded, a decrease of 60%! During these years, the overall success rate for all investigators declined from 31.4% to 22.6%, but the total numbers of individual research proposals (R01, R23, R29) submitted increased 14%, from 18,803 to 21,506. Much of this increase resulted from submission of revised proposals. In 1993 NIH (excluding NIAAA, NIDA, and NIMH) received 10,114 new R01 proposals; 6,945 were original first submissions. The success rate of these was 11.5%. First revisions numbered 2,342; these had a success rate of 21.4%. Second or third revisions numbered 881; and these had a success rate of 29.4%.

The relative number of revised competitive renewal R01 proposals in 1993 was even higher. Of 4,525 competitive renewal proposals received, 2,627 were original and 1,898 (42%!) were revised. The success rate of the initial submissions was 38.4% (competitive renewals always do better in review); that for first revision was 32.7% and for second revision, 35.7%. Some proposals endured as many as seven revisions in order to achieve funding.

There is wide recognition of the increasing importance of grantsmanship. Revised proposals are usually improved (in the perception of the reviewers) by attention to the suggestions of the reviewers. With the submission of so many revisions, proposal standards have reached a new high. The young investigator must submit a very strong proposal in order to be competitive. This is only possible with a base of knowledge about how the system works and how it is changing. This second addition is much improved in providing additional insight into the NIH grant system that we believe to be essential for the beginning proposal writer.

T. E. Ogden

Preface

It is still true. The basics of good grantsmanship do not change. The NIH is still the main supporter of non-directed life-science research, and the R01 grant is still the gold standard of research support. Technology does change. The Internet has drastically improved access to technical papers and government information. The advent of molecular studies culminating in gene array analysis and gene therapy has moved the frontiers of science far and fast. Studies at the molecular level abound and even the clinician must speak molecularese to stay on the "cutting edge". So, like the second edition, this third edition differs from the others mainly in the details of proposal preparation and review.

Recent changes have resulted in shortening of some chapters and the addition of others. The modular budget is here to stay. Annual budgets under $250,000 are considered in "modules" of $25,000, without itemization or justification of supplies, travel or other expenses. Individual salaries are not stated. This makes the budgeting process much simpler. By the time this edition is published, electronic submission of proposals will probably be general. The trend to the necessity for revision continues, although the approval rates are better with about 25% of new proposals making the funding level on the first try.

Triage, or "streamlining," also is here to stay. Those proposals that the reviewers consider to be in the bottom half of the group are not reviewed by the Study Section. They are returned without a priority score, but with critiques. We have enough experience with this system to be able to assure investigators that triage is not disapproval. Chances for funding of a triaged proposal are excellent, and we know of at least one triaged proposal that received the best priority score of the group when it was revised and resubmitted.

A major change in this edition is the omission of the data concerning Study Sections. These are available on the Internet; we provide the addresses. Since use of the Internet is as basic to good grantsmanship as use of a word processor, references to it occur throughout the book.

xv

The competition is still keen. Standards are higher than ever. Successful proposals are usually well written with hypothesis based, scientifically sound experiments and strong Preliminary Data for support. However, even if revision is necessary, prospects for funding have never been better!

T. E. Ogden
I. A. Goldberg

Part One: Beginning Grantsmanship

The 19 chapters that comprise Part One present discussions of funding sources for which research proposals should be designed, the nature of a strong proposal, and the process of peer review. We believe that the successful proposal is written with an eye to the perspective of the reviewer, and that the review process must be considered as the proposal is composed. Following these introductory chapters, each section of the NIH R01 PHS 398 form is discussed in detail.

1

The NIH and Other Sources of Research Support

This manual is all about raising money for research in the life sciences. Any quest for funds must begin with detailed knowledge of the possible sources of those funds. There are five primary sources of biomedical research support in the United States. Historically about one-third of support has come from the 22 grant-making components of the National Institutes of Health (NIH), and about 10% from other federal sources, such as the National Science Foundation (NSF) and the military. Today, more than half of the dollars spent on biomedical research in the United States comes from industry, and about 10% comes from all other sources, primarily private foundations. Entry into the NIH and the NSF systems is easy since all procedures are standard and the nature of the required proposal is specified exactly. All that is required is to obtain an application packet either directly (see Appendix A) or through your university.

Many military programs support research, but these are difficult to find and the proposal format may not be obvious. Individual Program Directors must be contacted. Ideas for proposals should be discussed with the appropriate director and a proposal submitted only if one is requested. Identification of the appropriate director can involve a good deal of legwork. Similarly, although there are thousands of philanthropic foundations in the United States, few of them support biomedical research projects and many of them do not accept unsolicited proposals. Many will fund specific pieces of equipment, however. Direct contact with a member of the foundation selection committee very substantially increases the likelihood of success, but this also will entail considerable effort for relatively small returns. Industrial support of research is generally highly goal oriented. Drug companies sponsor much of the clinical research done in medical school departments of medicine. Investigators may be approached by a company with a defined study in hand. A contract is negotiated with the institution, and no proposal is needed beyond that required by the Institutional Review Board (IRB) or Institutional Animal Care and Use Committee (IACUC). Basic scientists may find it possible to fund a technician's salary from industrial sources in exchange for service, and this may strengthen a laboratory. Scientists fortunate enough to work in fields with commercial relevance may be able to support their laboratories from royalties. Unfortunately most industrial support for research is expended in-house and is not available to researchers at academic institutions.

Since the vast majority of investigator-initiated, competitively funded biomedical research is supported by NIH grants, and these are obtained using the PHS 398 proposal packet, this book is largely devoted to the perfection of the R01 grant proposal. The basic principles of grantsmanship, however, apply to virtually all research proposals:

- An obviously qualified, expert, productive investigator
- A proposal tailored to the funding source, and its review
- A literate, focused, well-organized, interesting proposal
- Important hypotheses, effectively tested
- State-of-the-art science

NIH ORGANIZATION

Understanding the organization of the NIH is an essential part of success in this system. Both the Center for Scientific Review (CSR) and a NIH Institute are involved in the awarding of research grants (Figure 1.1). Scientific merit is evaluated by peer review groups called Study Sections. These are part of the CSR. The reviewed proposals, ranked according to merit, are then sent to one or more Institutes for funding. The proposals are reviewed again by the Institute Scientific Advisory Council. This body evaluates whether the Study Section review was fair, and whether the proposed work has high program relevance. The council then recommends funding, usually in accordance with the Study Section ranking. Thus, there is a dual review, and administrative separation between scientific merit and funding decisions.

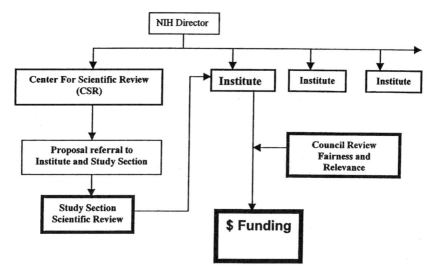

Figure 1.1. NIH dual proposal review system.

NIH CENTER FOR SCIENTIFIC REVIEW (CSR)

R01 proposals are reviewed by Study Sections that are constituted by the CSR. These Study Sections also review other types of proposals. Some of the other grant programs, such as the Program Project, are usually reviewed by Study Sections constituted by the Institute that would be involved in funding the project, as shown in Table 1.1.

The administrators of the Study Sections are concerned primarily with the scientific merit of the proposal under review. They have nothing to do with the funding of the grant and may not be very knowledgeable about the funding priorities of a particular program. Information about the nature of the proposal and questions about its review are the concern of the CSR personnel and should be addressed to the Study Section Scientific Review Administrator (SRA). The SRA is the person to call when late material needs to be added to a proposal or when there is a question concerning the review process or deadlines. Thus, until it is reviewed, an individual research proposal is the responsibility of the Study Section. After it is reviewed, the responsibility for a proposal is passed to an Institute, and questions about it should be addressed to Institute personnel. About 6 weeks after the submission deadline, a notice will be received

Table 1.1 *Peer Review of NIH Grants: A Partial List of Grant Types*

	Reviewed by Center for Scientific Review		Reviewed by Institutes
R01	Research Grant	P01	Program Project Grant
P01	Program Project Grant	P20, P30, P50, P60	Center Grants
F32, F33	Postdoctoral Fellowship Individual NRSA	K01, K02, K05, K07	Career Development
		K08, K23, K24	Mentored Clinical Scientist Development Awards
R15	Academic Research Enhancement Award		
S10	Instrumentation Award	T32	Institutional Training Grants (Institutional NRSA)
R43, R44	Small Business Innovation Research (SBIR) Award		
		T35	Institutional Short-Term Training Grant
R41, R42	Small Business Technology Transfer (STTR) Award	K12	Mentored Clinical Scientist Development Program
		R01	Requests for Applications (RFA)
		R03	Small Grants
		R13	Conference Grants
		R21	Development or Planning Grants
		U10	Cooperative Agreement Awards for Clinical Trials
		N01	Contract Awards, Requests for Proposals (RFP)

Application Type	Activity Code	Awarding Unit	Serial Number	Year of support	Suffixes
1	R01	HL	12345	01	A1
New grant application	Regular Research	NHLBI	12,345th NHLBI proposal	First year	First amended proposal

Figure 1.2. The components of an example NIH application number: 1 R01 HL12789-01A1.

identifying the Study Section and Institute(s) to which the proposal has been assigned. The telephone numbers of the SRA and the CSR are also provided, and the proposal is assigned a number.

The assignment notice should be carefully scrutinized to make sure that the proposal has been assigned to the appropriate Study Section and Institute (Figure 1.2). The proposal number will indicate whether the pro-

Table 1.2 *Institute Abbreviations*

AA	National Institute on Alcohol Abuse and Alcoholism	NIAAA
AG	National Institute on Aging	NIA
AI	National Institute of Allergy and Infectious Diseases	NIAID
AR	National Institute of Arthritis and Musculoskeletal and Skin Diseases	NIAMS
AT	National Center for Complementary and Alternative Medicine	NCCAM
CA	National Cancer Institute	NCI
DA	National Institute on Drug Abuse	NIDA
DC	National Institute on Deafness and Other Communicative Disorders	NIDCD
DE	National Institute of Dental and Craniofacial Research	NIDCR
DK	National Institute of Diabetes and Digestive and Kidney Diseases	NIDDK
ES	National Institute of Environmental Health Sciences	NIEHS
EY	National Eye Institute	NEI
GM	National Institute of General Medical Sciences	NIGMS
HD	National Institute of Child Health and Human Development	NICHD
HG	National Human Genome Research Institute	NHGRI
HL	National Heart, Lung and Blood Institute	NHLBI
LM	National Library of Medicine	NLM
MH	National Institute of Mental Health	NIMH
NR	National Institute of Nursing Research	NINR
NS	National Institute of Neurological Disorders and Stroke	NINDS
RR	National Center for Research Resources	NCRR
CT	Center for Information Technology	CIT
TW	John E. Fogarty International Center	FIC
	Center for Scientific Review (formerly Division of Research Grants, or DRG)	CSR

posal is new (Type 1), a renewal (Type 2), or a supplement (Type 3). The grant type (e.g., R01), the funding Institute (using the two-letter initial shown in Table 1.2), and the identification number are also shown. The support year (01 for a new proposal) and an abbreviation showing if the proposal is amended (revised) from, or a supplement to, a previous submission (A1 for a first revision) complete the number.

NIH PROPOSAL ASSIGNMENT

Upon receipt of a proposal, an Assignment Officer of the CSR makes a decision concerning its categorical nature and assigns it to a particular Study Section and to an Institute. The assignment is made largely according to key words in the proposal title, the Abstract, and the Specific Aims. These assignments are thus sometimes inappropriate and may not be in the interest of a fair review. For instance, a primarily clinical project that involves a small amount of basic research will do much better in a primarily clinical Study Section. The importance of the work may be clinical and not appreciated by nonclinical basic scientists who might well regard the basic science part of the proposal as uninteresting—"not on the cutting edge." If such a proposal were assigned to a basic science-oriented Study Section, the investigator should contact the SRA and request that the proposal be transferred to a section with a stronger clinical orientation. The request probably will be successful if there is another Study Section with sufficient expertise in the area of the research proposed, and if that Study Section is not already overloaded with proposals.

To ensure that proper assignment has been made, the investigator must be familiar with the members of the assigned Study Section. This information is available in the NIH publications on the Internet (<www.nih.gov>). About 25% of the members of a Study Section are new each year, and each session may have a number of additional ad hoc members. Thus, the SRA is the only person with up-to-date information about the membership of the Study Section for any given review. A request should be made to the SRA for a copy of the current roster if the Internet posting is not current. If there is likely to be a choice made between two Study Sections that could review the proposal, the covering letter sent to the CSR with the proposal packet should specifically request the Study Section preferred by the investigator. Provide an explicit explanation for your request. These requests are generally honored, if appropriate, and actually assist the Assignment Officer.

If the constitution of the Study Section seems weak or biased in the area of your proposal, and it cannot be reassigned to a more appropriate Study Section, you should request that an outside reviewer be used. Suggest several names of appropriate reviewers who are at institutions other than yours (and whose surnames and affiliations differ from yours). The SRA may also opt to add an ad hoc reviewer with expertise in your area for this one meeting, if there are several such requests. The SRAs are very sensitive to charges that a review was in any way unfair, and make every effort to avoid this. They are usually responsive to requests for changes if such can be incorporated into the regular budget of a scheduled meeting.

If satisfaction in assignment is not obtained, the appropriate Program Director of the Institute that would fund the research should be contacted and asked to intervene. A call from a Program Director (or Institute official) to the CSR will sometimes get attention and could produce the desired results. Many proposals could be funded from any of several Institutes. For instance, an R01 proposal concerning the molecular biology of

Table 1.3 *Institute FY 2000 Award Rates for All Grants and for R01 Grants (%)*

Institute	R01	All awards
NEI	43	42
NHGRI	42	43
NIDCD	41	40
NINDS	37	37
NIDA	37	38
NIGMS	37	37
NINR	35	32
NIAAA	35	31
NHLBI	33	35
NCCAM	32	29
NIAID	31	36
NIEHS	30	29
NIMH	29	29
NIAMS	28	27
NICHD	28	29
NCI	27	26
NIDDK	27	28
NIA	26	26
NIDCR	25	27
NCRR	15	18
Award rate for all of NIH	**31**	**32**

pulmonary endothelial cells could be funded by the NIGMS (37% award rate), or it could be funded by the NHLBI, which had an award rate of 33% in 2000. Obviously, there is an advantage in assignment to the NIGMS. As shown in Table 1.3, R01 award rates for the different Institutes varied from 43% (NEI) to 15% (NCRR) in fiscal year (FY) 2000. You must be familiar with the general funding status of your Institute and with the members of your Study Section to ensure that you have the best review circumstances. Finally, it may be advantageous to have a proposal assigned to more than one Institute, and this may be requested. In the case of such dual assignments, if the first Institute does not fund the proposal, it may be passed to the second for funding. Thus, for instance, an excellent proposal on the optic neuropathy associated with cancer not funded by the National Cancer Institute (NCI) because the appropriate program was oversubscribed might be picked up by the National Eye Institute (NEI) for funding. Dual assignment can increase the probability of funding.

INSTITUTES AND CENTERS

The grant-making part of the NIH consists of 22 Institutes or Centers and the National Library of Medicine. They are identified by a two-letter initial in official communications and grant numbers, and by a three- to five-letter initial in the literature (Table 1.2).

The Fogarty International Center makes grant awards, but does not use the R01 mechanism. Other governmental agencies that support individual research grant or contract programs are the National Centers for Disease Control (CDC), the Occupational, Safety and Health Administration (OSHA), and the Agency for Healthcare Research and Quality (AHRQ). Their programs are smaller than those of the NIH and have a slightly different form of review, but do use the PHS 398 application kit.

The mission of the Institutes is to promote research for the prevention and cure of human disease. However, most diseases are incurable in our present state of knowledge. Prevention and cure can be achieved, but only with a fundamental knowledge of all aspects of human biology. This fact justifies NIH funding of a variety of basic research projects in biology and all related disciplines such as bioengineering, behavioral sciences, and biomaterials. Human models of many diseases are not appropriate as research tools, so a number of animal or *in vitro* models are used, including invertebrate and computer models where appropriate.

Each NIH Institute has a budget with a number of line items, each funding a categorical program. The funds within that program are distributed as different types of grants, with a substantial fraction going to the R01 individual research grant. Larger or smaller amounts, varying with the Institute, go to support Program Project Grants, Career Awards, fellowships, contracts, etc. As an example, the major categorical programs of the NEI are six: Lens and Cataract; Corneal Diseases; Glaucoma; Retinal and Choroidal Diseases; Strabismus, Amblyopia and Visual Processing; and Collaborative Clinical Research. The NIAID, in contrast, has some 30 separate programs of research support. Funds may be transferred among the programs, in proportion to the number of proposals submitted. Prospects for funding are best in programs that receive the fewest good applications relative to the size of their budgets.

The extramural grant programs of the NIH are described in Internet publications of the NIH, and the categorical programs of all of the Institutes are summarized there (<www.nih.gov/icd>). It is essential that researchers be familiar with the programs and the Program Directors (Health Scientist Administrators) of the Institute that could fund their research. The NEI has published and widely distributed a detailed plan of vision research priorities with information concerning the number of currently funded grants in a program, recent accomplishments, and important research questions to be addressed. This publication was developed by the National Advisory Council of the NEI. It is a great help in targeting relatively undeveloped areas of research. The NEI is the only Institute with such a detailed publication. Information concerning the programs of other Institutes must be gleaned from a variety of sources. Brochures, the Institute Program Directors, colleagues who are familiar with a particular program, Program Announcements (PAs), and notices or Requests for Applications (RFAs) published on the Internet are helpful. The NIH Guide (<http://grants.nih.gov/grants/guide/index.html>) may also be helpful. It is updated on a weekly basis.

Some of the many types of NIH research grants are listed in Table 1.1. The various Institutes frequently fund research grants through RFAs, using funds set aside for specific areas of research targeted by their councils. These mechanisms of support are discussed in later chapters. The NIH also occasionally solicits Research and Development contracts for specific research projects. These Requests for Proposals

(RFPs) are advertised on the Internet and in the *Commerce Business Daily*. Proposals relevant to these different mechanisms are reviewed by Study Sections of either the CSR or the Institute responsible for the funding (see Table 1.1). *Of these programs, only the R01 grant is likely to be useful for long-term support of the beginning investigator in a university setting.*

Most, but not all, grant mechanisms use the standard application package (PHS 398) that can be obtained from the Grants and Contracts Office of your university in hard copy or computer friendly format. The entire application kit, and forms suitable for electronic submission, can be obtained from the NIH in PDF format at <http://grants.nih.gov/grants/forms.htm> or in Word/Excel format from <http://tram.east.asu.edu>. If the latter is used, be sure to scroll down to "NIH" on the Agency Forms page, and click on "Mac" or "PC" to obtain the appropriate pages. Before submitting an application in any program for the first time, the Program Director of the appropriate Institute should be contacted. The Internet lists the officers of every NIH organization and identifies contacts in each Institute designated to answer a variety of specific questions. Follow the links to home pages of the various Institutes and Centers at <www.nih.gov>. These program officers are very interested in promoting their programs and in increasing the numbers of submitted applications that qualify for their programs. Their advice concerning details of the proposal is usually very good and they are often generous with their time in helping a new investigator. When appropriate Program Directors have been identified, call them and request that they look over your Biosketch and a brief summary of your proposed research. Ask for some advice concerning the most appropriate funding mechanism or other more appropriate funding sources. You have nothing to lose and everything to gain by being proactive.

Advisory Council

The NIH uses a dual system of review designed to provide balance and prevent conflict of interest (Figure 1.1). While the Study Section evaluates the proposal for scientific merit and the appropriateness of the budget, it is involved in the decision of whether or not to fund only in the sense of a triage. Thus those proposals designated "not competitive" will not be funded. The recommendation for funding of the remainder comes from the Advisory Council of the Institute that will provide the funds. The various Institute councils usually meet about 3 months after the Study Sections. Their charge is to evaluate each proposal for *relevance* to Institute programs and *fairness* of review, and to recommend whether or not it should be funded. In fact, the councils concur with the Study Section recommendations by *en bloc* action in over 95% of the R01 proposals, and it is estimated that over 98% of decisions concerning funding of R01s are based on Study Section priority scores. The relative ranking (percentile) of a proposal may be improved at the discretion of the council if the proposed research has high program relevance in an area that is underfunded. This will greatly improve prospects of funding. The council also evaluates the adequacy of the review. They may request a rereview if they feel the Study Section lacked adequate expertise or was biased in its judgment. The council may also recommend that budget changes suggested by the Study Section be rescinded. The specific recommendations of the council to the Institute staff are almost always followed to the letter.

Advisory Councils are also impaneled to make recommendations to the Institutes concerning strategic planning and identification of future areas of important research, preparation of Institute budgets for congressional action, and general matters of policy. Subcommittees of some Institute Advisory Councils may be delegated the task of reviewing special categories of proposals such as those for Center grants, Training grants, and grants for clinical trials or facility construction. The councils of the NIDDK and NHLBI have subcommittees to review proposals in each major division or program (digestive diseases, lung diseases, etc.). Institute council members, like Study Section members, are appointed to staggered 4-year terms. Council members tend to be senior scientists and clinicians, and often chairpersons of their respective university departments. The councils also include two or more nonscientist members of the public.

NATIONAL SCIENCE FOUNDATION

The NSF, through its Directorate for Biological Sciences, also funds bioscience research programs—if the subject is sufficiently basic, and has no direct relation to medicine or disease. Generally, funding is at a much lower level than that with the NIH. The NSF has an annual budget of about $4 billion, of which about 10% ($414 million in 2000) is used to fund research in biological sciences. In 2000, $34 million was used for bioengineering and environment sciences, $45 million for research in behavioral and cognitive sciences, and $61 million for social and economic sciences. The peer review system used by the NSF differs fundamentally from that of the NIH and it makes very good sense to submit proposals to both organizations, tailored to the requirements of either the NSF or the NIH. Duplicate or similar proposals will be accepted from beginning investigators but not from scientists who have already received federal grant support. It is not that uncommon for a proposal to receive a poor priority score from one group and a fundable score from the other.

Medical Research Is Ineligible

However, many of the basic science proposals submitted to the NIH could also be submitted to the NSF. It is only necessary that they be rewritten to emphasize their basic importance and deemphasize their clinical or health-related relevance. An example is an NIH-type study of the distribution of nerve fibers of various sizes within the optic nerve. Such a study is of importance to understanding the pathogenesis of nerve fiber loss in glaucoma. It might involve a primate model with experimentally induced ocular hypertension. As an NSF alternative, however, the same study could test hypotheses concerning the origin of retinotopy and guidance of developing axons to target organs. The latter study could involve any species, including the primate. Details of NSF applications and programs are available on the Internet (follow the links at <www.nsf.gov>).

The NSF Guide to Programs (NSF 01-2; available at the NSF website) states,

> The foundation considers proposals for support of research and education in engineering and any field of science, including but not necessarily limited to astronomy, atmospheric sciences, biological and behavioral sciences, chemistry, computer sciences and engineering, earth sciences, information science and engineering, materials research, mathematical sciences, oceanography, physics and social sciences. Interdisciplinary proposals also are eligible for consideration. Research with disease-related goals, including work on the etiology, diagnosis or treatment of physical or mental disease, abnormality or malfunction in human beings or animals,

is normally not supported. Animal models of such conditions, or the development or testing of drugs or other procedures for their treatment also are not eligible for support. Research in bioengineering, with diagnosis or treatment related goals, however, that applies engineering principles to problems in biology or medicine while advancing engineering knowledge is eligible for support. Bioengineering research to aid persons with disabilities also is eligible for support.

Since many projects are suitable for either NSF or NIH funding, beginning investigators should submit proposals to both agencies at the same time, particularly if prospects for NIH funding are marginal. The box "Beginning Investigator" on the cover sheet (Form 1207) should also be checked. Those who have previously held a federal research grant cannot submit simultaneous proposals to both agencies.

The same principles of grantsmanship apply to both NSF and NIH proposals. The Research Plan section of the NIH proposal [25 pages long and containing (a) Specific Aims, (b) Background and Significance, (c) Preliminary Studies/Progress Report, and (d) Research Design and Methods sections] can be used virtually as is in the NSF proposal, but must be reduced in length from 25 to 15 pages. Thus, the labor of duplicating a proposal for the NSF is minimal, and well worth the result of possibly doubling your chances of funding. NSF programs are headed by Program Directors who can and should be contacted before an application is submitted. The Program Directors will provide essential assistance concerning the appropriateness of the research and the budget. The latter is particularly important since the NSF budget is smaller than the NIH budget and the probability of funding is somewhat dependent on budget size. *Typical NSF research budgets in Biology range from $50,000 to $150,00 in total costs per year for 3 years.*

Reviewers used by the NSF are experts in their field of fundamental biology. Most or all of them will be funded by NIH grants and many will have been members of NIH Study Sections. They are accustomed to seeing R01-type proposals and will appreciate adherence to that format. The 10-page difference in length must be absorbed by the Preliminary Studies and Methods sections. The reviewers must specifically comment on "the effect of the activity on the infrastructure of science, engineering and education," as well as its broad impact on society. In most biomedical research, this impact should be shown not in relation to health issues, but rather in relation to the field of study.

To take full advantage of the possibility of NSF support, the various

Table 1.4 *2000 NSF Funding for Biological Sciences (Dollars in Millions)*

Molecular and Cellular Biosciences	105
Integrative Biology and Neural Sciences	95
Environmental Biology	90
Biology Infrastructure	65
Other	59
Biological Sciences Total	**414**

Source: Fiscal Year 2001 NSF Budgetary Request.

programs must be understood. The best information about each program, particularly whether it is over- or underutilized, can be obtained in direct conversation with the Program Director.

The distribution of funds among the various components of the NSF Biological Sciences Program (Table 1.4) is instructive of where emphasis is placed.

NSF proposals are classified as new, renewal, or equipment. Submission is by institution, and any group qualified for an NIH submission is eligible. In addition, the NSF will accept proposals from unaffiliated individuals, who ordinarily may not apply to the NIH. Such individuals should contact an NSF official before applying.

Instrumentation grants are an excellent way to fund expensive core equipment such as computer systems, DNA synthesizers, electron microscopes, and confocal microscopes. The equipment should support a multidisciplinary group doing funded research in one or more NSF-supported areas. The comments of Chapter 25 on NIH instrumentation grants apply equally to those from the NSF.

Small Grants for Exploratory Research (SGER) may be requested. These are limited to $100,000 for 1 year and use an abbreviated proposal subject to administrative review only. The individual Program Manager must be contacted. These grants are designed to support pilot studies leading to full grant proposals.

Deadlines are announced but are not always observed by most NSF programs. The review process generally takes about 6 months.

MILITARY SOURCES

The Army, Navy, and Air Force each have a program for review and funding of unsolicited proposals involving biomedical research. Preproposal letters are accepted at any time. Success relates directly to the relevance of the project to well-defined, but often changed, service interests. It is essential that a preproposal letter be sent in first, that the appropriate program officer be identified and contacted, and that a proposal be requested by the officer. There is a good probability that requested proposals will be funded. Once established, military support is often long-term and levels of support can be negotiated at any time. These are a stable and generous means of support. Unfortunately, these grants also are limited in number and can be obtained only by those whose research is related to a military objective. Uncertainty about the programs mandates close contact with the program managers.

Occasionally, military biomedical research programs are mandated by Congress to address politically "hot" topics such as AIDS or breast cancer, or to support specific research at a specific institution in a senator's state or a congressman's district. Some of these initiatives allow neither open competition nor peer review, some require peer review but are noncompetitive, and others may be so public and extensive that open competition and scientific peer review must be carried out. An example is the annual appropriation, beginning in 1993, of more than $200,000,000 for the US-AMRMC to conduct research on breast cancer. The Army Medical Directorate wisely sought the advice of the Institute of Medicine of the National Research Council on how best to distribute this bounty, and an openly competitive, peer-reviewed program was initiated. In 2001, these Congressionally Designated Medical Research Programs also included prostate cancer and other research areas, for a total of $400 million. Unless your institution is actively lobbying for your research program, or is unusually fine-tuned to congressional "pork barrel" projects, the best source of advance information about such programs is the News section of *Science* or *Nature*.

It is also possible to obtain research support in the form of individual research contracts with investigators who are stationed within military laboratories. Such arrangements are based largely on personal contacts, common scientific goals of the two laboratories, and the ability of the military researcher to convince superiors in the chain of command that a research contract is needed.

U.S. Army

The most recent description of army research programs appears in the Broad Agency Announcements of the USARO.

U.S. Army Research Office
P.O. Box 12211
Research Triangle Park, NC 27709-2211
<www.aro.army.mil>
Biological Sciences Division: 919-549-4230

In addition, the Army conducts peer-reviewed research programs in the areas of breast, prostate, and ovarian cancer, and neurofibromatosis, women's health, and osteoporosis through the Congressionally Directed Medical Research Programs of the U.S. Army Medical Research and Materiel Command (USAMRMC/CDMRP). Write to

Attn: MCMR-PLF
Fort Detrick, MD 21702-5024
301-619-7079
<http://cdmrp.army.mil>

U.S. Air Force

The Air Force Office of Scientific Research (AFOSR) manages all basic research conducted by the USAF. It does this through grants to university scientists, contracts for industrial research, and direct support of Air Force laboratories. AFOSR is particularly proud of its success in transferring extramural research results to the exploratory development programs of USAF laboratories and the close relationship between grantees and those laboratories. Information about "Research Opportunities" and "How to Apply" can be obtained from the following address:

Air Force Office of Scientific Research (AFOSR/AFRL)
801 North Randolph St., Rm. 732
Arlington, VA 22203-1977
703-696-9513
<www.afosr.af.mil>

U.S. Navy

The Office of Naval Research (ONR) supports considerably more biomedical research than do the other branches of the military. Its programs and contact persons are described at the web site of the ONR. Follow the links to the Broad Agency Announcement, and to the biomedical programs and staff listed under "Science and Technology, Human Systems."

Office of Naval Research
800 North Quincey Street
Arlington, VA 22217-5660
703-696-4501
<www.onr.navy.mil>

PRIVATE FOUNDATIONS

About 11% of support for biomedical research in the USA comes from private foundations, of which there are over 24,000. A handful, such as the American Cancer Society, the American Heart Association, and the American Diabetes Association, are large and have formalized proposal procedures, deadlines, and peer review, and make substantive grants for research support. Applications can be obtained in University Offices of Contracts and Grants. The smaller foundations are difficult to penetrate, and often have a private agenda and clientele. Success may be largely dependent on personal contacts with foundation officers. The numerous foundations are listed in several compendia with descriptions of their areas of interest and their recent gifts. A letter of intent should be sent to the foundation initially and a proposal sent only if requested. If the foundation is interested, every effort should be made to establish personal contact with the appropriate officer.

The URLs of some of the larger foundations are:

American Heart Association: <www.americanheart.org/research>
American Cancer Society: <www.cancer.org>
American Diabetes Association: <www.diabetes.org/research>
Juvenile Diabetes Research Foundation International: <www.jdf.org>
Alzheimer's Association: <www.alz.org/research>
National Parkinson Foundation: <www.parkinson.org/grants.htm>

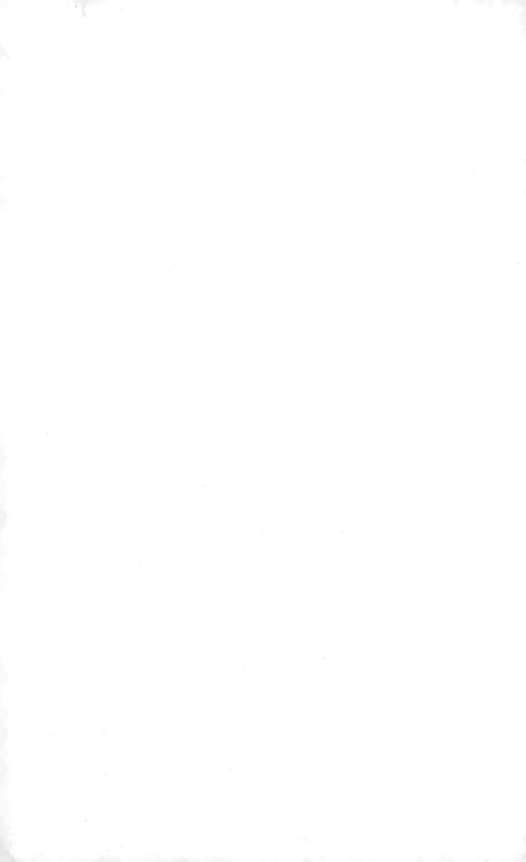

2

A Strong Proposal

Experience with the vagaries of federal funding may lead to growing cynicism about the system, despite strong feelings of loyalty and support for it. This is, after all, an age of realism. The "operational definition" of scientific merit is the priority score given to a proposal by a Study Section; the pragmatic definition of a strong proposal is simply any proposal that is funded. Explanations for success or the lack of it are legion. Unfortunately, good science does not always lead to a successful proposal, although badly written proposals are often funded if their science and the Principal Investigator's (PI) background are sufficiently strong. On the other hand, proposals based on faulty science are hardly ever successful. Between these extremes lies a group of proposals whose science is sound and with Principal Investigators that are well trained and productive. Some will be funded, others will not. It is for this latter class of proposal, lying as it does in the "gray zone" of funding, that this book is dedicated. Without exception these proposals could be stronger (get a better priority score) if they were better written. By "better written" we mean easier for the reviewer to read and to understand.

APPEARANCE

The gold standard of proposal writing is exemplified by any article in the *Scientific American*. These are written for readers who are scientists but are unfamiliar with the area of the particular article. The prose is kept simple, specialized words and abbreviations are avoided, and every page has at least one diagram or figure. A well-written proposal is written to communicate with all the reviewers, not just those with expertise in the field. The first impression a reviewer gets of a proposal is when it is lifted off an 18- to 24-inches-high stack of other proposals. If it contains 2 pounds of appendixes in addition to its 25 pages of text, that impression

21

is bad. If it is 60 pages long because it has the Biosketches of 20 Co-Investigators, the impression is bad. If there is obvious cheating through the use of a small type font with crowded pages, the reaction is likely to be very negative. There is nothing more discouraging to a tired reviewer than to open a proposal and see every possible space covered with type. No double spaces, no indentations, no figures, and no titles—nothing but little tiny words crawling like so many ants across the page.

A word processor is as basic a piece of equipment to a present-day researcher as a typewriter was 30 years ago. A research proposal written in longhand in the 1970s was no more acceptable than a proposal written without a word processor is today. Proper use of the computer should eliminate typographical errors from the text. Desktop publishing programs and ordinary word processors produce publication-quality text in publication-quality print. Anything less is simply substandard. Remember, grants are awarded in a competition, and the competitors submit proposals that are publication-quality documents. You can do no less and hope to be successful.

Every page of a proposal should have the same general appearance. It is poor grantsmanship to use different fonts or to insert obviously photocopied pages from other proposals. It makes a bad impression, for instance, to include a Biosketch photocopied from a previous submission. This is a common failing of collaborative projects in which the Co-PI hands the PI a Biosketch prepared several years previously, obviously for a different purpose. This indicates to the reviewer that the collaborator does not take the project seriously enough to update the Biosketch. It speaks poorly for the success of the collaboration. Similarly, all statements in a proposal, including those of the Biosketch, must be accurate and consistent. There must be no internal contradictions. These suggest poor quality control. The proposal is taken as an example of the product to be expected from the investigator. Since it is read very carefully, it may have an even greater impact on the reviewers than published papers.

Good Writing Is Brief

This is a challenge that will pay great dividends. Reduce the text sufficiently that the page limitations can be met with at least a size 12 font. Double-space between paragraphs and use 1.2 line spaces between lines.

Use diagrams to reduce narratives, and paragraph titles to facilitate skimming. Do not force reviewers to read something they already know by submerging it in essential text. A strong proposal will give the appearance of being well organized and readable at first glance. It will stand out from its fellows and the reviewer will look forward to reviewing it with pleasant anticipation rather than dread. What a pity such writing is rare!

Proposal guidelines must be followed. These are specific for each different funding program. Any deviation from page restrictions, Biosketch format, section order, IRB or IACUC requirements, etc., may result in a worse priority score or even cause the proposal to be returned without review. Reviewers expect a specific order of presentation and length. They resent having to read extra pages or search for information they usually find in a specific section. They do appreciate innovative grantsmanship, but insist that its expression remain within the bounds set by the guidelines.

Review Criteria

The typical NIH Study Section has 15–20 members. No more than 3–4 members are assigned to and actually read a given proposal. *But they all vote on it.* Although the assigned reviewers will read the proposal in detail, most of the remaining reviewers will merely flip through it looking for red flags. The most important of these are found in the budget and in the Biosketch.

The budget must be reasonable at a glance. What is reasonable is discussed at some length in the chapters on budgets and budget justification. The "reasonable threshold" varies greatly among institutes and different types of research. The average NIH-wide R01 award in 2000, however, was $210,000 (direct costs). Among institutes the average award varied from $285,000 (NCRR) to $170,000 (NIDCR; see Table 2.1).

The *Biosketch* should indicate, also at a glance, solid training, steady productivity, and recent publications pertinent to the proposed research. The reviewer must be given the impression that the investigator is absolutely capable of carrying out the proposed research and that there is a high likelihood of success and significant publications.

The *Specific Aims* section of the Research Plan is the most critical page of the entire proposal. Failure of the reviewer to understand the Specific

Table 2.1 *Average First-Year Direct Cost[a] of NIH Awards by Institute in FY 2000*

Institute	All	New	Renewal
NCRR	285	260	300
NHGRI	240	205	320
NINR	235	230	270
NIDA	235	245	210
NIA	225	220	225
NIAAA	220	210	235
NHLBI	215	210	225
NINDS	215	205	235
NIEHS	215	220	205
NIMH	215	210	225
NIAID	205	205	205
NICHD	205	200	220
NCI	205	200	205
NIDCD	205	195	210
NCCAM	200	200	—
NEI	200	175	215
NIAMS	200	190	210
NIDDK	195	190	195
NIGMS	180	160	195
NIDCR	170	165	190
Total NIH	210	205	215

[a]Approximate dollars times 1000.

Aims presages disaster for the review and is always the fault of the investigator. It is an insurmountable red flag.

Diagrams are a must. A well-designed diagram in the Specific Aims or the Background and Significance sections may reveal at a glance general theory, what is already known, and hypotheses and their tests. It will be much appreciated by the nonassigned Study Section members. Reference to any issue of the *Scientific American* will demonstrate the effectiveness of a diagram in communicating complicated ideas. If the labels of the diagram coincide with those used in Specific Aims and Experimental Design, the logic of the proposal will be established and understanding will flow smoothly as the reader advances through the proposal.

Showing raw data of the "Oh, wow!" variety in the preliminary data section may make a good impression on the reviewers. Although mostly for the benefit of the nonassigned reviewers, such figures must be able to withstand a careful scrutiny by the assigned reviewers. The figures should be attractive, clear, and simple to understand without reading a long legend.

There is a danger for computer users—the availability of fancy borders and icons may tempt the investigator to produce an illustrated reader rather than a research proposal. The effect of such gratuitous artwork is unpredictable and depends on the idiosyncrasies of the reviewer, who may not like it at all. In preparing a proposal, as in many things, it is wise to avoid extremes.

The more substantive aspects of a strong proposal are likely to be appreciated only by the assigned reviewers who read it carefully. They are required to address specifically (1) research significance; (2) research approach; (3) innovation; (4) investigator; and (5) environment. In a good proposal, exposition is clear, logical, and brief. There are no typos. The science is as close as possible to state-of-the-art. Novel methods are supported by solid preliminary data. The problem is important and interesting. The investigation is directed at fundamental mechanisms that are basic to normal function or a disease process. Specific hypotheses about those mechanisms are presented, and feasible tests of the hypotheses are suggested. Data sought are quantitative and subject to statistical validation. The Principal Investigator has a proven record of success with the techniques proposed, is well equipped, and is a member of an established group with which collaboration is productive.

A clear deficiency in any of these areas will weaken the proposal. They are considered in detail in the following chapters.

Hypotheses

Probably the most common weakness of proposals that are based on good science but are poorly written is failure to identify and test important hypotheses. This failure gives rise to a common criticism: "the proposal lacks focus and is diffuse." This weakness will be apparent immediately to a critical reviewer who expects to find hypotheses stated in the Specific Aims. Hypotheses are statements of new ideas. Research that cannot be expressed in terms of hypotheses, or of testing alternative hypotheses, is only a data gathering exercise and cannot be evaluated statistically. Such research may be very important, but often is not perceived to be very interesting. But such data gathering enterprises can almost always be presented in terms of interesting hypotheses that reflect the imagination and insight of the investigator. Thus to set a goal of "understanding the function of the vitronectin receptor on a retinal pigment epithelial cell" is much weaker than to hypothesize specific functions for the receptor (mechanisms) and then to suggest experiments to test the hypotheses. In the first case the study may be construed to be a fishing expedition. The latter case states a specific goal that can be evaluated and suggests that the investigator knows what to look for, i.e., knows the field better than anyone else (except the reviewer, of course). In actuality, a great deal of research is of the "look-see" variety. The researchers have a number of hypotheses in mind but simply lack enough data to choose among them. This is particularly true with basic studies of molecular cellular mechanisms. It requires some effort to formulate such basic studies in terms of hypotheses, but it can always be done and the effort pays off in terms of a stronger proposal.

Quality Is a Must

A proposal cannot be strong unless its scientific content is strong. Strong science in this context implies inherent scientific validity as well as relevance to targeted areas of research. It also implies use of state-of-the-art techniques and experimental designs. Forty years ago there was a resurgence of interest in use of the Golgi stain for studies of neuronal structure, and many projects based on this procedure were funded. Today this procedure has been largely supplanted by immunohistochemical stains and single-cell injections. Golgi studies are passé, although fully capable of providing excellent new data in many preparations. A proposal based on the Golgi stain alone will have difficulty attaining a fundable priority score. One of the reviewers will likely comment on a "traditional study which ignores modern technology," or "unfortunately, more powerful state-of-the-art procedures are not proposed." A simple criterion of what constitutes "state-of-the-art" is simply what the best of the competition is doing, as perceived by the reviewer. An investigator who identifies proliferating retinal pigment epithelial cells on the basis of appearance in the light microscope is not in the same league with a colleague who bases the identification on staining with a monoclonal antibody specific for the cells.

First Person or Passive Tense Writing

It is inevitable that investigators write about their own work and the work of their laboratory. They must decide to whom they will attribute the work ("I," "we," or "the PI") and then be consistent. Do not let false modesty interfere with identification of achievement. On the other hand, few, if any, investigators are solely responsible for their own success. We, personally, are somewhat put off by a proposal with too many "I" references. Yet to use indirection (e.g., "The PI has shown. . . .") is cumbersome and interferes with readability. The best approach is probably the one most often used: the pronoun "we" (e.g., "In our past studies, we have shown. . . ."). This helps to alleviate the impression of egomania.

PROPOSAL PROBLEMS

At an NIH-sponsored meeting on grantsmanship, the 10 most common reasons for proposal failure were listed:

1. Lack of original ideas
2. Diffuse, unfocused, or superficial Research Plan
3. Lack of knowledge of published relevant work
4. Lack of experience in essential methodology
5. Uncertainty concerning future directions
6. Questionable reasoning in experimental approach
7. Absence of acceptable scientific rationale
8. Unrealistically large amount of work
9. Lack of sufficient experimental detail
10. Uncritical approach

Items 2, 3, 5, and 7–10 represent a failure to communicate; they result from flaws in grantsmanship. Although all the items may simply reflect a poorly prepared investigator, they more often result from sloppy writing. "New ideas" are often those presented at the latest meetings and are hardly ever truly original. Publications are widely available, and "lack of knowledge" often really means failure to cite. Lack of experience with methodology can be corrected by creative use of collaborators and consultants; this is basic to good research as well as to good grantsmanship. Flaws in experimental approach represent failure of communication, poor use of consultants, or failure to obtain a knowledgeable review from a colleague prior to submission. Thus every one of these deficiencies is attributable, at least in part, to poor grantsmanship.

HOMEWORK FOR BEGINNERS

A strong proposal, in the best of worlds, is written from a background of knowledge about who will be the likely reviewers, what their biases are, what type of research they do, and what kinds of procedures they use. This information is available on the Internet and in their publications, which, hopefully, will be cited in the proposal. A major difference between experienced and new investigators is that the former are probably personally acquainted with at least some of the reviewers; they know how the system works and they use this hard-won knowledge to their advantage. Novices must: (1) determine which Study Section (<www.csr.nih. gov/review/irgdesc.htm>) and Institute (<www.nih.gov/icd>) will get their proposal; (2) talk to the Institute Program Manager about their budget and Specific Aims; (3) review the funded grants of the Study Section members using CSR rosters (<www.csr.nih.gov/ASPDocs/Committees/ rosterindex.asp>) and the grants database CRISP (<https://www. commons.cit.nih.gov/crisp/>); and (4) get their proposal reviewed by a colleague before it is submitted.

In summary, the appearance of the proposal, how it is assembled, its neatness, and how closely it resembles published material all have an impact on the way an investigator is perceived by the nonassigned reviewers. It is well worth the extra trouble necessary to deliver a professional looking document that *meets the expectations of the reviewer.*

3

Proposal Review

THE NIH PEER REVIEW SYSTEM

Unsolicited research proposals submitted to the NIH are reviewed for scientific merit by a Study Section. The flow of the review process is diagrammed in Figure 3.1. If found competitive for funding, proposals are referred to an institute and reviewed again by the Institute Council for fairness of review and program relevance, and then funded or withdrawn by the Institute. NIH proposals probably receive a more searching scientific review than do those submitted to any other funding sources. The Study Section is a legally constituted body of the Center for Scientific Review (CSR). Besides scientific merit, the section must also judge the significance of the proposed study and to what degree it represents the state-of-the-art in its chosen area. An important judgment is whether or not the Principal Investigator has been and is likely to continue to be productive, and whether the proposal is "competitive" for funds, i.e., in the top half of the proposals reviewed.

The *streamlining system* (also called "triage") is a recent and drastic change in NIH peer review. Congress directed the NIH to "reinvent" its procedures with a goal of increased efficiency at reduced cost. It is unfortunate that NIH targeted the most sensitive aspect of its function for change. Under the triage system, every proposal receives a full review by at least two assigned reviewers who decide whether or not it is "competitive." If all reviewers agree that the proposal is not in the top half, it is withdrawn without further discussion (streamlined). The written reviews are returned to the investigator immediately (in theory) to facilitate revision, but the proposal is not presented to the committee, thus saving perhaps 10–15 minutes of meeting time per proposal. Most Study Sections attempt to eliminate the bottom half of proposals from consideration by the full committee. This is reasonable because the Institutes

29

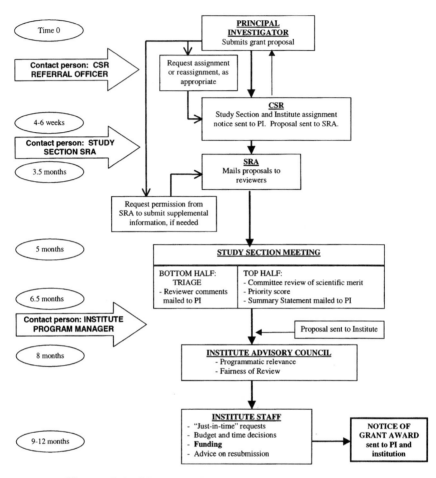

Figure 3.1. Diagram of the proposal review process.

consistently fund fewer than half of the proposals submitted, due to funding limitations.

It was hoped that the triage system would lead to more relaxed meetings and thoughtful discussion of the remaining more competitive proposals, since the meeting would handle about half as many applications. But the Study Sections work as they always have, and the meetings last 2 days instead of 2–3 days, with a paltry dollar savings. The assigned reviewers have to do just as much work to produce the reviews, and the fate of a project hinges even more heavily than it has in the past on the biases of two or three individuals. It is not clear that triage has done anything toward solving the problems that cause applicants to write and rewrite multiple proposals, nor the problems of younger investigators.

It is not a disaster to have your proposal triaged! Do not fall into the trap of believing that triage is the same as disapproval. Senior investigators may take triage as a slap in the face, but beginners should not take it personally. The only meaning of triage is that the reviewers agree your proposal is not in the top half, *in its present state*. There may be many reasons for this judgment. A common reason is that the reviewers would like to see additional data or clarification before supporting a fundable priority. You are in good company with more than half of your equally brilliant and qualified competitors. Be responsive to the critiques, and get a revision submitted as soon as possible. If you follow their directions, the reviewers now become coauthors of your proposal. Award rates of revised proposals are much higher. Trust us—this is how the game is played!

Following presentation of the written reviews at the meeting, the budget is considered. The budget may be accepted as proposed or cut in specific areas. Cuts in the budget must be justified and this always involves some kind of negative comment. Each member then assigns a priority score to the proposal with 1.0 being perfect and 5.0 being barely worthy of consideration for funding, although, theoretically, triage should remove scores from 3.0 to 5.0. Because of the funding crunch, Study Section members are asked to use tenth points in assigning priority scores. The average of all these scores is the priority score of the proposal. The score values are then combined with the scores rated at the previous two meetings and translated into a rank percentile that establishes the position of the particular proposal within the population of recently competing proposals. Combination of the score with the previous scores purports to compensate for the inevitable fluctuations of Study Section mood that are characteristic of human behavior.

What ranking is fundable for an R01 varies among the Institutes, among programs, and from year to year. What priority score corresponds to a particular percentile also varies among Study Sections and from meeting to meeting. Success is better considered in terms of award rates: the percentage of submitted proposals that achieve funding. This was 31% overall for R01s in fiscal 2000. Thus, it can be predicted that about two out of three proposals reviewed will not be funded. Competing renewal proposals do much better (50%) than do new proposals (26%).

This represents a continuing catastrophic situation for biomedical research since the majority of those who fail to get funds will be young investigators. The poor award rate has been exacerbated by the mandate of Congress that the average length of NIH grants be reduced to 4 years. This has effectively increased the pool of competing renewal applications from established investigators. The lack of support for recent trainees today will translate into future shortages of qualified academic scientists, particularly those trained in the new technologies.

NIH administrators have been concerned about a reduction in the number of proposals submitted by young investigators. In 1985, 3000 proposals were submitted by investigators whose age was 37 or less; 1308, or 43%, of these were actually funded. In 1993, 527 proposals from young investigators were funded, despite the fact that the total number of proposals reviewed by NIH doubled between 1983 (19,000) and 1993 (38,000). The situation has improved in recent years. In 1998, 4765 of 26,493 awards went to investigators aged 40 or less. The total numbers of proposals submitted annually to the NIH dropped almost 30% from 1993 to 1998. This may reflect disenchantment with prospects for success. However, the funding picture is not one of gloom and doom, if you take advantage of the opportunity for revision. With revision, awards rates for new proposals approach 50%. This is as good as it has been since the 1960s. Another good sign for the success of the young investigator is the intent of Congress to double the NIH budget. This has led many Institutes to increase emphasis on funding of young investigators and more innovative projects.

Study Sections usually contain 15 to 18 regular members and often as many as 5 or 6 ad hoc members. The regular members serve for staggered terms of 4 years; approximately 4 retiring members are replaced by newcomers every year. Most sections meet three times a year on the NIH campus in Bethesda, Maryland, or nearby. They may review from 50 to 120 proposals. Members are paid $200.00 per meeting day plus expenses. This is minimal compensation considering the large amount of time spent in the review of proposals and in the preparation of written comments. A typical conscientious Study Section member devotes a substantial part of the work year to this process, for which the compensation is a paltry $1200! Fortunately, for most reviewers, this is truly a labor of love.

Study Sections are staffed by a Scientific Review Administrator (SRA) and a Grants Technical Assistant assigned by and responsible to the CSR. The SRAs are usually professionals, often with research experience, but may or may not have expertise in the subject of the Study Section. Members and the chairpersons of the Study Sections are chosen by the SRAs, usually upon the advice of past members and occasionally as the result of input from Institute program staff. Virtually all members are currently funded with R01 grants, since it is awkward, to say the least, to have a member who is unsuccessful in the system. The chairperson is usually someone who has previously served on a Study Section, has senior status in the field, and has reasonable leadership skills. The SRAs impose order and a characteristic personality on their sections. Some manage the affairs of the section more than others do, but all can have an impact on the success of individual proposals. They are the arbiters of appropriate discussion and can cut off comments from reviewers that are inappropriate or possibly self-serving.

If the discussion of a proposal was very negative, but the assigned reviewers were positive, or vice versa, the critiques may not reflect the priority score very accurately. This leaves the Principal Investigator in a quandary as to why the proposal fared so poorly. In such instances, the SRA should be contacted; sometimes they can provide additional information about what happened. You need to know your SRA. NIH bureaucrats attend national meetings in order to meet the investigators with whom they deal. You must seek them out, introduce yourself, and apprise them of your research intentions or problems. Give them a face to accompany your next proposal. They are in a position to be very helpful to you. You need this person.

Proposal Submission

The process of proposal submission and review is illustrated in Figure 3.1. The details of submission are discussed in Chapter 17. When received by the CSR, the proposal is assigned to a Study Section for review and one or more Institutes for funding. Questions about assignment and permission for late submission should be directed to the CSR Assignment Officer (telephone: 301-435-0715). About 3 weeks after the deadline, the proposals are transferred to the Study Section SRA, who will manage the scientific review. Sometimes the constitution of the assigned Study Section may seem weak or biased in the area of your proposal. If it cannot be reassigned to a more appropriate Study Section, you should ask the SRA to assign the proposal to an outside reviewer. Suggest several names of appropriate reviewers who are at other institutions than yours (and whose surnames and institutions differ from yours). The SRA may also opt to add an ad hoc reviewer with expertise in your area for this one meeting, if there are several such requests. The CSR staff are very sensitive to charges that a review was in any way unfair, and make every effort to avoid this. They are usually responsive to requests for changes if they can be incorporated in the regular budget of a scheduled meeting.

Four to six weeks before the Study Section meeting, the proposals will be sent out to the reviewers. Supplementary material will usually be accepted by the SRA at any time prior to this mailing (see Chapter 17). The Study Sections meet about 5 months after the submission deadline, and the results of the review in terms of the priority score are generally mailed to the PI about 1 week later. The Summary Statements are mailed out about 6–8 weeks later. The responsibility for the proposals is transferred to the appropriate Program Managers of the various Institutes at the end of the review. The Program Manager typically will know your score and have your Summary Statement only a few days before you do. The proposals are reviewed again, usually *en bloc* by the Institute Scientific Advisory Councils, about 8 months after the deadline. The Program Managers usually can give you a rough idea about the likelihood of funding, once they know the priority scores. They can certainly tell you if you must revise and resubmit. They are bombarded by telephone calls, of course, but they are used to it.

Questions concerning the review should be put to the SRA. The SRAs can be very helpful in providing guidance and insight into the failings of a particular proposal, but they have nothing to do with funding and cannot tell you whether a given percentile is fundable. The name and telephone number of the SRA will be found at the NIH web site (<www.csr.nih.gov/ASPDocs/Committees/rosterindex.asp>) and on the application receipt letter, together with the Study Section and Institute assignment (Appendix B). Sometimes it is desirable to include with your proposal figures that you want all members to be able to see. Call the SRA and ask permission to send 20 copies of your proposal for direct distribution to all the Study Section members, instead of the usual (poor quality) photocopies. This request will usually be granted. Your copies must be two-sided, but can include color photos.

Questions about funding go to Institute Program Managers. They often attend Study Section meetings, and may be helpful in interpreting critiques. Your SRA can tell you if your Program Manager was present during the review. Managers expect to be contacted by PIs and usually take notes, particularly when there is division among the reviewers and much discussion during the review. They also have a good idea of what is a fundable and what is not a fundable (i.e., revision needed) priority score or percentile. They will not give you a firm answer about funding until they are certain. However, usually they will give an indication. "It looks very good" probably means you will be funded. "It is not clear at this time" probably means you are in the gray zone; get busy on your revision.

The Review Process

In most Study Sections, each proposal is assigned to a primary reviewer, one or occasionally two additional reviewers, and a discussant. They must read the proposal in detail and, excepting the discussant, write a two to four or more page review that follows a standard format. The chairperson calls up each proposal at the beginning of the meeting and asks the reviewers if it is competitive (top 50%). If all reviewers agree that it is not competitive, it is triaged, and the written reviews are given to the SRA for incorporation into the Summary Statement. If even one reviewer puts the proposal in the top half, it is not triaged. After removal of the triaged proposals, the rest are reviewed in order. The written reviews follow a set pattern. Following presentation of the research problem and the methods to be used, usually lifted largely from the Specific Aims or Abstract of the proposal, a critique is presented stressing its strengths, weaknesses, and innovation. This is followed by a short review of the research environment, and the qualifications of the research team. The secondary reviewers may write only a critique section. You should assume that *only the assigned reviewers read your proposal.* Most of the members look at a given proposal carefully for the first time as it is presented in the meeting. Their scrutiny is superficial to say the least, and is limited to about 10 minutes while the reviews are being read. Their scores, in aggregate, carry five to six times more weight than the informed scores of the assigned reviewers. They base their scores largely on what they hear, but they are influenced strongly by the factors discussed in the previous chapter: general appearance, a reasonable budget, strong Biosketch, and effectiveness of the Specific Aims.

During the reading of the reviews, the nonassigned members generally browse through the proposal in an attempt to stay awake. Most glance at the budget and look carefully at the Biosketch of the PI, looking for red flags. Then in the remaining time they look at the Abstract or Specific

Aims. After the reviews are read, the proposal is open for discussion. Any member who is an expert in the area of the proposal or is familiar with some aspect of it or with the PI is likely to comment on its value, often to support or disagree with a comment of one of the assigned reviewers. Other members may question the reviewers concerning perceived red flags, the most common of which are an overpriced or inadequately justified instrument, a weak Biosketch, a request for too many technicians, or poor productivity.

The chairperson then calls for a discussion of the budget and recommendations as to cuts or, very rarely, to increases. In some Study Sections, specific scores are not stated in the reviews, to provide more freedom for the other members of the Study Section and to prevent everyone from assigning the identical score. Reviewers use a well-publicized code to indicate what they think the priority score should be: "outstanding" (1–1.5), "excellent" (1.5–2), "very good" (2–3.0), "good" (3.0–4.0), and "acceptable" (4.0–5.0). In other Study Sections, specific scores are stated by the reviewers. It is the responsibility of the SRA and the chairperson to make sure that all members of a section use the same criteria and speak the same language in referring to the value of a proposal. Scores that are well outside the window delineated by the assigned reviewers are rare and are considered biased; they may be excluded from the average by the SRA.

It is not uncommon for the assigned reviewers to differ in their assessment of a proposal. In some Institutes, a priority score of 1.8 is fundable, but a score of 2.3 is not. If these are the scores suggested by the assigned reviewers, the rest of the group will certainly assign scores within this window. But, how will they decide between 1.8 and 2.3? They are all professionals, with professional-class egos. They are not rubber stampers. They know that their vote may make a difference. If they are impressed with what they see, and if they can read and understand the logic and hypotheses of the Specific Aims in about 3 minutes, they will award a better score, perhaps 1.8 or 1.9. If they are not impressed, or they find a red flag, or cannot understand the Specific Aims, their scores will tend toward 2.3 and funding may be missed. *This is why a successful Specific Aims is the single most important page in a proposal.*

Action can theoretically be deferred for future review if more information is required, but this is a rare event in recent years. In unusual instances some members may object to the majority opinion sufficiently to vote against it, in which case they must generate a "minority report." The priority score is recorded by each member on pages provided by the SRA; these are gathered and tabulated at the end of the meeting. The priority score assigned to the proposal is the average of all of the reviewers' scores (multiplied by 100). In cases of a split vote, the council scrutinizes the review very closely and may call for a rereview, although it usually concurs with the majority opinion.

The meetings usually are attended by Program Directors from Institutes concerned with the subject matter of the proposals. It used to be common for this person to be questioned closely by section members about funding levels in an attempt to ascertain what priority score is likely to be funded. The members are also concerned about prospects for future funding of their own grants. Since funding is now based on percentile rank rather than priority score, and the relation of score to percentile rank changes with every meeting, the relation of the two is less clear and there is less of a tendency for members to assign scores on the basis of a desire to see a particular grant funded. At least that is the theory of the percentile arrangement. Although previously every attempt was made by the CSR to discourage the assignment of priority scores according to a "fund or no fund" basis, this was happening regularly. Members who wanted a proposal funded assigned it a score better than its science merited and gave other proposals proportionately worse scores. This resulted in a bimodal distribution of scores. The new system has done much to correct this, or at least cause the scores to have a more even distribution. But it does not completely overcome the tendency for clustering that causes the fundable proposals to be separated by hundredths of a point, a meaningless distinction on which to decide the future of many research projects.

Consider the plight of the reviewers. Each is assigned 10–15 proposals to review, about 6 weeks before each of the meetings. A careful review, with preparation of a report, and perhaps some literature work, takes about a full day. Reviewers are busy, productive scientists with heavy demands on their time. They do not like to waste time. When they have finished a review on a proposal they like, they want to see it get a fundable averaged priority score. They become its protagonist so their time will not have been wasted and tend to inflate its score. They protect a favored proposal in the open review by deflating the scores of its competitors. Of course everyone does this to some degree.

Flaws of the peer review system are many and it is constantly under review by the NIH. The sections are generally conservative, representing as they do the current wisdom of successful science. Radical ideas do not do well in review. Established investigators have a psychological advantage over other scientists, particularly those at the beginning of their careers. The Study Sections attempt to take into consideration the inexperience of the young investigator, but competing renewal proposals consistently score about two times better than new applications. Obviously such proposals must have received a rating of "outstanding" or "excellent" in a previous review in order to be funded, and this approbation tends to carry over to the current review.

Many Study Sections are called on to review proposals for which their expertise is thin or not current. An attempt is made to correct this by addition of ad hoc members, but these members are not always entirely appropriate. They may be unknown to the regular section members, who also will be unfamiliar with the ad hoc members' criteria of review and distrustful of their comments. Thus the severe criticism of a new reviewer may be attributed to the personality of the reviewer and taken with a grain of salt. A more destructive circumstance is that of a hypercritical ad hoc reviewer whose personality is unknown to the section and whose damaging comments about a perfectly good proposal are taken too seriously.

Every Study Section has a unique group personality, often shaped by a few strong members. The bane of the SRA is the member who feels compelled to argue at length with other members. Such are often quietly removed from the section roster. The members learn to evaluate the comments of each other with an adjustable rule. Some are excessively optimistic about the merits of all their assigned proposals; others nitpick strong proposals to destruction. After a period of acclimation, the section achieves a certain balance. But woe unto the proposal whose assigned reviewer is, unbeknownst to the rest of the Study Section, an ego-tripping nitpicker! There is no mechanism other than rereview to repair the damage done by intemperate and undeserved criticism. Thus the weaknesses of the peer review system of the NIH are obvious and it has its detractors, but no one has come forward with a better system of review!

It is unusual for more than two or three members of a section to have expertise in exactly the same area, and it is common for a single reviewer to be the only available expert on a specific topic or method. The other reviewers will rely heavily on the analysis of the assigned reviewers, weighted by their opinions of possible reviewer bias. Because the rest of the section members far outnumber the assigned reviewers, and are essentially uninformed about the proposal, their reaction to the reviews and a brief glimpse of the proposal will determine its success. For this reason, it is worth repeating, the Abstract and Specific Aims of the proposal are extremely important. These two pages are the only parts of the proposal that are sure to be read by most of the members! A successful Specific Aims can influence the enthusiasm of the unassigned reviewers.

Study Section members suffer some privation for the privilege of serving. Their own research proposals cannot be reviewed by a section on which they serve, yet that section is probably the one most qualified to provide the review. Assignment to an alternate less-informed section may result in a poor review. An ad hoc section may be called to provide the review, but such sections do not perform on a predictable basis and their priority scores may be based on criteria that are different from those of the regular section, making integration into the funding ranks difficult. The Institutes attempt to overcome this but must avoid all suggestion of favoring Study Section members.

Conflict of interest is difficult to avoid in a relatively small group of interacting individuals. The burden of avoidance is placed on the members, who are required to leave the meeting room when a proposal from their own institution is presented or whenever they feel they have a conflict of interest. Proposals submitted by members' past fellows who have moved to other institutions are not considered to be a conflict if the member is no longer collaborating with the fellow. However, a member should never be involved with a review of a proposal from someone with whom there is recent collaboration since it is essential to the health of the peer review system that even the appearance of a conflict of interest be avoided.

Advisory Council

As described in Chapter 1, the NIH uses a dual system of review designed to provide balance and prevent conflict of interest. While the Study Section evaluates the proposal for scientific merit and the appropriateness of the budget, and identifies noncompetitive proposals, it is not involved in the decision of whether or not to fund the competitive proposals. The recommendation for funding comes from the Advisory Council of the Institute that will provide the funds. The various Institute councils usually meet about 3 months after the Study Sections. The councils also evaluate the adequacy of the review. They may request a rereview if they find that the Study Section lacked appropriate expertise, or was biased in its judgment. The council may also recommend that budget changes suggested by the Study Section be rescinded. The specific recommendations of the council to the Institute staff are usually followed to the letter.

Appeal

If the PI, after reading the Summary Statement, strongly feels that the review was unfair, biased, or otherwise severely flawed, the appropriate Institute Program Manager should be contacted and a request for special scrutiny by the council discussed. A letter is then sent to the Manager presenting the problem. This is presented to and considered by the Institute Scientific Advisory Council, which may call for a rereview or may alter the priority score without rereview. There is a downside to rereview. In this case, no changes in the proposal are permitted. It is generally handled again by the same Study Section, but may go to a new one. This takes a complete review cycle. If the rereview is unsuccessful, the revision, which would probably do much better than the original, is delayed about half a year.

NSF PROPOSAL REVIEW

Each proposal in the Biological Science program of the NSF is mailed to from six to eight reviewers, some of whom may be suggested by the Principal Investigator. The reviewers are asked to submit a written discussion of the scientific strengths and weakness of the proposal, and its broad impact on education and society, and to indicate a rating of excellent, very good, good, fair, or poor. These "scores" and the written reviews are considered by a Study-Section-like panel that ranks the competing proposals and segregates them into three groups. The "outstanding" group is the top 10%, and is given a high priority for funding. The next 30–35% are a "fund if possible group." The rest are considered a low priority for funding. The bottom 10% are disapproved for funding. One or two panel members also may write reviews of each proposal. The administrators, particularly the individual Program Directors, exercise rather more free agency than do their NIH counterparts in deciding which proposals should be funded.

The NSF generally funds at a much lower level than the NIH and a Program Director is likely to suggest to the PI who has submitted an

NIH-type budget that it is inappropriate. It must be determined by the PI whether a smaller award can be productively used. Typical NSF project awards range from $50,000 to $100,000 *total costs* per year for 3 years. Thus, direct costs available will be about 60% of this, depending on the indirect cost rate of your institution. These awards are of particular benefit to investigators who experience interruption of their usual funding since NSF funding may be offered for a year or two to bridge the gap. Strong proposals may be considered worthy of support by both the NIH and the NSF. There is good communication between the agencies and both will not fund the same project. Also it is forbidden to submit the same proposal to both agencies at the same time, unless the PI has never before been awarded a federal research grant. The NIH award is usually accepted since it is likely to be larger.

NSF reviews are probably more helpful than those of the NIH, since as many as six or seven verbatim reviews are sent to the Principal Investigator. Also, reviews depend largely on the luck of the draw: the particular group of reviewers asked to review a proposal. Highly innovative projects probably receive a more sympathetic reading from NSF reviewers than from NIH Study Sections, and we are personally familiar with one proposal that was disapproved on the basis of lacking all scientific merit by an NIH Study Section but was approved with very high scores and funded by the NSF! On the other hand, the NSF budget for biological research is very small compared with that of the NIH. However, its award rates are about the same.

NSF proposals should follow the same format as NIH proposals, with minor modifications appropriate to a budget about half the size of an NIH budget. The appropriate Program Directors are often very helpful in judging the proper scope of the project and arranging for a sympathetic review. They should be contacted for advice before the proposal is submitted (follow the links under "Guide to Programs" at <www.nsf.gov>). Like the NIH, the NSF generally funds down the ranked proposals until funds are exhausted. However, your prospects for funding are dependent on the reviews, tempered to a great extent by the categorical needs of the program as evaluated by the administrators.

MILITARY REVIEWS

There is a great deal of variability in the method of review of proposals submitted to the various military agencies. Many funding decisions are the prerogative of the administrative head of a particular program, others involve reviews by a few individuals, and many are subjected to an in-depth review by a board of peers. Information about the review process for a particular program should be solicited from the program contact officer. Every effort must be made to identify the individuals responsible for the programmatic decisions. These individuals should be contacted if it is at all possible. The best approach is a direct meeting and presentation. Sometimes these can be arranged through the auspices of a member of Congress.

Military research is highly goal specific and awards may be made more on the judgment that a particular proposal meets program criteria rather than that it is imbued with great scientific merit. It is not always easy to discover just what the goals of a particular program are, and thus the importance of contacting the responsible officer. By law, all Requests for Proposals (RFPs) or Requests for Application (RFAs) issued by government agencies must be advertised in the *Commerce Business Daily*. Unfortunately, this is somewhat less than useful information since the proposals in this publication are often couched in terms appropriate for a preselected contractor and sometimes list deadlines that only someone already informed about the contract could meet.

PRIVATE FOUNDATIONS

There are over 24,000 private philanthropic foundations in the United States. About 1 in 20 of these will give operating funds (salaries and supply budgets) to support research projects. Many will provide funds for the purchase of equipment or for construction and renovation of research facilities. The proposal review process of private foundations seldom is informed in the scientific sense, although major foundations such as the American Cancer Society, Juvenile Diabetes Research Foundation International, and the American Heart Association have proper peer reviews. Decisions for funding are more apt to be made on the reputation of the applying institution/university and on familiarity with the researcher, the researcher's preceptor, or an officer of the applicant's institution. Direct contact with foundation officers is virtually mandatory to secure funding from the smaller private foundations. Every effort should be made to talk at length with the responsible parties, and, if it is feasible, the foundation headquarters should be visited and a personal relationship established.

In summary, the mechanics of proposal review must be understood if the system is to be bested. Particularly, the Study Section that will review a given proposal must be identified and the work of the members reviewed. Thus proposals can be written with a background of knowledge of the biases of the likely reviewers. One of the major reasons that experienced investigators are successful in review is simply that they know their Study Section and its members, and use this knowledge in structuring their proposals. Young investigators can acquire this important data from their mentors and older colleagues, and by use of the Internet.

The NIH has posted on the Internet a short commentary presenting their view of the proposal assignment process. This is presented in Appendix B-6.

4

The R01 Research Grant

The NIH supports about one-third of the biomedical research done in the United States. A large part of this support involves R01 grants, so called because the alphanumeric "R-zero-one" precedes the assigned NIH proposal number. These grants are unsolicited, i.e., investigator initiated. They are designed to support discrete projects performed by the named investigator. Much of the funding allocated to each NIH Institute is expended as R01s. The proportion varies from Institute to Institute and is under administrative control according to the advice of their respective councils and congressional mandates. In fiscal year 2000, the NIH awarded 44,363 grants, of which 24,499, or 55%, were R01s. Of the total appropriation of $17.8 billion, $14.8 billion, or 83%, went to the research grant programs, including $7.1 billion for R01 awards. This was 48% of all grant funds and 40% of the NIH budget. In fiscal 2001, Congress awarded $20.3 billion to NIH programs, and the President's requested budget of $23.6 billion for 2002 proposed is a 15% increase over this amount. The requested budget for 2003 ($27.3 billion) is an additional increase of almost 16%. There should be proportional increases in R01 awards each year.

DIRECTIONS

The application packet for the R01 grant carries the identifier "PHS 398." It should hardly be necessary to advise that this packet must be read cover to cover, but, in fact, very few investigators take the time to do it. The entire application kit can be obtained on the Internet at <http://grants.nih.gov/grants/forms.htm>. The directions for the Research Plan (pages 15–28) are explicit and clear and must be followed. This can be done without impairing the scientific freedom of the writer because the directions, especially for the key scientific sections (Sections *a* to *d*, pages 16–18), are reasonable. Even the most complex of projects can be described in the allotted space if the effort is made to be concise.

The PHS 398 packet requests that

> the Research Plan should include sufficient information needed for evaluation of the project, independent of any other document. Be specific and informative, and avoid redundancies. Organize *Items a-d* of the Research Plan to answer these questions:
> 1. What do you intend to do?
> 2. Why is the work important?
> 3. What has already been done?
> 4. How are you going to do the work?

Freedom of Information versus Privacy

Information in a research proposal is privileged—as much as any document given to 15–20 interested scientists can be privileged. At the close of every Study Section meeting there is a great show of tossing the reviewed proposals into waste bins. However, some Study Section members have been observed to keep a few of particular interest, usually those with a good review of some topic close to the member's heart. Certainly Study Section members benefit and learn from their participation in this quasi-academic process. There probably have been instances where a member has actually been in a position, because of funded research capability, to quickly capitalize on someone else's ideas. Fortunately this seems to be very uncommon. Such behavior would be catastrophic to the applicant and would be a disaster for the peer review system. Protection of proprietary information presents the researcher with a quandary. One author of this book, Goldberg, feels that details must be presented or there is a risk that funding will be missed. Study Section members are quick to find fault with new ideas unless they are truly great, in which case they give credit where it is due. Ogden, being older and perhaps more cynical, suggests that applicants working in a highly competitive field, such as the molecular biology of AIDS, would be wise to use restraint in putting too many proprietary secrets in a research proposal. This boils down to a value judgment; the bottom line is that enough information must be provided to secure funding.

The PHS 398 packet states that the information of the proposal may be used for auditing and lists eight general circumstances in which federal agencies may review the proposal. The following paragraph from the packet should be considered carefully:

> The Freedom of Information Act and implementing DHHS regulations (45 CFR Part 5) require the release of certain information about grants, upon request, irrespective of the intended use of the information. Trade secrets and commercial, financial, or otherwise intrinsically valuable information that is obtained from a person or organization and that is privileged or confidential information may be withheld from disclosure. Information, which, if disclosed, would be a clearly unwarranted invasion of personal privacy, may also be withheld from disclosure. Although the grantee institution and the principal investigator will be consulted about any such release, the PHS will make the final determination. *Generally available for release, upon request, except as noted above, are: all funded grant applications including their derivative funded noncompeting supplemental grant applications; pending and funded noncompeting continuation applications; progress reports of grantees; and final reports of any review or evaluation of grantee performance conducted or caused to be conducted by the DHHS.* Generally, not available for release to the public are: competing grant applications (initial, competing continuation, and supplemental) for which awards have not been made; evaluative portions of site visit reports; and summary statements of findings and recommendations of review groups. [Emphasis added.]

The Freedom of Information Act is used by antivivisection organizations to identify sensitive research, and the activities of these organizations can be detrimental to biomedical research and individual researchers. The sensitivity of animal research will be discussed in a later chapter. Here it is appropriate to emphasize that the investigator must be certain that the descriptions of experiments in the proposal are in accordance with federal guidelines for the care and use of experimental animals. *Animals should not be mentioned in the titles of proposals.*

Page Limitations

Page limitations must be followed. Section 1 of the application concerns the budget and budget justification, for which there are no page limitations. Note, however, that severe restrictions are placed on justification content, in the case of modular budgets. The Biosketch is limited to 4 pages and includes 2 pages for research projects and support during the past 3 years. Resources and Environment usually do not require additional pages but are, in fact, not limited. *The limitation for Sections* a *through* d *of the Research Plan is 25 pages.* It is wise, but not mandatory, to follow the recommended allotment (Specific Aims, 1 page; Background and Significance, 2 to 3 pages; Progress Report/Preliminary Studies, 6 to 8 pages; Experimental Design and Methods, 13 pages). Additional material concerning progress or methods can be conveyed through the publications or full-page diagrams in the appendix, but only the assigned reviewers will see them. Appendix material is not copied, so the other 15 or so Study Section members will not see it unless it is passed around at the time of the meeting. The instructions state, *"Do not use the appendix to circumvent the page limitations of the research plan"* (emphasis added). To cheat with an extra half-page here and there, or to use small type, is to run the very real risk of degrading the priority score. In the extreme, such proposals may be denied review. During February–March 2001, the CSR Referral Office returned ~200 proposals to investigators, requesting resubmittal for a future deadline in the proper format.

The assigned reviewers actually get the proposal copies that are submitted. The other members are given photocopies, often of dubious virtue. If color photographs or high-quality photographs are essential to the proposal and should be seen by all the members, submit 20 copies of the proposal and ask the SRA to distribute these to the Study Section. It is not wise to try this dodge with the appendix material (except perhaps a single page) because the size of the resulting packet will have a negative impact on the Study Section members.

The sections of the application concerning (*e*) Human Subjects, (*f*) Vertebrate Animals, (*h*) Consortium/Contractual Arrangements, and (*i*) Consultants have no page limitations, but must provide the requested information while being kept as short as possible. Material concerning animals or human subjects that is discussed in detail in the Research Plan should not be repeated, but should be summarized briefly with reference to the pages where it is presented. The focus should be the specific information requested. Section g of the application is Literature Cited. It is not limited as to pages (but see Chapter 14).

Project Title

Page one of the application form is filled out by the business office in most institutions. Instructions for each item are explicit on pages 6–10 of the General Instructions portion of the application packet. The most sensitive part of this page is the proposal title, which must be limited to 56 typewriter spaces. Longer titles will simply be truncated and may become meaningless. Titles should be as general as possible since it is hoped that they will be carried on through several competing renewal cycles. It is inevitable that a specific title such as "Vitrectomy treatment of ocular trauma" will no longer describe a project that, over 10 years, evolved to studies of cellular proliferation in the vitreous of the eye. Fortunately, it is permissible to change the title of a proposal in order to maintain relevance to a continuation of support for an evolving series of investigations.

The instructions state,

A new application must have a different title from any other PHS project with the same principal investigator/program director. A competing continuation or revised application should ordinarily have the same title as the previous grant or application. If the specific aims of the project have significantly changed, choose a new title. A supplemental application must have the same title as the currently funded grant.

A significant change in Specific Aims can be interpreted to be a new project, so care must be taken to make it perfectly clear that the proposed work is a natural outgrowth and logical extension of the funded project. Some investigators who have preferred not to run the risk of being classified as a new project, and simply kept the original title, although it no longer described the proposed research, have been criticized by their Study Section. If the title is changed, care must be taken to ensure that the grant number is not, that the research is continuing, and that the proposal is not classified as new. Competing renewals clearly have an edge over new proposals in funding, as do amended proposals. This may be crucial for proposals with a marginal priority score. The considerations involved in the decision to submit either a new or a competing renewal proposal are discussed at length in Chapter 15.

The title of a proposal is very important to the CSR Referral Officer. It has a direct bearing on the Study Section chosen to review the proposal and the Institute assignment. If the word "AIDS" is in the title, the proposal will go to an AIDS Study Section regardless of the research proposed. If you want your proposal to go to the NEI, do not use the word "Age" in the title. That might cause it to be assigned to the NIA. Obviously, you must decide ahead of time which Institute you wish as your patron, if you are to avoid misdirection.

Grant Types

New investigators are often undecided about which of the several NIH grant programs is appropriate for their initial request for funds (see Chapter 18). The R01 mechanism is the primary method of support of individual research projects. It should be used by virtually all qualified investigators. The NIH played with the R29 "FIRST" award for about 10 years. It was discontinued when it was realized that it provided little benefit and perhaps harmed some of the recipient young investigators. One problem with this First Independent Research Support and Transition award was the confusion as to what was meant by "independent" and what was meant by "transition." Many starting investigators hoped that this was an easy 5-year grant for the inexperienced; however, the NIH intended it as "the first award for an investigator who was already appointed to an independent position." The reviewers were almost schizophrenic in applying the guidelines. A more serious problem was that the ceiling amount of $70,000 per year was not adequate for an independent research project and could not be supplemented with NIH funds. Most devastating was that after 5 years of NIH R29 support, some of the independent scientists were downgraded by their promotions committees for not having an R01! So, it is worth repeating that the R01 mechanism is the primary method of support of individual research projects. It should be used by virtually all qualified investigators. Anyone who is overqualified for a postdoctoral fellowship and who has an independent academic or research position is qualified to receive an R01 grant.

There are other possible choices for an initial application that are intended for starting scientists who have a clinical degree. The K08, Mentored Clinical Scientist Award is designed to develop the fundamental laboratory research ability of clinicians with little research training. The K23, Mentored Patient Oriented Research Development Award is designed to provide newly trained specialists with support for research training and career development in clinical science. These awards are not for everyone; they require that the newly trained academician devote at least 75% of effort, under the guidance of a more-senior mentor, for up to 5 years, to the research project.

Small Grants-in-Aid are made by some but not all Institutes. These are usually limited to $100,000 per year for 2 or 3 years and are designed for pilot (R03) or developmental (R21) studies. Some institutes award K01 grants to new investigators with the Ph.D. degree and postdoctoral training in a basic science. They must be willing to devote the 5 years to developing their research career in a specified area of interest determined by the Institute. These "starter" grants are usually advertised in RFAs and Program Announcements (visit the relevant Institute home pages at <www.nih.gov/icd>). Unfortunately these awards do not have the status of R01s in university circles.

The rationale for these various grant mechanisms is that their design may in some way ease the entry of new and inexperienced investigators into the research business. Criteria for review of these proposals were intended to be more relaxed than those for the R01 proposals. Unfortunately, this is a subjective adjustment required in many instances of the same reviewers involved in R01 review. Proposals that are actually weaker than an R01 rarely receive a fundable priority score. The decision as to which mechanism to use should be made after talking with the appropriate Institute Program Director. In the final analysis, however, the R01 is the benchmark of a successful investigator. It must be mastered to secure stable support in the academic environment.

Writing the Proposal

If writing is easy for you, you will simply sit down and dash off the proposal. Unfortunately, it may not have the thought put into it that goes into the proposal of someone who is less gifted, but struggles slowly through the process. The real work of writing a successful proposal is done during the planning/outlining stage. If this is done properly, the proposal will be succinct, logical, clear, persuasive, and, what is really important, easy to read and understand.

If writing is difficult for you, it is probably only because you lack practice. Writing is a skill that really does become easier as you do more of it. Beginning investigators, despite 10 or more years of training, often have had little occasion to practice the fine art of the English language. Most have to teach themselves by emulating the styles of their successful peers. Unfortunately, you will probably make little real progress until you find someone who knows English writing to carefully edit your work. If you are lucky, that person will be an experienced scientist in your department (the availability of such a person is a good reason to choose a particular department). If you lack departmental access to a good editor, seek one out anywhere you can. Graduate students in the English

Department of your university are often willing to edit papers for a nominal fee. This is a good investment, particularly if you are willing to learn from the experience (see Chapter 18).

A weak Biosketch is the dilemma of the young investigator. Minimum qualifications to obtain funding are adequate training and expertise, and clear evidence of productivity. For someone emerging from postdoctoral training, the latter means at least 4–5 publications, with several as first author. These fetal Biosketches are scrutinized very carefully for evidence to indicate that the investigator can function independently. If the Biosketch is weak, as is often the case with new investigators, it can be bolstered by a paragraph in the Budget Justification section emphasizing the previous independent activities of the PI and a letter from the previous mentors to the same effect. New investigators should also make free use of whatever collaborations they can engineer to strengthen their credibility in areas in which they may be viewed as weak. Proposals from new investigators to continue work in or near their (predoctoral or postdoctoral) mentor's laboratory are probably doomed to fail. They will be viewed as extensions of the mentor's laboratory and research rather than an independent initiative.

STARTING A NEW PROPOSAL

A few words of advice about the process of starting a new proposal are in order. For those who have difficulty starting a new project, there is a simple trick that works very well. Simply write down what is to be accomplished. This usually is framed in terms of a hypothesis, which is first expressed as a question. An example might be, "Are large fibers of the optic nerve selectively destroyed in glaucoma?" This question leads to several more specific questions (corollaries of the hypothesis). These are very likely encompassed within the former. The specific questions should suggest experiments, and the general question is a rudimentary Specific Aim. This thoughtful exercise may take several weeks or even months, and will probably require some literature review, during which the project becomes delimited. At some point, enough work for two projects should be outlined, then trimmed, and combined to provide three or four clearly defined Specific Aims related to specific corollaries of the unifying hypothesis.

Having defined a project that is of interest, the Specific Aims page for a proposal should be crafted. The missing ingredient is usually an experimental model that logically combines the hypotheses and corollaries. It is irrefutable that the scientific method is the basis of good research, and that the scientific method is based on the generation and testing of specific hypotheses. One should start with an important hypothesis, choose the most powerful experimental approach, and design experiments to critically test the hypothesis. In the real world, however, most of us start with limited experimental tools and are most challenged by the need to find a worthwhile hypothesis upon which we can apply our expertise.

At any rate, once the Specific Aims section is written, the rest is easy. We suggest that beginners read through Part I of this book, and then reread each chapter as the appropriate part of the proposal is tackled. The chapters are replete with little gems of grantsmanship that eventually become second nature to the successful grants applicant.

The use of outlines makes the process of proposal preparation much less threatening. Start each section with a basic outline of what should go into that section. This is presented in detail in each chapter. Your task, then, is to translate these basic outlines into a form appropriate for your project. Once the outline is written down, and each paragraph specified as to content, it only remains to fill in some words. The skilled grant writer crafts a logical outline and retains the shell of it in the proposal. This not only assists the reviewers but also gives them an appreciation for your logical mind.

Advice for Beginners

Researchers are human, and humans are born to procrastinate. Researchers work to meet deadlines. This behavior leads to last minute writing, insufficient editing, and inadequate review. A wonderful prescription for failure! As noted above, a common failing of neophytes is a thin Biosketch and a disinclination to write. In fact, most fail to recognize that they have elected to be professional writers (see Chapter 19). The NIH deadlines are very real. If they are your personal deadlines, you will never deliver a proposal that is your best effort. Commit to deadlines that precede the NIH dates by at least 2 months. Produce a complete proposal by that date, and then get it reviewed by an appropriate expert.

You Must Think Ahead

Every researcher should be thinking about their next proposal/projects. The computer should contain several Specific Aims and papers at all times. Ongoing research is the Preliminary Data for a new proposal. This has a large amount to do with the success of established investigators. They use currently funded resources to gather data in support of their next proposal. If this lifestyle is adopted, the computer will always hold several papers and proposals in various stages of gestation. As deadlines approach it is a simple matter to put the finishing touches on, add the finished data, get a knowledgeable review, and send it off.

5

The Abstract
and Specific Aims

The Abstract and the Specific Aims are combined in this chapter because they are very similar. The Specific Aims should be written first to fit within one page, and then trimmed as necessary to fit within the Abstract box and augmented with brief statements of significance and experimental methods. Do not squeeze it into the box by using a smaller type font. The instructions on form page 2 of PHS 398 specify,

> State the application's broad, long-term objectives and specific aims, making reference to the health relatedness of the project. Describe concisely the research design and methods for achieving these goals. Avoid summaries of past accomplishments and the use of the first person. This abstract is meant to serve as a succinct and accurate description of the proposed work when separated from the application. If the application is funded, this description, as is, will become public information. Therefore, do not include proprietary/confidential information. *DO NOT EXCEED THE SPACE PROVIDED.*

The Abstract and Specific Aims are the two most important pages in the proposal. One or the other of these pages may be the only part of the proposal that some of the reviewers will read. Consider again the scenario of the Study Section meeting. The members are seated around a large table. Two of them are the assigned reviewers who have studied the proposal in detail and who will read their written reviews to the group. These presentations take 5–10 minutes each, and during this time the other 15 or so members will browse through the proposal. If any part of the proposal is actually read it is probably the Abstract or the Specific Aims, and it is more likely to be the Specific Aims that is read because of its larger format. It is also common for members generally familiar with the area of the proposal, but not actually assigned to review it, to read its Specific Aims before the Study Section meeting, in order to be better prepared to discuss it.

Study Section members have their own styles of review, but most probably start by quickly scanning the Specific Aims. Thus, this section also has a major impact on the primary reviewers and ultimately on the priority scores. If the Specific Aims are tightly written and beautifully logical and informative, they give a very good first impression of the proposal.

THE SPECIFIC AIMS

Preparation of a research proposal should start with the Specific Aims; the rest of the proposal merely amplifies what is presented there. After reading a well-written Specific Aims, an experienced reviewer will understand the problem addressed, the hypothesis being tested, and the feasibility and power of the experimental approach, and will have a feeling about their importance. If the Specific Aims fails to communicate these ideas, the reviewer is left frustrated and depressed by the realization that this essential information will have to be forcefully extracted from the depths of the proposal.

Failure of the Specific Aims has a devastating and cascading effect on the review. After struggling with it, the reviewer goes on to the Background and Significance section. The review of the literature and discussion here may be pertinent but lost on a reviewer who does not understand what the proposal is all about. As reviewers, at this point we usually abandon any attempt to follow a line of logic and turn to the Experimental Design and Methods section to see if we can at least figure out what will be done. Sometimes it is necessary for a reviewer to list proposed experiments, and assign them to a Specific Aim in order to understand the thinking of the investigator. Then the Background and Significance section is reread in search of that elusive thread of logic one hopes is there. All in all, it is very difficult for mere science to overcome such a psychological handicap imposed on the reviewer. The proposal with a poorly written Specific Aims will surely not receive the priority score it might merit on the basis of its science. The PHS 398 guidelines say, "List the broad, long-term objectives and what the specific research proposed in this application is intended to accomplish, e.g., to test a stated hypothesis, create a novel design, solve a specific problem, or develop new technology. *One page is recommended.*"

We prefer to write a Specific Aims page in four pieces, which are then perfected, trimmed, and merged. These are roughly: (1) general goal/ significance, (2) a theoretical framework or model, (3) hypotheses, and (4) tests of the hypotheses; this last is the actual Specific Aims.

General Goal and Significance

The problem is stated and is shown to be important. This must be done in one or two sentences. It is not necessary to belabor the obvious. For instance, the mere mention of AIDS is sufficient to establish significance; save the gruesome statistics for the Background and Significance section. An indication of the direction of the study is expressed in the goal statement. This should be broad enough to give the impression that this study is part of a larger research plan that will continue beyond the bounds defined in the Specific Aims. A long-term goal might be identified generally as simply the alleviation of the problem.

Example

> Macular degeneration is the most common cause of lost reading vision in the elderly. The pathogenesis of this disease is poorly understood but involves the development of subretinal neovascularization and changes in the choroidal circulation. Our long-term goal is to develop methods for the prevention and treatment of macular degeneration based on understanding of molecular mechanisms that are the basis of the pathology in the retina.

This example identifies the problem, its significance, the field of study, and the long-term goal in only 67 words. It also provides a basis for assignment of the proposal to the National Eye Institute or possibly to the National Institute on Aging, both of which have better funding rates for R01 grants than do some other NIH Institutes. The problem is important by definition, since the NEI has identified it as an area where research is needed.

In making this opening statement it is essential to avoid abbreviations. When we first saw this paragraph it read, "ARMD is the most common cause of decreased VA in the elderly. The pathogenesis of this condition is poorly understood but involves the development of SRN and changes in the choroidal circulation. . . ." Although the primary reviewers undoubtedly would know the meaning of these abbreviations, many of the other Study Section members might not. The effect of this is to dissuade the latter from reading further in the Specific Aims. Instead they will use the time to prospect for red flags.

It is equally useless to simply list a series of experiments, or even worse, a series of methods, as the Specific Aims without providing enough background for the reviewer to understand the problem being studied. A well-written Specific Aims section informs as it goes along, so that no questions essential to its understanding are left unanswered.

A Theoretical Model

Having identified the problem, present a broad theoretical construct or model to which the problem can be related. In disease-related research, the model usually pertains to pathogenesis and will probably logically connect several different hypotheses. It may be difficult to generate such a model in some types of research that are still in a descriptive phase of development, but theory can add great depth to the proposal. Its absence is a blatant red flag, and alerts the reviewer to the possibility that the proposal will lack focus and depth.

A possible model for the above example of subretinal neovascularization (SRN) is,

> Factors released by degenerating retinal pigment epithelial cells (RPE) lyse the underlying basement membrane, exposing the choriocapillaris, and attracting macrophages. These release angiogenic factors to cause endothelial proliferation and migration and so stimulate the choroidal vessels to invade the subretinal space. The SRN amplifies the RPE degeneration.

This theory is actually a set of causally related hypotheses, one or more of which can be the subject of the proposal.

Diagrams are rarely seen on Specific Aims pages. This is unfortunate, because a diagram is sure to catch the eye of the nonassigned reviewers. Better yet, a Specific Aims that is sufficiently brief to accommodate a diagram is very well written indeed! A possible diagram of this model is shown in Figure 5.1.

The theory must be plausible, and it is useful if it has been around long

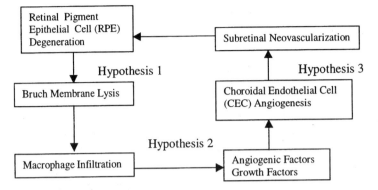

Figure 5.1. Diagram of a SRN theoretic model.

enough to generally be accepted. But many theoretical models are much too broad to be a suitable subject for research. However, any of the several hypotheses in such models could well be the focus of a study. To investigate all parts of a broad model would result in an excessively broad project that might well be downgraded in review because of lack of focus.

One of the most common complaints about weak proposals is that they are too "diffuse." This usually means that the Specific Aims are not sufficiently closely interdependent. A diffuse proposal is usually superficial, since several different investigations cannot be pursued efficiently and in depth within the usual allotted time. Diffuse proposals often lack a theoretic framework that would serve to keep the work focused. Having expressed a basic theory, the temptation to study all parts of it at the same time should be avoided. It is, after all, the path along which you will continue your research after the successful conclusion of the present study.

Interdisciplinary research is also in great demand by the NIH Institutes because it is a good way to foster the application of new technologies to old problems. It is difficult to write an interdisciplinary proposal that is not diffuse. A neuroscientist interested in the biology of transmitters may enlist the aid of a molecular biologist to generate some oligonucleotide probes for specific transmitter receptor genes. What transmitters of the 20–30 possibilities should be studied? As few as possible! Also it would be catastrophic for the proposal to suggest that the work be done in nervous tissue of Alzheimer patients, as this would shatter the focus of the study. Problems of particular interest to the molecular biologist must not be allowed to surface in the proposal, as this will decrease its focus.

Obviously a great deal of diplomacy is required to set up a strong, focused multidisciplinary study.

Another catchphrase of the NIH Institutes is "clinical relevance." There is a great temptation to combine clinical and basic science studies in the same proposal, probably due to a general perception that clinical relevancy increases the prospects for funding. Such a study is by definition diffuse, and great care must be taken to convince the reviewer that each part of the study goes into as much depth as possible with the material at hand. It is certainly true that the Institute Advisory Council, based on high program relevance, may elect to improve the priority score assigned to a proposal by the Study Section. But this is not done often and usually happens only when research is proposed in a relatively unfrequented area. High program relevance does not automatically lead to increased scores if the area is already being studied adequately. It is much more common for a proposal to suffer the stigma of being diffuse because an attempt at clinical relevancy was forced.

Hypotheses

Having established the problem and a logical structure within which it can be considered, one or more specific hypotheses should be stated. This is the most important part of the Specific Aims section, and is often missing or stated in such general terms as to be useless. Unless a specific hypothesis can be stated and tested, research is nothing more than a fishing expedition. Admittedly, descriptive research begins the study of a new field and is essential as a base for in-depth studies, but there are very few such new fields of study. A trap that awaits us all is the "interesting observation" that beckons to us like the Sirens of Ulysses. Research that is designed to investigate something just because it is there may be very interesting to the PI, but rarely to enough of the Study Section to generate a fundable priority score. Phenomenological proposals are weak and tend to end up on the rocks. It is worth repeating that a proposal is strengthened if a hypothesis is clearly identified, if it relates logically to a broad theoretic model, and if the proposed experiments will actually test it.

Some hypotheses are hardly worthy of the name. "Colorectal cancers are detected more often with the flexible sigmoidoscope than with the rigid sigmoidoscope" is a hypothesis of sorts, but is trivial and hardly worth a research effort to test. It was proposed as the basis for a retrospective study of data from over 800 sigmoidoscopies in a large county hospital. The flexible instrument reaches higher into the colon than the rigid sigmoidoscope. The difference in detectability could be related to variation of the incidence of cancer with position along the colon, a possible problem of epidemiology. This proposal was greatly strengthened when it was rewritten as an epidemiological study to test the hypothesis that the incidence of high colonic cancer in men is reduced by long-term use of a high-fiber diet. The same data were used for the study, but the approach was changed.

We live in an age of powerful experimental tools. The availability of a technology has the tendency to stimulate research that uses it. Proposals that are based on technological advances rather than on important hypotheses cannot help but be weak. A good example was the introduction of a powerful procedure used by molecular biologists called the polymerase chain reaction, or PCR. This procedure amplifies minute amounts of DNA in a tissue section, thereby permitting the recognition of virus particles. With the emphasis on AIDS research, there was a rush to seek evidence of HIV in a variety of different tissues. "The hypothesis to be tested is that HIV is present in the [you name it] of patients with AIDS Related Complex" was a formula for far too many studies, some of which were actually funded since the NIH was compelled to use the funds given to it by Congress for AIDS research. A hypothesis is not strong unless it is related to a significant theoretical model of the disease.

A hypothesis worthy of consideration can be tested directly or gives rise to corollaries or predictions that can be tested. Untestable hypotheses are worse than useless; they are destructive in that they may consume time and effort without a concomitant advance of knowledge.

Excessive listing of hypotheses signals lack of focus. A single important hypothesis is best; most proposals list two or perhaps three (four is one too many).

Specific Aims (Tests of the Hypotheses)

Specific Aims are then stated. These are the tests of the hypotheses presented in terms of experiments or groups of experiments. These should be listed numerically and should be reiterated verbatim and in order in the Experimental Design and Methods section of the proposal. The Specific Aims should be just that, specific. They must be brief and indicate the general nature of the technology used (but should not include discussion of the actual methods). This section usually fills about a third of the page. The reason for each of the aims should be obvious from consideration of the hypotheses and their corollaries. There is never enough room on this page to really explain the rationale of each aim. But this is done in exhaustive detail later in the proposal. It is only necessary that each aim fit within the structure of the theory. Avoid editorializing: "These studies may lead to the development of novel strategies for the treatment of whatever." Do not cite references. If the reviewer has to look up a reference in order to get through the Specific Aims, it is a failure. Three Specific Aims are usually enough!

Example

The following Specific Aims was submitted to the NIH. It is instructive for several reasons. You might wish to evaluate and rate it before reading the critique of it.

Alzheimer's disease (AD) is a dementing disorder of unknown etiology. The diagnosis of "presumed" or "probable" AD is made through clinical diagnosis, in recognition that AD can only be definitively diagnosed histopathologically. Characteristically, memory is initially impaired, followed by visuo-spatial deficits, and, finally, involvement of all cognitive functions (Hutton, 1987).

We hope to address a number of Specific Aims by the completion of this project:

1. Is there selective involvement of a particular component or class of cells in the visual system of AD patients? If so, can this be related to the pathophysiology of AD in the rest of the brain? If there is a predilection for loss of a class of ganglion cells in AD, this may yield insight to the reasons for predominant degeneration of large neurons in other areas of the brain (Terry et al, 1981).

2. Can visual testing be used, in conjunction with present neurological and psychometric evaluations, as a screening procedure to identify AD?

3. Can visual testing or histopathological assessments of the visual system be used to identify subtypes of AD? If so, this might provide insights leading to possible management and treatment strategies for AD.

4. We will gain insights into both anatomical and functional AD subgroups through correlative histopathological and clinical assessments of the visual system in the age-matched controls (normals) used in this study.

5. Significant new data relevant to the effect of age on the visual system will be gathered.

Critique

This is a weak Specific Aims. The first line is excellent, but the rest of the opening paragraph is fluff without a clear relationship to the proposal.

The brief description of the defects of AD speaks down to the reviewers, who are certainly well informed about it. The reference is superfluous.

There is no hypothesis or theory offered.

To write, "We hope to do this or that," is weak. It may be honest, but it is bad grantsmanship. It leaves room for doubt as to whether what follows will be achieved. A major concern of the reviewer is the question of what the PI will have left if part of the proposal does not work. The Specific Aims should never contain anything that is controversial, equivocal, or negative.

Aim 1 could have been stated as a hypothesis and test combined. "We will test the hypothesis that large neurons are selectively destroyed in AD by measuring the sizes of ganglion cells in the retinas of AD patients and of age-matched controls." The rest of Aim 1 is editorializing. The suggestion that this retinal study might be correlated with the results of other research on brain tissue is speculation. Such correlations are notoriously difficult, and to throw one in here seems to be window dressing. Speculations in the Specific Aims are very destructive since they interfere with its purpose, which is to provide an executive summary of the project. Speculation is by its very nature weak and argumentative. The less of it in a proposal the better.

Specific Aim 2 is clearly a non sequitur. What does a screening procedure have to do with large cell loss? Actually there is an association, but it is speculative. There is a suggestion that visuomotor skills are dependent on large ganglion cell input from the retina to the brain. The investigators hope to find visuomotor deficits in AD patients, and if these can be seen early in the disease, the tests could be used for screening. Unfortunately, the opening paragraph states that memory loss is the initial event in AD, and loss of visuomotor function comes later. Clearly a test of memory loss would be a better screening procedure. This is not suggested since there is no apparent correlation between memory loss and large cell loss.

Specific Aim 2 could have been stated thus: "A corollary of this hypothesis suggests that large ganglion cell dependent visuomotor function of AD patients should be defective. We will test this with eye track recordings in patients and age-matched controls."

Specific Aim 3 is combined speculation and window dressing. What is meant by "subtypes of AD"? At present, as stated in the opening paragraph, we cannot even diagnose AD without histopathology, so how can we talk about clinical subtypes? Of course diagnosis by histopathology cannot help "management and treatment strategies of AD." This aim is best eliminated.

Specific Aim 4 assumes that Aim 3 was successful, and is otherwise editorializing, as is Aim 5. Both should be eliminated.

A restructuring of this Specific Aims could be built around the following, excerpted from above and expanded:

> Alzheimer's disease (AD) is a dementing disorder of unknown etiology. Recent studies have shown that AD is associated with loss of larger brain cells and with optic nerve degeneration. Since the retina is actually part of the brain and has been studied in far greater functional and anatomic detail, it may provide an ideal model in which to investigate the relationship of a cell's size to its susceptibility to damage in AD.
>
> Specific Aims:
>
> 1. We will test the hypothesis that large neurons are selectively destroyed in AD by measuring the sizes of ganglion cells in the retinas of AD patients and in age-matched controls.
>
> 2. A corollary of this hypothesis suggests that large ganglion cell dependent visuomotor function of AD patients should be defective. We will test this with eye track recordings in patients and in age-matched controls.

This is considerably less than a full page. It should be expanded to emphasize the desirability of a collaborative study involving a basic scientist and a clinician, and the availability of a large patient base. Ideally, the theoretical model would contain hypotheses about the functional relations between AD etiology and neuron size, or about the mechanisms that drive these relations. These should lead to the prediction that there should be a predilection of AD to affect large rather than small neurons.

A successful Specific Aims section can be read in about 3 minutes. It leads the reader to understand the goals of the project and its importance, the theory behind the study, the hypotheses to be tested, and the tests to be used.

The following is a relatively well-written Specific Aims:

> A number of clinical diseases have been associated with disorders of retinal pigment epithelium (RPE) transport and barrier function. The long-term goal of this research is to fully characterize these properties of human RPE to facilitate treatment and perhaps prevention of these diseases.
>
> During the last period we also developed and standardized a new method by which fluid fluxes can be measured directly rather than calculated from isotope fluxes, which are subject to cumulative experimental errors. We plan to incorporate this method into our proposed studies, to test the following **hypotheses:**

a) Cultured fetal human RPE, under normal conditions, transports fluid from its apical side to its basal side utilizing a $Na+$, $K+$, $Cl-$ cotransport system as well as a $Na+$, HCO_3- cotransport system.

b) The activities of these transport systems are modulated by intracellular cAMP concentrations.

c) Cultured fetal human RPE mediated transepithelial fluid movement is modulated by beta adrenergic agonists, histamine, prostaglandin E1, and vasoactive intestinal peptide (VIP) that alter intracellular cAMP concentration. In addition, agents that alter intracellular cAMP metabolism, such as the phosphodiesterase inhibitor isobutylmethylxanthine (IBMX), also alter human RPE mediated transepithelial fluid movement.

To test these hypotheses, we propose studies with the following specific aims:

1. To characterize cultured fetal human RPE transepithelial transport by extending Ussing chamber studies using pharmacologic probes, ion manipulation, and isotope flux studies.

2. To determine how cultured fetal human RPE transepithelial transport is modulated by intracellular cAMP.

3. To determine the degree to which cultured fetal human RPE transepithelial transport may be regulated by extracellular receptors (such as those to beta adrenergic agents) and to determine the degree to which cultured fetal human RPE transepithelial transport is affected by agents (such as IBMX) that alter intracellular cAMP metabolism.

In the original, this Specific Aims section just filled one page. The hypotheses could be improved by deleting the phrases about methods and emphasizing the hypothesized movement of fluid in real life. The Specific Aims themselves could be improved by eliminating the editorializing, since these comments are repeated in the Methods section. This was for a competing renewal proposal, so reference to past productivity and continuity of work is good.

THE ABSTRACT

The Abstract (called "Description" in PHS 398) should contain (1) the essence of the Specific Aims; (2) a few short sentences concerning the health relatedness of the research; and (3) its scientific significance in terms of its long-term goals. Such statements are often added to the Specific Aims as well. This is useful, provided that the essential parts of the section are not shortened to make room for this addition.

The following is an acceptable abstract in that it expresses a hypothesis and states the experimental approach to its testing. The significance of the proposed work is also presented. But it fails the appearance test. There are no spaces. Hypothesis, Method, and Significance are not highlighted. It is jammed into the box.

Magnesium (Mg) deficiency may play an important role in the pathogenesis of enhanced vascular reactivity in hypertension. The overall hypothesis to be evaluated is that Mg deficiency caused by glucose intolerance, insulin resistance, or other factors in hypertensives leads to increased vasomotor tone via altered release of vasoactive cycloxygenase and lipoxygenase products of arachidonic acid and enhanced angiotensin II (AII) action. To evaluate the effects of Mg deficiency in normal subjects we will induce the condition by administration of a low Mg diet. Vascular and adrenal sensitivity to AII, platelet aggregation, and eicosanoid levels will be studied prior to and after Mg deficiency is established. Since evidence suggests that Mg deficiency can modulate insulin action, the effect of this deficiency on glucose tolerance will also be studied. In another project the effect of insulin on intracellular Mg levels will be studied using a new fura 2 Mg dye technique. These studies will be performed in groups of subjects with varied blood pressure and insulin levels. Also the effects of acute intravenous and chronic oral Mg loading on the above parameters will be studied in similar subject groups. We will directly study the effect of Mg on AII, insulin, and insulin-like growth factor action in isolated and cultured adrenal glomerulosa cells. Concentration of Mg will be varied and signal transduction and steroidogenic effects will be evaluated. These studies will provide insight into mechanisms important to the pathogenesis of altered vascular reactivity of subjects with hypertension or hyperinsulinemia.

An Abstract that completely fills the box, without line spaces or indentations, affords a repulsive aspect for a tired reviewer, who may well decide to skip it. An Abstract of three or four paragraphs separated by line spaces and containing the words "Hypothesis" and "Specific Aims" in bold, on the other hand, catches the eye, promises interesting informative reading, and has a positive impact on the reviewer (see below).

Magnesium (Mg) deficiency may play an important role in the pathogenesis of enhanced vascular reactivity in hypertension. The overall **HYPOTHESIS** to be evaluated is that Mg deficiency caused by glucose intolerance, insulin resistance, or other factors in hypertensives leads to increased vasomotor tone via altered release of vasoactive cycloxygenase and lipoxygenase products of arachidonic acid and enhanced angiotensin II (AII) action.

Specific Aims: (1) Determine the effects of low Mg on vascular and adrenal sensitivity to AII (platelet aggregation and eicosanoid levels, and glucose tolerance). (2) Determine the effect of insulin on intracellular Mg levels (fura 2 Mg dye technique). These studies will be performed in subjects with varied blood pressure and insulin levels. (3) Determine the effects of acute intravenous and chronic oral Mg loading on the above parameters. (4) Determine the signal transduction and steroidogenic effects of Mg on AII, insulin, and insulin-like growth factor action in isolated and cultured adrenal glomerulosa cells.

Significance. These studies will provide insight into mechanisms important to the pathogenesis of altered vascular reactivity of subjects with hypertension or hyperinsulinemia.

6

Background and Significance

The PHS 398 application form directions state,

BACKGROUND AND SIGNIFICANCE. Briefly sketch the background leading to the present application, critically evaluate existing knowledge, and specifically identify the gaps that the project is intended to fill. State concisely the importance and health relevance of the research described in this application by relating the specific aims to the broad, long-term objectives. *TWO TO THREE PAGES ARE RECOMMENDED.*

To receive a fundable priority score, a research project must be perceived by the reviewers to be important, interesting, and likely to succeed. Having digested a well-written Specific Aims, the reviewer approaches Background and Significance with a general idea concerning the scope of the project, the technology involved, the logic of the experimental approach, and, it is hoped, the general hypotheses to be tested. These ideas were presented as unsupported statements in the Specific Aims, so it is the purpose of the background section to provide the missing support through expansion and judicious reference to the literature. Section *b* (Background and Significance) must establish three things within the confines of not more than three pages.

1. *The project is important.* It relates to a significant deficit in our knowledge of human disease or an important biologic process. The results of the hypothesis tests will have a predictable impact on theory and/or ultimately lead to improvement of the human condition.

2. *The science is interesting.* The study can be related to a general theoretical model that is the subject of widespread interest; important areas within the model that are unproven, controversial, or ambiguous are addressed.

3. *There is a high probability of success.* Specific hypotheses to be tested can be identified as part of the theoretical model; tests of the

hypotheses (Specific Aims) are feasible, definitive, and within the range of the PI's apparent expertise.

Styles of writing vary greatly; the product of good writing, however, always satisfies the basic requirements of journalism. It is essential that this section be outlined before it is written. The three pages will accommodate no more than 12 paragraphs. If diagrams are used, and this is often very helpful, each will occupy the space of one or more paragraphs. The outline should provide titles for most paragraphs. When the outline is complete, there should be an obvious logical connection from one paragraph to the next. The logic of the connection is stated in a sentence that should be added to the outline. These sentences may eventually appear in the finished document as transition sentences between paragraphs. If you do not like to outline, go ahead and write up the section. Then make an outline of what you have written. Look at it critically for logic, flow, and transitions, and correct it accordingly. Then rewrite the section.

Example 1: Writing the Background Section Outline

The following is a sample outline developed for a proposal concerning studies of the biology of subretinal neovascularization, the growth of abnormal blood vessels beneath the retina that occurs in a variety of eye diseases. It assumes 12 paragraphs.

1. Subretinal neovascularization (SRN) contributes to age-related macular degeneration, the most common cause of loss of reading vision. [*Importance.*] The new vessels develop from the choroid as the result of some unknown stimulus such as an angiogenic growth factor. [*Transition.*]

2. Chemical factors cause the growth of blood vessels. These factors must be present in the subretinal space in relation to the retinal pigment epithelial (RPE) cells, which have been shown to be phagocytic and to produce certain cytokines. [*Area of focus and transition.*]

3. RPE cells may elaborate cytokines that are angiogenic under pathologic conditions such as inflammation, but suppress endothelial cell growth under normal conditions (see diagram). [*General theory.*]

4. In disease states, RPE cells transform to macrophage-like or fibroblast-like cells and are capable of generating a number of cytokines or angiogenesis factors when activated. [*Review of known RPE cell function.*]

5. However, much of the biology of RPE cells is not understood, such as their response to a variety of cytokines or their ability to produce cytokines that might be mitogenic for endothelial cells. [*Knowledge gaps.*]

6. Angiogenic factors are probably present in the subretinal space to stimulate the growth of SRN. [*Review of cytokines associated with angiogenesis.*]

7. SRN develops as a result of release of factors from RPE cells activated by common cytokines (e.g., interleukin-1 and complement) associated with inflammation. [*Hypothesis.*]

8. Review of pertinent work for or against the hypothesis.

9. The supernatant of activated RPE cell cultures should cause endothelial cell proliferation in vitro. Interleukin-1 should cause RPE cell activation, and should be present in the subretinal space in conditions leading to SRN. [*Rationale for hypothesis corollaries to be tested.*]

10. Results of in vitro studies that support the hypothesis will provide the basis for in-depth studies of an animal model; review literature of SRN model. [*At the time of this proposal, use of transgenic animals was very innovative.*]

11. The biology of RPE cell activation in animal models of different retinal diseases associated with SRN can be explored. [*Direction of future research.*]

12. SRN growth may be inhibited pharmacologically by specific antagonists of RPE cell activation or RPE cytokines. [*Translation to the human.*]

Below, the concepts to be developed in this section will be explored more fully.

IMPORTANCE

Evaluation of importance is a value judgment that the nonassigned panel members make based on past experience and the impact of the assigned reviewers' personalities and reports. Research that is perceived to be unimportant will receive a worse priority score. Some NIH Institutes have developed plans for research support that describe in detail the views of their Advisory Councils concerning what is important. The 5-year plan of the National Eye Institute, for instance, identifies vision research in a variety of different areas that need emphasis (<www.nei.nih.gov>). Other Institutes release Program Announcements that highlight targeted areas of research interest. These guidelines are used extensively by the Institute staff to evaluate the progress of NIH programs. Research that can be related to these plans or announcements is significant by definition, and this will be accepted by many of the Study Section members.

Although some Institutes have not developed and published as clear guidelines as others, all have some sort of research goals. The bounds of the established Institute areas of interest should be carefully observed. Follow the links to "extramural funding" or "grants" within each Institute home page at <www.nih.gov/icd>. To deviate from Institute goals is to risk being considered outside the mainstream of important research, and to risk loss of priority because section members consider the proposed work relatively trivial.

Unfortunately, publications of the Institutes are outdated before they are in press. Also, some areas earmarked for additional development may have been inserted for political reasons and may be of no interest to Study Section members. For instance, one item in an early NEI plan called for more research on techniques of noninvasive evaluation of the visual system. This sounds fine but most section members had no interest in this area and very few proposals to develop new tests were funded.

The most knowledgeable source of wisdom concerning the importance of a project is the Institute Program Manager of the categorical program that would fund the work. Program Administrators should be consulted if there is any question about the importance of the aims of a proposal. These people also know how many other proposals in the same area have been submitted or are actually funded. (Follow the links within the home page of each Institute to listings of extramural programs and staff).

Importance is subjective. Researchers usually consider anything they are interested in to be important. This is a trap waiting for all of us. What is important for a proposal is not what the investigator thinks is important, but what the Study Section thinks is important. This can be easily determined if the identity of the section members is known. A quick computer search of the publications during the past few years of key section members will show very clearly what they think is important. It will also show which of the many possible experimental approaches they consider most useful. For instance, a section that has five or six members that include immunohistochemistry in their research will appreciate studies using the same procedures, providing, of course, that they are well done.

Section members will not just accept the word of a consultant for a project about the importance of a study unless they are unfamiliar with the area and the consultant is very well known. This is rarely the case. The assigned reviewers generally are familiar with an area even if they are not experts, and their decision about its importance is probably mostly reflex or personal bias. Members may be strongly impressed by the bias of other section members. On several occasions, Dr. Ogden was the only medically trained scientist present at a Study Section meeting. If a question came up concerning the relevance of a proposal to some disease process, it was inevitable that he was asked to pontificate—and it was a bit disconcerting to witness the solemnity with which his words were considered. Members who were better scientists than he and who knew more than he about the research under discussion were all too ready to accept his opinions concerning the clinical significance and importance of a project.

If, in evaluating the members of a section that will review your proposal, you find insufficient expertise in your research area, you should contact the SRA or the CSR assignment officer and request assignment to a more appropriate Study Section. For example, a colleague submitted a proposal concerning immunotherapy for ocular choroidal melanoma. It was reviewed by one of the many cancer Study Sections and assigned to the NCI for funding. The Study Section did not contain an ophthalmologist and downgraded the proposal on the basis that the disease is too rare to merit support and is not targeted for study by the NCI. On resubmission, after numerous letters and telephone calls, the proposal was assigned to a visual sciences Study Section and to the NEI for funding. It received a sympathetic review from panelists who were appreciative of the importance of ocular melanoma as an eye disease and the proposed studies were funded.

In the ideal proposal, importance is inherent in the subject matter and it is simply not necessary to belabor the issue. In fact, it is a mistake to place heavy emphasis on the importance of a study that all present would accept as important. This uses valuable space in the proposal and may appear to be "talking down" to the Study Section. It will certainly aggravate the reviewer who has to wade through unnecessary journalistic hype.

It is not easy to categorize types of research as to importance, and there are many exceptions to any rules that might be stated. With this apologia, consider research directed to the study of basic mechanisms related to normal function or pathogenesis more important than that directed to the study of phenomena. Applied research is less important than basic research. A study of the cellular mechanisms involved in glucose regulation is more important than a study of the modulation of blood glucose levels by diet. A study of membrane charge carriers in cerebral neurons is more important than a study of the electroencephalogram in certain diseases. A study of potassium flux through the membrane of a cardiac cell is more important than a study of changes in the EKG caused by different blood levels of potassium. A study of the mechanisms of transfection with HPV is more important than a study of the incidence of carcinomas of the cervix having HPV transfected cells.

Phenomenological research is rarely funded. Without a statistical study to prove it, our impression is that such studies are viewed by Study Sections as less exciting, and accordingly receive poorer priority scores. What should matter is the standard of research in the particular field, but it is hard to stimulate the interest of 18–20 Study Section members by a descriptive study when there are so many mechanistic, hypothesis-testing proposals going unfunded. Some areas of research simply have not progressed beyond the descriptive stage. But if some researchers in the field have progressed beyond the descriptive, descriptive studies will not be competitive.

Quantitative research is clearly more important than qualitative. Many investigators do research that is qualitative; they avoid quantitative approaches because of a weakness in mathematics or perhaps a preference for studies that are experimentally less arduous. Our impression is that the qualitative workers outnumber the quantitative. What is certain is that a proposal that involves quantitation and that is reviewed by a section member whose own work is qualitative will probably do all right. A proposal that is qualitative and that is reviewed by a member whose work is quantitative will almost certainly suffer. Quantitative work is more arduous and those who do it are convinced the effort is worth it. It is natural for such a person to feel that a proposed qualitative study would be better if it were quantitative. This attitude will permeate the review consciously or subconsciously, and may influence the rest of the section members to degrade their scores. For the strongest possible proposal, as much quantitation as possible should be included.

Disease-related basic research is generally perceived to be more important than studies with little clinical relevance. Despite this obvious truth, clinical research projects are treated so badly by regular Study Sections that separate review mechanisms must be used to justify funding. This results from the tendency of Study Sections to be composed of basic scientists who have little sympathy for the limitations on experimental design imposed by the use of human subjects. Clinical studies always lack the rigor of well-designed laboratory studies, and a special effort must be made to make their design as tight as possible. Studies that combine clinical and laboratory experiments are likely to be considered more important than studies that are purely clinical. Conversely, a laboratory study that includes a direct clinical application may be considered more important than without the clinical arm. These generalities apply only if the clinical study is good. A poorly designed clinical study cannot be salvaged by some laboratory work. It may destroy what might otherwise be a strong basic science project.

A useful test of importance is to ask, "What impact will the results of this research have on other research in the field or on our understanding and treatment of disease?" If there is not a clear answer to the question, the work may not be perceived as very important.

INTEREST

An important project may not be very interesting. This is perhaps the problem with clinical projects that involve nothing more than how many people with cancer of the lung smoke tobacco. It is a challenge to make such studies interesting to the reviewers so that they get excited about the study and actually become its protagonists in the meeting. The best thing that can happen to a proposal is for the assigned reviewers to become so enamored with it that they actively try to sell it to the rest of the section. Their enthusiasm will be contagious and a better priority score will result.

Interest is also subjective, and different things interest different people. What can be said generally is that something that is new is more likely to be interesting. New ideas are interesting: new experimental approaches, new hypotheses, new interpretations of old data. These are interesting. They are also probably controversial, but controversy is interesting. Diagrams enhance interest, if they are easy to understand and are done well. Color enhances interest (particularly of the assigned reviewers), and should be used freely. But be careful that a black and white photocopy of your colored figures is legible. Recently, use of a two-column page has become more common. This certainly sets a proposal apart, and it enhances readability and interest. The importance of interest cannot be overstated. Study section meetings get immensely dull after a day or so, and a great effort is required to keep one's concentration on the proceedings. Anything remotely interesting or novel is very welcome and will be rewarded, provided the interest is not overly centered in controversy.

Innovation creates interest. The reviewers are now required to make a specific statement concerning innovation in a proposal. Every effort should be made to persuade the reviewer that some part of your proposal is innovative. This is often not easy. Most research is, in fact, not innovative. It uses approaches that have proven to be useful in other situations. For instance, a cytokine shown to be important for maturation of alveolar cells might be studied in relation to renal tubular cells, to see if it had the same effects. This study, if new for the kidney, might be well worth undertaking, but it would probably not be considered innovative. A study using a new method to produce a highly specific knockout mouse for testing a hypothesis about the function of a newly identified protein would probably be considered innovative (in the year 2002). In general, innovation involves a new conceptual, methodological, or design strategy that surmounts an (heretofore) insurmountable barrier to acquisition of new information.

Everyone loves a good story. The proposal that unfolds a complicated theoretical model like a storybook, bringing the reader along in logical steps, posing interesting questions, offering exciting insights, and suggesting clever tests, will fascinate the reader. It will not be overloaded with trivial detail. Every sentence will pull the reader along another step. In our collective experience as Study Section member or chairman, NIH administrator, or Grants Counselor, we have carefully read and critiqued many hundreds of proposals. Only a handful were written in a way to enhance interest. What a pity!

SUCCESS

The Background and Significance section should present the problem to be studied in a way that leaves the reviewer optimistic about the prospects for success of the project. This feeling will be based on the clarity of the presentation, its sharp focus on an important problem, a clearly defined experimental model, and a few specific, testable hypotheses. Diffuse, poorly focused proposals do not forebode success. The statement that "very little is known about (whatever)" identifies a gap in knowledge, but suggests that the problem is being approached from a base of ignorance. Even if this is true, it is a negative attitude that bespeaks failure, as does any project that can be construed to be a "fishing expedition" because specific hypotheses are not stated. This section establishes the depth of the PI's thinking and knowledge. Every paragraph, every sentence, and every reference should be necessary and should contribute *in a positive way* to the whole. Do not raise problems with the project in Background and Significance. They must be put to rest, of course, but the place to do this is in Research Design and Methods. Discussion of competing hypotheses or arguments for or against your own pet hypothesis is not necessarily negative. Present the discussion in the positive light of your ability to test the alternatives.

SIGNIFICANCE

The significance part of this section should be addressed in a last *short* paragraph that points out how the research will advance knowledge perhaps by removing a barrier in the field, or enhance knowledge or treatment of disease. Since the significance of the work had better be very obvious to the reviewers by the time they get this far into the proposal, a specific statement of significance is probably optional. It certainly does not warrant more than a few lines.

Example 2: Unifying the Background Section

The following is the Background and Significance section from a competing renewal proposal for a study of subretinal neovascularization. It is relatively well written and addresses the difficult problem of integrating in a logical manner a series of 16 experiments. How each of the experiments relates to an overall theory of angiogenesis is also shown. This proposal received the best priority score among the set of 78 proposals considered by the Study Section at that meeting. References have been deleted.

Subretinal neovascularization (SRN) is the common denominator of a number of different disease processes and the determinant of the disciform response. In a case-controlled clinical study, Hyman found SRN and the disciform response to be responsible in 83.5% of cases of significant visual loss secondary to macular degeneration, which is the leading cause of central or reading vision loss in the United States and the United Kingdom. The resultant great human and economic loss has led the National Eye Institute (NEI) to designate macular degeneration a high priority area for research. The pathogenesis of SRN and the disciform process remains poorly understood. There is a need for extensive studies of this important process under controlled laboratory conditions. [*Comment:* This paragraph forcefully establishes the importance of this particular area of research, and cites the NIH plan for emphasis.]

In our experimental model, intense argon laser photocoagulation is applied at eight separate macular sites. The burns cause breaks in Bruch's membrane and retinal necrosis. Histologically detectable SRN occurs in 76% of lasered eyes. In those eyes that develop SRN, the "active" (38%) lesions show leakage and pooling of dye on fluorescein angiography. The remaining "inactive" lesions do not exhibit leakage and pooling of dye but morphologically do exhibit subretinal neovascularization. They are characterized by an absence of serous retinal detachment and an active proliferation of the choroidal stroma and RPE. [*Comment:* Although the transition is rough, this paragraph indicates the familiarity of the researchers with SRN and indicates they have a good experimental model with which to study it.]

Our experimental model of SRN (Fig. 6.1) is characterized by an immediate coagulative necrosis of the retina, RPE, choroid, and variable subretinal detachment (Fig. 6.1—Laser). This is followed by an inflammatory response with infiltration of PMNs and fibrin into the serous retinal detachment at 48 hours. Macrophage infiltration begins slightly later on day 3, but increases as the number of PMNs decreases (Fig. 6.1—Inflammation). Our **hypothesis** is that macrophage infiltration is necessary to proceed to the next stage of proliferation. The RPE is seen to be proliferating by day 8, followed by new vessel formation and fibroblast proliferation (Fig. 6.1—Proliferation). Active (Fig. 6.1—Active) or inactive (Fig. 6.1—Inactive) new vessel formation is usually complete by day 14. The active vessels grow into the serous retinal detachment and the inactive vessels are enclosed by RPE. The active vessels involute at varying times over the following weeks. Our second **hypothesis** is that the RPE proliferation is responsible for this involution. [*Comment:* This paragraph further describes the experimental SRN and suggests several testable hypotheses concerning its pathogenesis, and is illustrated by a diagram that accompanies this section. Since this diagram represents progress as well as proposed experiments, it could have been presented in the Progress Report. The advantage of placing it in the Background and Significance is that the proposed model of pathogenesis is shown early in the proposal.]

The actual stimulus to angiogenesis is unknown, although Ben-Ezra has suggested that macrophage-derived prostaglandin E-1 may have a strong neovasculogenic potential and Polverini has demonstrated that extracts of activated macrophages have angiogenic activity. Penfold, and Grindle and Marshall have emphasized the importance of the macrophage in the development of SRN and, more recently, Penfold, Killingsworth and Sarks have described the role of the macrophage and other inflammatory cells in the breakdown of Bruch's membrane. Studies of the late repair process and phagocytic response in the photocoagulated retina have demonstrated cir-

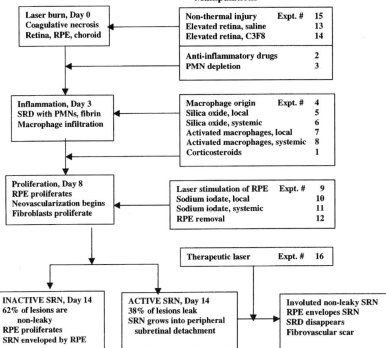

Figure 6.1. Diagram of laser-induced subretinal neovascularization (SRN) model. Sixteen experimental manipulations are indicated by experiment number as they relate to different stages in the development of the process.

culating monocytes to be the main source of phagocytic cells. [*Comment:* In this paragraph the literature concerning theories of SRN pathogenesis is reviewed with emphasis on angiogenic factors.]

Both active and involuted SRN have similar endothelial cells with fenestrations and tight junctions. They differ in that the RPE surrounding the vessels of the involuted lesion seems to provide a barrier to the diffusion of fluid into the subretinal space. The RPE proliferates in many retinochoroidal diseases and may have a papillary form in which sequential layers of RPE are laid down as tubes. Tubules of RPE may enclose the proliferating blood vessels. Both types of RPE proliferation occur in our model. As the RPE proliferates, recovery is both anatomical and functional. [*Comment:* This paragraph offers some ideas about the differences between "active" and "inactive" SRN, a clinically important distinction. It refers to the second paragraph and is something of a non sequitur in this location. It is a very interesting subject for several clinicians on the Study Section who were targeted as potential reviewers and was probably inserted to underline the clinical relevance of the project.]

Our experimental model is reproducible and has been utilized by others. Although it differs from senile macular degeneration (SMD) in many aspects, it does have features in common with many diseases characterized by the disciform response. Like the clinical disease, it shows many variations and presentations, and leads to serous detachment, spontaneous hemorrhage, and cicatrization as part of its involution. In addition, the development of SRN in man after therapeutic laser photocoagulation correlates closely with our model. Also, the disciform response in myopia may run its course from first symptoms to cicatrization within eight weeks, which is in keeping with the time course of our experimental model. [*Comment:* Clinical relevance is hammered home. A common complaint about animal models is that they have little relevance to clinical disease. It is hoped that this paragraph will blunt this criticism.]

Our model of SRN shown in Fig. 6.1 invites manipulation at a number of points. These are indicated in the boxes on the right which propose specific interventions in the pathogenesis of SRN. We have already shown experimentally that high-dose corticosteroid infusion from the time of laser photocoagulation significantly reduces subretinal neovascularization. In addition, we have developed a chronic indwelling vitreous cannula, which can be used without adverse effects in monkey eyes for up to 1–1/2 years. This allows us to deliver agents directly to the retinas of animals with developing SRN. [*Comment:* A complex theoretical model of SRN pathogenesis was presented in a full-page figure (Figure 6.1). The diagram is sufficiently self-explanatory that there is very little in the way of legend needed. The goal of the study is therapeutic intervention and the diagram indicates the rationale for 16 different experiments, each designed to test a particular hypothesis or interfere with a particular process thought to be essential in SRN pathogenesis.]

Each intervention attempts to enhance or depress a specific postulated pathogenic mechanism. The results of the study may reveal the relative importance of each of these wound-healing responses to the development of SRN. This knowledge will ultimately lead to a more rational and effective approach to SRN therapy. [*Comment:* This last boilerplate paragraph sums up the logic of the significance section and the rationale for the particular experimental strategy outlined in this proposal.]

This example shows very clearly that no matter how good the priority score, any proposal can be improved. The success of this section was based largely on the use of a full-page diagram that presented a basic theory of pathogenesis and indicated the relationship of the Specific Aims and the individual experiments to the theory. The animal models were innovative. No attempt at an exhaustive review of a very large body of literature was made. The PI had numerous publications in the field, and could afford to be quite sketchy in the presentation of this section, which could have been much more tightly written. The strength of the section was its success in orienting the reader in a painless manner to a complex new theory of SRN pathogenesis and to show very simply a long list of experimental manipulations. This particular approach to grantsmanship involves provision of necessary background for each experiment in the Research Design and Methods section. It would have been a disaster to include all the necessary background and literature review for so many experiments in the significance section. Although it was successful in this case, the Background and Significance sections of most proposals focus on basic mechanisms rather than experiments. The diagram of Figure 6.1 took an entire page, yet the section was still limited to three pages.

Times change. Technology advances. This project would probably be considered diffuse now because it involved many different mechanisms of pathogenesis. The studies would certainly be considered superficial by today's standards since signaling pathways were not to be studied. It is a severe challenge for professionals to keep abreast of the rapidly changing technical advances in their fields. This hard fact of life explains the failure of many M.D./Ph.D. training programs, in which 2 years of medicine are followed by 3 years of graduate training for the Ph.D., and then by the final 2 years of medicine, internship, and residency. At this point a career decision must be made. An additional 2–3 years of fellowship training is mandatory for a university career. If the fellowship is clinical, it is anathema for basic research. The techniques and thinking experienced during the Ph.D. training will be nearly 10 years out of date. On the other hand, if a research fellowship is done, the individual is probably not qualified for a clinical research position in many specialties.

Example 3: Diagrams in the Cause of Brevity

The following example is the Background and Significance section of another successful proposal. It shows the power of diagrams to reduce verbiage and to explain complex relationships. This was a competing renewal application, so a few words about the successes of the initial grant period were appropriate. The subject is uveitis and a new theory of pathogenesis incorporating a number of hypotheses was presented. The logic of experimental intervention is immediately apparent from consideration of the diagrams. The section reads like it was excerpted from a textbook. It is easy to appreciate the basis of its success—it is simply well written.

The references have been removed to facilitate reading. The paragraphs are numbered here for convenience of discussion; they were not numbered in the original.

1. Uveitis is one of the major causes of legal blindness in this country. In over 70% of the cases, the pathogenesis remains obscure, even after extensive clinical and laboratory investigations. Visual prognosis is worse in cases that present with severe intraocular inflammation, and this poor prognosis is due to retinal tissue damage in the form of vascular leakage, cystoid macular edema and other alterations. In such inflammations, even though T- and B-lymphocytes initiate the process, amplification, perpetuation and tissue damage are mediated by polymorphonuclear leukocytes (PMNs) and macrophages. Others and we have shown the significance of oxygen metabolites released by PMNs and macrophages in amplification of intraocular inflammation and tissue necrosis, but there has been no systematic study of the mechanism(s) leading to retinal damage by these toxic metabolites. Such systematic studies must be performed in well-defined animal models of uveitis. [*Comment:* The first paragraph indicates the importance and need for systematic studies of uveitis, and expounds a general theory of its pathogenesis: tissue damage in uveitis is a result of the action of oxygen metabolites released by inflammatory cells. It states that the mechanism of action of these metabolites needs to be determined and suggests that the proposed studies will test possible mechanisms. The transition sentence here concerns oxygen metabolites. Unfortunately, the last sentence is a non sequitur about their animal model.]

2. Inflammatory Mediators: In uveitis, retinal damage is caused by chemical mediators derived from plasma proteins or inflammatory cells. These include arachidonic acid metabolites, proteolytic enzymes and oxygen metabolites. Arachidonic acid metabolites are primarily involved in vascular permeability, chemotaxis and amplification of inflammation; however, it is difficult to explain acute inflammatory cytolysis on the basis of proteolytic enzymes alone since the reaction constants of proteolytic enzymes are relatively low; proteolytic enzyme deficient animals appear to have no diminution of the acute inflammatory response; enzyme inhibitors do not reduce acute inflammation; and addition of proteolytic enzymes does not increase inflammation. Thus, it is apparent that reactions other than those mediated by proteolytic enzymes account for the early tissue damage in uveitis. Attention has recently been directed to reactive oxygen metabolites released by PMNs and macrophages during the initial phase of inflammation. We have shown the significance of these molecules in amplification of uveal inflammation and in acute retinal damage. Our pilot data clearly implicate these toxic metabolites as the principal cause of acute retinal damage. [*Comment:* The second and third paragraphs amplify the assumption that the oxygen metabolites are the cause of tissue damage and establish the contributions of the PI.]

3. Oxygen Metabolites and Free Radicals: It has been documented that, upon phagocytosis or exposure to certain membrane-active agents, PMNs and macrophages undergo a "respiratory burst" characterized by increased consumption of oxygen, increased utilization of glucose via the hexose monophosphate shunt, and release of reactive oxygen metabolites, the principal product being superoxide anion, an inorganic free radical. The superoxide radical itself is poorly reactive in aqueous solution, and the tissue damaging effects are from more reactive derived products, including hydrogen peroxide, HOCl and hydroxyl radicals (see Fig. 6.2).

4. PMNs and macrophages, on stimulation, discharge lysosomal granules containing myeloperoxidase, along with hydrogen peroxide, into the phagocytic vacuole or into the extracellular milieu. In the presence of

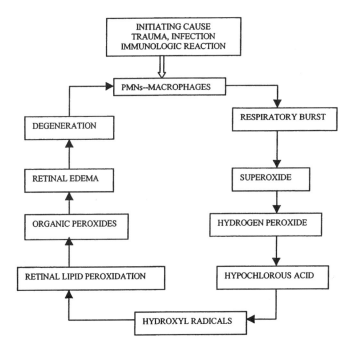

Figure 6.2. Schematic representation of oxygen metabolite generation and its effect on the retina. Once the phagocytic cells are activated by one of the initiating causes, superoxide is generated along with hydrogen peroxide. These, in turn, form other reactive products, resulting in retinal lipid peroxidation. Chain reaction of this peroxidation leads to formation of organic peroxides, and eventually results in retinal edema and degeneration. Degenerated products attract phagocytes and these cells are also recruited by lipid chemotactic factors generated during the tissue damage.

hydrogen peroxide, myeloperoxidase catalyzes the oxidation of the halides, such as chloride, to form HOCl. This acid is a potent oxidant that can react with a wide variety of biologically important molecules. Furthermore, HOCl can react with other oxygen metabolites derived from the superoxide to form hydroxyl radicals. Even though in vitro studies have documented the potent oxidant nature of this acid, there have been no studies to evaluate the role of such acids in mediation of ocular tissue damage in uveitis. [*Comment:* A specific knowledge gap is identified in paragraphs 3 and 4.]

5. The hydroxyl radical is an extremely powerful oxidant that can interact with various organic and inorganic molecules. In addition to the above-mentioned source, it is believed that hydroxyl radicals are formed primarily from interaction of superoxide and hydrogen peroxide (Haber-Weiss reaction). This reaction, although energetically favorable, occurs at very slow rates. The presence of iron salts and their complexes has been shown to catalyze effectively the interaction between superoxide and hydrogen peroxide (iron-catalyzed Haber-Weiss reaction). [*Comment:* Paragraphs 3, 4, and 5 present a detailed theoretical model. It is a linked series of hypotheses that suggest the mechanism of metabolite induced damage, and refers to a figure that is virtually self-explanatory, but which has an excellent legend that summarizes the essence of the model succinctly.]

6. We found that treatment of uveitis in rats with the iron chelator, deferoxamine, resulted in significant reduction in uveal inflammation as well as in the formation of lipid peroxidation products. Treated animals showed a relatively well-preserved retina when compared with untreated controls. These studies suggest that free iron and hydroxyl radicals can cause retinal damage; however, there is no study utilizing hydroxyl radical scavengers at various stages of uveal inflammation, particularly in the initial and late stages, to detect the role of these radicals leading to retinal damage by lipid peroxidation. [*Comment:* Paragraph 6 reviews past experiments and the literature to delineate another specific gap in our knowledge of the pathogenesis of uveitis, i.e., the effects of using oxygen metabolite scavengers to reduce tissue damage in uveitis.]

7. The above oxygen metabolites and free radicals have been observed in vitro to exert direct cytotoxic effects, including lipid peroxidation of cell membranes, inactivation of intracellular enzyme systems (oxidation of -SH groups), DNA damage, injury to tissue, structural proteins and proteoglycans, and generation of lipid chemotactic factors. We have elected to study lipid peroxidation of cell membranes, as the visual loss in humans with uveitis occurs mainly from retinal tissue damage, and we hypothesize that such damage may result from free radical-induced peroxidation of lipid-rich retinal cell membranes). Even though there are no studies addressing lipid peroxidation in uveitis, formation of various lipid peroxidation products in vivo has been demonstrated in other systems, such as in complement activated pulmonary edema. [*Comment:* This is a transition paragraph to a second study.]

8. Lipid Peroxidation: Lipid peroxidation represents one form of early tissue damage. It can be initiated by oxygen or its metabolic products. In vivo, it provides a steady supply of free radicals since it is a chain reaction leading to the formation of organic peroxides. The accumulation of such peroxides and oxidation of lipid membranes can have a devastating effect on cellular vitality, leading eventually to degeneration and necrosis. Lipid peroxidation is known to disrupt cell membranes and intracellular organelles, with subsequent release of their compartmentalized contents. Such damage to lysosomal membranes could amplify the destructive process by release of hydrolytic enzymes, thus perpetuating the inflammation and tissue damage. Products of lipid peroxidation consist of hydroperoxides, CD, MDA, and other aldehyde products, some of which yield fluorochromic proteins containing amino phospholipids and proteins cross-linked intermolecularly with characteristic conjugated Schiff base structures. Several investigators have outlined a possible scheme of events in lipid peroxidation, the initial step being hydrogen abstraction resulting in the formation of a CD. This is followed by formation of a lipid peroxide, hydroperoxide or MDA.

9. Our preliminary experimental studies in animals with S-antigen induced uveitis are required to detect the lipid peroxidation products present at the various phases of intraocular inflammation and at the different stages of severity in uveitis. [*Comment:* Paragraphs 7, 8, and 9 identify a second cause of tissue damage: the metabolites of lipid peroxidation of membranes. The logic of assaying the uveitis afflicted retina for the presence of these metabolites is presented and the essential nature of the author's animal model indicated.]

10. Specific intervention at various stages of free radical generation: Recently, we and others attempted to modulate the inflammatory process noted in the experimental forms of uveitis by antioxidants and hydroxyl radical scavengers. The early treatment of animals with lens-induced uveitis by enzyme antioxidants produced a reduction in the severity of ocular inflammation and tissue damage associated with the inflammation. The enzymes studied included SOD and catalase. Similar antiphlogistic effects of these enzymes were also found in the retinal S-antigen induced uveitis in guinea pigs and uveoretinitis in rats. Such protective effects of antioxidant enzymes were also noted in pulmonary and renal inflammation. However, there has been no in-depth study of the biochemical and morphological alterations produced by the free radicals and/or the prevention of such alterations by specific interventions at the various stages of free radical generation (Fig. 6.3).

11. There have been no systematic studies to evaluate the roles of various oxygen metabolites in the perpetuation of retinal tissue damage, and in the formation of lipid peroxidation products in uveitis. Such studies should include blocking the generation of superoxide by adenosine, scavenging and converting already generated superoxide to H_2O_2 by SOD, converting H_2O_2 into nontoxic products by catalase or glutathione

Stages of Free Radical Generation

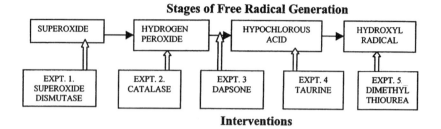

Interventions

Figure 6.3. Specific intervention therapy by antioxidants and free radical scavengers at various stages of free radical generation.

peroxidase, blocking the enzymatic action of myeloperoxidase by dapsone, inhibiting the effect of HOCl by taurine and neutralizing the formation and effects of hydroxyl radicals by deferoxamine or other agents such as DMTU. Furthermore, effects of the above specific intervention therapy on immunopathogenicity of uveitis in general, and on T- and B-cell functions, chemotaxis, complement activation, and changes in arachidonic acid metabolites in particular, have not been evaluated. There has been a report suggesting changes in some of these immunological functions when intervention therapy was used. Such immunopathologic studies in uveitis could provide insight into the in vivo specificity of antioxidants and hydroxyl radical scavengers in suppression of oxygen free radical-induced amplification and perpetuation of ocular inflammation, and the role of these anti-inflammatory agents in modulation of the immunopathologic process. [*Comment:* The last two paragraphs present the logic of uveitis therapy based on interruption of oxygen metabolite formation. This is very clearly supported by a second diagram that indicates the site of action of a number of putative therapeutic drugs along the path of free radical formation.]

This Background and Significance section was generally very well written, and it was greatly strengthened by its figures. However, it shows poor balance between oxygen metabolite production (the subject of the initial grant) and lipid peroxidation by oxygen metabolites (the subject of this competing renewal proposal). The concepts are presented well but the allocation of space fails to properly emphasize the current interest in lipid peroxidation. This section occupied only slightly more than two pages of the submitted proposal. It would have been appropriate to expand the lipid peroxidation parts by another two or three paragraphs. Finally, the use of abbreviations in this section is unnecessary and detracts from its readability. The frequent references to the "unknown" have a negative connotation. They should be replaced with statements about alternative possibilities or reasonable expectations.

LITERATURE CITATIONS

This should consist of no more than 30–50 entries. Small font superscripts for references conserve space. It is not good grantsmanship, however, to make a statement and then list 10 or more references by number, e.g., "15–25," even though there is plenty of room to do so; this is obvious padding and does not reveal any ability to discriminate among the pertinent publications. It is particularly important for new investigators to be discriminating in their literature review. All of the papers cited must be carefully read and understood. They should be of excellent quality and not controversial. It is a serious mistake to cite a reference listed in another paper without reading it carefully; it may be of poor quality or have been shown to be wrong. Nothing is as disastrous as a statement from a reviewer that "the PI seems unfamiliar with the literature and has cited inappropriate references." Excessive referencing gets in the way of readability. It will irritate some reviewers and does nothing to convince them that you are anything other than a beginner.

The most current research is discussed among researchers at meetings following presentations. Often the state-of-the-art has not been published, but knowledge of it may distinguish the experts from the novices. Reference to unpublished work is useful, only if it is not contested by a reviewer. Before using such references, a new investigator would be wise to discuss the material with colleagues; controversial material should not be used without discussion of the controversy, and this takes valuable space, and will probably not be germane to the proposal.

The literature review must include reference to previous studies that are similar or identical with those proposed. It is very damaging if the reviewer is aware of a similar study and it appears that the PI is not. This leads to comments like, "The work proposed has been described in the paper by Jones, but this is not cited and it is not clear that the proposed research will break any new ground." Such comments result in poor priority scores. Additional comments about references will be found in Chapter 14.

George Eaves[1] lists seven basic questions about a research proposal on which most reviewers base their evaluation. The reviewers should have answers to four of the questions when they have finished the Specific Aims and Background sections:

1. Are the aims logical?
2. Is there a valid hypothesis to be tested?
3. Are feasible tests of the hypothesis possible? Would such tests produce new data?
4. What is the significance and originality of the proposed research relative to its scientific field?

The reviewer should also have formed a strong impression about a fifth question: is the PI qualified and competent in the field? This question will not be fully answered until the Progress Report and Preliminary Data are reviewed, but how the Background section is handled will reveal much about the depth of the PI's thinking.

Some years ago, the logic of the Specific Aims was discussed in a section entitled "Rationale." This application label caused a great deal of confusion and was eventually deleted from the PHS 398 form. What is wanted is essentially a statement that the proposal represents the juxtaposition of an important problem, a qualified investigator, appropriate technology and facilities, and an environment that will lead, through accomplishment of the Aims, to solution of the problem, given the necessary funds.

HYPOTHESES

It is worth repeating that hypotheses should be the basis of all but frankly descriptive research, but there are interesting and important hypotheses and there are many more that are trivial. Of course hypotheses may be invalid if they are based on demonstrably false assumptions. Trivial hypotheses are common. They represent poor grantsmanship and weak analytical thinking. They also result from traditional thinking about problems or attempts to force a hypothesis into a project that is phenomenological. For example, it may be hypothesized that a test of blood alcohol

---

[1]Out of print NIH Publication "Preparing a Grant Application to the National Institutes of Health. Selected Articles, 1987."

can be based on analysis of expired air, but this is a trivial hypothesis. The research to prove the hypothesis may be important for various social or clinical reasons, but is scientifically trivial. Important hypotheses relate to basic mechanisms, the understanding of which advances science. With some thought it is almost always possible to transform a study based on trivial or phenomenological hypotheses into one involving basic mechanisms and scientifically important hypotheses. In the above example of testing for blood alcohol, a hypothesis relating to the transport of alcohol through the lipid bilayer of alveolar membrane might address basic mechanisms but involve the same research. This more basic perspective will greatly strengthen the proposal.

7

Preliminary Studies

Section *c* of the Research Plan of an application for an R01 Individual Research Grant is called Preliminary Studies if the proposal is new and Preliminary Studies/Progress Report if the proposal is a competing renewal or an application for supplemental funds. This chapter will focus on Preliminary Studies and is relevant to new and competing renewal proposals. Chapter 16 includes discussion of the Progress Report in the context of the competing renewal proposal.

INTRODUCTION

Start with an introduction that lists the figures or data to follow and explains the purpose for which each is included. It is frustrating for a reviewer to find pages of data that may appear to be unrelated to the project. Preliminary Data has never been published. It is new and provides proof that the PI has an active laboratory and is currently working on the project. Do not waste space and burden the reviewer with irrelevant data or any data that are included in the appendix in publications or manuscripts. The assigned reviewers will read the papers. It is good, however, to point out important findings or conclusions and refer to specific sections of a paper in the appendix. The exception to this advice is the truly awe-inspiring figure that might interest the nonassigned reviewers. Certainly important published findings should be discussed briefly if they support the current proposal.

PURPOSE

The Preliminary Studies has several well-defined purposes, the accomplishment of which will have a great impact on the eventual success

91

of the proposal. Its main purpose is to persuade the reviewers that the PI is expert in all of the procedures proposed for which there is direct responsibility. The second purpose is to establish beyond a reasonable doubt that the proposed studies are feasible in the hands of the PI. This includes presentation of data in support of any component of a theoretical model for which published data may be lacking, and pilot data that at least suggest that the PI's hypothesis will be supported. A third important purpose is to show that a proposed collaboration actually functions to produce usable data. Thus this section, if successful, will provide support for any weakness in the proposal. Competing renewal proposals are funded at about twice the rate of new proposals. A large part of the difference in success may be attributed to the Preliminary Studies. An established researcher has the facilities and funds to obtain good data and the opportunity to demonstrate support for possible weaknesses. This is a difficult challenge for the newcomer.

The PHS 398 instructions state,

> For new applications, use this section to provide an account of the [PI's] preliminary studies pertinent to the application information that will also help to establish the experience and competence of the investigator to pursue the proposed project.
>
> Peer review committees generally view preliminary data as an essential part of a research grant application. Preliminary data often aid the reviewers in assessing the likelihood of the success of the proposed project. . . .

BREVITY IS IMPORTANT

This section should be limited to no more than 8 pages. The distribution of pages within the research plan is not fixed, but the total number of pages is: 25 pages are the limit. This includes all pages of illustrations submitted as part of the Preliminary Studies. If this section is expanded, it is at the expense of some other section. Up to 10 reprints of publications and manuscripts accepted for publication may be submitted in support of the proposal, as an appendix. This material will likely be seen only by the assigned reviewers, while material submitted within the Preliminary Studies section can potentially be seen by all members of the Study Section.

EXPERTISE

It is not necessary to establish proof of expertise in areas where the credentials of the PI will not be questioned. Thus a practicing cardiologist need not show expertise in the interpretation of the EKG, as this would certainly be assumed. A cardiologist who proposed to use the electroretinogram (ERG) to evaluate visual function in animals with induced atheromata would need to show expertise in recording and interpreting the ERG response. Appropriate expertise can be established by submitting publications of the PI in which the procedure was used, or by enlisting the collaboration of someone who is qualified. Alternatively, data actually obtained by the PI in a manner similar to that to be used in the proposed study may be submitted as direct evidence of expertise. If this is done, it is essential that the data be absolutely splendid.

The Preliminary Studies section should be written *after* the Methods section is finished. The proposed methods should be carefully scrutinized and every proposed procedure listed. An honest self-appraisal for each procedure should ask, "Am I perceived by my peers to be expert at this?" This perception will be based on training, experience, and publications. If the answer is unclear or in the negative for any procedure, evidence must be provided in this section that the procedure can be done expertly by someone on the research team.

The most convincing data are photographic or actual chart recordings. Tabular data are less convincing since they are more readily manipulated, and do not directly demonstrate technical expertise. Photomicrographs, electron micrographs, pictures of gels, spectrophotometer traces, electrical recordings, angiograms, etc., are best. These data should be of absolutely spectacular quality. Avoid showing data that are not impressive to the casual observer, even if they are as good as the procedure can provide. For instance, the quality of electron micrographs obtainable with EM immunohistochemistry is poor at best. Such figures may be misinterpreted by casual reviewers, suggesting to them that expertise in EM is lacking.

Recall the mechanics of review. The assigned reviewers have all the appendix material, and can judge competence in a procedure. They will understand even the most complex illustrations in this section. The rest of the reviewers, however, do not have the appendix material and will only glance through the section. They will not have time to read lengthy legends. These reviewers are the ones to impress with spectacular data. But the data must be easily comprehensible and obviously of high quality. Tabular data require too much time for analysis to be much help in communicating with these nonassigned reviewers.

The proposal given to the nonassigned reviewers is a photocopy. Figures in the Preliminary Studies section often copy very badly. Line drawings and tracings do well, but half-tone prints are a disaster. Shaded or colored areas come out black. If halftone prints or color photographs would substantially help your cause, there is a way to get them included in the proposal copy given every reviewer. With the permission of the SRA of the section, 20 or more copies of the proposal may be sent to the SRA in addition to the usual 6 submitted to the CSR. In this circumstance, the material actually submitted will be distributed to all members of the section. If this road is to be taken, the proposal should be copied on both sides of the paper and the figures must be reproduced by color Xerox or high-quality color printer. These should be on photo-quality, standard weight paper, and fit unobtrusively into the proposal. Such figures give the proposal a professional look, are quite adequate to show expertise, and are much neater than when photographs are mounted on pages. Reviewers appreciate efforts to make a proposal more readable. Examples of figures submitted in support of successful proposals are shown in Appendix C.

FEASIBILITY

Good research breaks new ground. It involves innovative experimentation, the feasibility of which is often less than obvious. It is a serious mistake to leave a reviewer with doubts that a particular experiment will work, or that any of the Specific Aims will not be achieved. Questions concerning the feasibility of the proposed work should be resolved in this section by presentation of solid, clean, and convincing pilot data. The data should establish that the approach is sound but should not answer the important research questions. Care must be taken not to give the impression that the proposed experiments have already been done! As an example, the effects of a drug on a new animal model of a disease may be the focus of the study. Data showing the validity of the model should be shown in detail. The model is, after all, only a research tool, but you have to have good tools in order to get good data. This is established with the pilot data. Present the model as a good tool, supported by pilot data, and propose experiments, for instance, drug dose–response studies, that make use of the model as a basis for in-depth studies to test specific hypotheses.

Preliminary data should always be supportive. Use wisdom in discussing the weaknesses of your proposal, and do not bring up any problem for which you have no solution. Generally there should be nothing negative in Preliminary Data. Problems and weaknesses should be fully dealt with in Experimental Design and Methods. For instance, if patient recruitment will be a problem, show data here to establish that in your hands, it will be no problem. If you do not have this kind of data, show in the Design section how the problem will be handled. Obviously, it is much stronger to have data showing you have already dealt with the problem.

AVOID DEVELOPMENT

You are asking for trouble if a substantial part of your project depends on the development of the model. Obviously if the model must still be developed, it is not known that it will work. If it does not work, there will be no study. Similar considerations apply to the development of diagnostic tests. Research involving the use of a new test is clearly not feasible if the test is not valid. The temptation is to propose validation of the test as the first stage in the project, but this clearly announces to the reviewers that the test at the present time is not valid. If the test cannot be validated for some reason, no studies based on its use are possible and the proposal should be disapproved on the basis of possibly lacking scientific merit. In actual practice, such proposals are usually not disapproved, but they get a sufficiently bad priority score to be comfortably unfundable. Tests and models must be shown, by hard data presented in this section, to be valid and usable. Studies based on them are then considered on their own merits.

Development of new procedures is, nevertheless, the subject of many proposals. These applications can be strengthened by establishing that the proposed approach to the problem is feasible. As an example, ocular melanomas may be treated with cobalt plaques rather than the traditional enucleation in an attempt to save a sighted eye. Evidence from other tissues shows that the effect of radiation on neoplastic tissue can be enhanced if the tissue is warmed. Perhaps warming of the ocular melanoma would permit treatment with lower doses of radiation and with less risk of radiation necrosis of the retina. A proposal to develop a method of localized heating of the tumor based on microwave radiation of the plaque would be much stronger if there were *in vitro* data showing that the susceptibility of ocular melanoma cells to radiation was increased with small increments of temperature. It would also help if there were pilot data to show that nondestructive and localized heating of the retina is possible with the proposed procedure. Given this established base, it can then be proposed to test hypotheses about the appropriate parameters of radiation and heat in a variety of situations. This would be vital data to support use of the procedure in humans.

Data on the feasibility of particular procedures may be required from the standpoint of survival of an animal model. A study of the role of the macrophage in wound healing might include the use of animals with reduced numbers of circulating monocytes caused by radiation-induced bone marrow depression. The care of such animals is notoriously difficult and a proposal to study healing of thoracic wounds over a 12-month period would raise doubts that survival could be prolonged to that extent. Pilot data showing longevity of the animals in the hands of the PI would allay this concern as well as show the investigator's concern with the problem. If the problem is ignored it is assumed that the PI is not well informed about the problems of the proposed experiment, and this is disastrous for the score.

Beginning investigators all too often propose studies that they think are sound from descriptions in the literature, but with which they have no actual experience. Such studies are very likely to contain unrecognized flaws that are laughable to informed reviewers. Examples are the proposal to administer a complicated questionnaire to patients admitted to the emergency room with an acute myocardial infarction; the proposal to obtain blood samples from the same HIV-positive patients in a large county hospital at weekly intervals over a period of a year; the proposal to administer a large battery of tests to acutely ill AIDS patients; and the proposal to obtain simultaneous intracellular recordings from adjacent neurons in the brain of the awake behaving monkey. It is unlikely that a proposal containing such difficult or logistically unlikely procedures would emanate from an experienced investigator or that credible pilot data could be produced in support of the studies. The way to avoid such bloopers is to have the proposal read by someone who is knowledgeable in the area prior to submission. In many institutions, the chairperson of a department must sign the proposal and there is a clear moral obligation attached to the signature that the quality of the proposal meets minimum standards. We feel that department chairs should take more interest in the proposals of their junior faculty, and assist them to obtain adequate help.

COLLABORATION

The above melanoma example describes a classic multidisciplinary study. The Preliminary Studies section offers the opportunity to establish that such collaborations, in this case involving a cell biologist, an oncologist, an ophthalmologist, and a specialist in nuclear medicine, actually work. In presenting the data, the contribution of each of the collaborators should be noted. It is not sufficient to support a claim to collaboration by only a form letter appended to the proposal, unless there is published evidence that the arrangement exists. Proposed collaborations are compelling when there are preliminary data to show that the collaboration works. Of course the data must be excellent in quality. It is not uncommon for the reviewers to encounter claims of collaboration that are hardly credible, and supported by no preliminary data and only a form letter. These are examined critically and may actually damage a proposal if they are considered padding.

HAPPY GRANTSMANSHIP

It is appropriate to expand on a philosophy of research that is actually a modus vivendi with the cruel necessity an investigator faces for self-support. It is also appropriate to place the discussion in this chapter since the Progress Report/Preliminary Data section is where the "buck stops." Preparation and planning are the names of the game. Research is not done in a vacuum. There must be preparation in the form of training, obviously, but also in the form of experience. Training should include exposure to the proposal process, but rarely does. Experience provides preparation for procedures and their use. Together they qualify a new investigator to do the same research as the mentor, but this is not enough for a new proposal. New investigators require some preliminary data and research tools they can call their own. These usually must be acquired after leaving the laboratory of the mentor, but it would be far better if they could be obtained during the training period when the facilities are readily available.

For those new investigators still in the laboratory of an adviser, make every effort to design the research for your first proposal now. Once you have the general outline of the research you wish to do, try to get some preliminary data in your current situation that will support your future proposal. Use discretion in discussing this proposed research with your mentor if it encroaches on the work of your current laboratory. It is far better, however, to choose a project that is not simply an extension of your mentor's work. The idea is obvious: you will be in a far better position to submit your own research proposal in the future if you start planning for it now.

The same philosophy carries far more impact when applied to the practicing investigator. Bear in mind that, as of this writing, only 51% of competing renewal R01 research project proposals are funded by the NIH on first submission; 35% of previously funded investigators who got continued funding in fiscal 2000 had to revise their proposals. This represents, at least in part, unwillingness to plan ahead and to devote the required resources and time for generation of a strong, well-written proposal the first time. As you work through your current projects you should be planning your next proposal. Every paper you write should be thought of as a progress report for your competing renewal. If you cannot state at this moment what your next project will entail, your vision is too limited. You need to expand your scientific horizons, and a good way to do this is to start writing your next proposal. This may require some reading in areas that are new to you. It should spur you to contact colleagues about collaborations, to visit their laboratories, to exchange seminars, and to discuss possible experimental designs over lunch. In short, development of your next Specific Aims can get you out of a research shell. Who can argue that facilitation of scientific interchange is not a good thing? That is the wonderful consequence of getting actively involved in development of your next project.

THE EVILS OF PROCRASTINATION

Effective preparation takes time. To begin preparation of a proposal 6 months before its deadline is to preclude the possibility of using the proposal to identify the need for pilot data, since the time will be too short to permit its acquisition. This short time also precludes adequate review of the finished proposal. Ideally, preparation for a new proposal starts with the funding of the current proposal, and the conduct of the current research is always with a mind to its support for the next proposal.

Lacking such a carefully planned existence, preparation for a new proposal should start at least 12 months prior to the deadline, or 18–24 months in the case of a competing renewal, where the preparation of manuscripts will provide important support. Sad is the investigator who uses the impending proposal deadline as a motivator to write some papers. The resulting manuscripts will be prepared hurriedly under pressure. There will not be time for their external review; their quality will be less than it might have been. If the future direction of your research is actually dependent on experiments you are doing only 6 to 12 months before submission of a new proposal, you cannot hope to generate a very strong proposal. Actually this rarely occurs. Most investigators have a very good idea of their experimental goals. The actual experiments may be subject to adjustment on the basis of experience, but this can be handled as a series of alternatives. If the Specific Aims can be stated, even with alternatives dependent on current research, 12 months before the due date, and if manuscript preparation has been kept up to date, ample time will be available to produce an absolutely first-rate proposal.

The final version of the proposal, including budget, should be completed 3 months before the deadline. This is the secret of success for a new investigator! This proposal should be sent to at least two reviewers who are knowledgeable and willing to spend some hours reading it carefully. If funds are available, offer the reviewers an honorarium of at least $350 and request a written report or a face-to-face or telephone interview. Do not hesitate to send the proposal to an acknowledged expert with whom you are not acquainted, particularly if you can pay for the service. Do not send the proposal to a member of the Study Section that will review it, as this will cause the reviewer to be disqualified from looking at it as a section member. *Actually it is very poor form to ever approach a sitting member of a Study Section that will review your proposal.*

Take the recommendations of your reviewers seriously. The more critical the reviewers, the more help for the proposal. Do not waste your time arguing or trying to explain your differences with the reviewers; rewrite any section considered unclear or confusing. If your reviewers misunderstand your writing, view this as your failure to communicate. Be particularly sensitive to the reviewers' reactions to the hypotheses stated and whether or not they are convinced that the tests of the hypotheses are valid. If suggestions are made for different experiments, try to incorporate them into the proposal, but only if the approach does not require additional pilot data.

Work is done to meet deadlines; it is usually done as a high-priority item immediately before the deadline. If you accept the deadlines set by the funding agency as your personal deadlines, you will fail to get the most out of your grantsmanship, and you will fight to complete the proposal a week or so before the due date. As a result, your proposal, lacking a considerate review, will be less than it might have been. The solution is obvious: accept a deadline 3 months before the due date with a full commitment to meet it. It may require only a bit more effort and pressure on laboratory and clerical staff to meet your advanced deadline than it would to meet the regular NIH deadline, but it will be well worth it. The extra 3 months for lcisurely review and correction will result in a better proposal that will very likely get a better priority score, and improved prospects for funding.

8

Research Design and Methods

The form PHS 398 instructions state,

Describe the research design and the procedures to be used to accomplish the specific aims of the project. Include how the data will be collected, analyzed and interpreted as well as the data sharing plan as appropriate. Describe any new methodology and its advantage over existing methodologies. Discuss the potential difficulties and limitations of the proposed procedures and alternative approaches to achieve the aims. . . . Provide a tentative sequence or timetable for the project. Point out any procedures, situations or materials that may be hazardous to personnel and the precautions to be exercised.

Research Design is very different from Method. Design is *what* will be done. Method is *how* it will be done. Design is interesting, logical, and organized. The design of a project involves conceptualization of a logical sequence of experiments that test specific corollaries of an important hypothesis. Designs of individual experiments can be clever or innovative, intuitive, powerful, straightforward or complex, naive or sophisticated, and effective or inappropriate. Experimental design reveals much about the depth of the thinking of the PI.

Methods are dry as dust. Methods are a cookbook recitation of the intimate details of a procedure. They are quantitative, precise, often repetitive, often completely familiar to the reviewer, and lengthy. Methods are absolutely necessary to answer simple but vital questions concerning technique that will come up as the proposal is reviewed.

From the standpoint of the reviewer, the proposal that mixes design with methods is frustrating and difficult to read. It is much more friendly to provide an initial Design section that communicates everything the reviewer needs about the logic and conduct of the project, including numbers and types of samples, animals, or experimental subjects and controls.

This should be written to be informative and to be scanned quickly. A following Methods section should provide all of the details about procedures listed in the design. The reviewer is thus given the option of not having to read the details of a procedure with which the PI seems expert. Nothing is more irritating to the reviewer than to be forced to wade through pages of details in order to ferret out the logic of a particular experiment.

DESIGN

The Research Design subsection should answer the question, "what will be done in order to accomplish the Specific Aims?" It is simply a list of procedures in the order in which they will be done. The goal of this section is to communicate this information in as brief and logical a sequence as possible. After a quick scan of Design, the reviewers should understand perfectly the logic, nature, and appropriateness of the proposed experiments. At this point in the review, they also will know whether the requested time is appropriate. Rigorously exclude any description of the methods by which things will be done.

It is essential that the Design follows the lead of the Specific Aims, and that the experiments be organized according to the relevant aim and hypothesis. If you have followed the suggested page allocation, you should have about 13 pages left for Design and Methods. Design should take only about 3 pages. We like the presentation of Research Design below.

Start the section with the statement, "Design will be outlined first, followed by detailed descriptions of the methods to be used." Having chosen a definite form for this section, stick to it for all specific aims and experiments. Divide your project into a number of experiments. This will greatly simplify the review. Ten experiments are workable. We have seen as many as 26, but this is awkward to say the least. An epidemiological project might have only 1 experiment. The individual Specific Aims and hypotheses are quoted verbatim for the convenience of the reviewers, so they will not have to look back in the proposal.

Specific Aim 1 (verbatim as in the Specific Aims)
Hypothesis (verbatim as in the Specific Aims)
    Experiment 1: Title
        Hypothesis corollary to be tested
        Rationale, if appropriate

  Design: list procedures
  Data expected, analysis, and interpretation
  Problems and solutions, if appropriate
 Experiment 2: Title
  Hypothesis corollary to be tested
  Rationale, if appropriate
  Design: List procedures
  Data expected, analysis, and interpretation
  Problems and solutions, if appropriate
Specific Aim 2 (verbatim)
Hypothesis (verbatim)
 Experiment 3: Title
  Hypothesis corollary to be tested
  Rationale, if appropriate
  Design: List procedures
  Data expected, analysis, and interpretation
  Problems and solutions, if appropriate

In Appendix D is an outline for the design of one experiment that some investigators have found useful. In following this form, the narrative parts should be kept to a minimum. This is a detailed executive summary of the project. If the reviewers are confident in your ability, this is all they will have to read and you have saved them from the labor of about 10 pages of a very boring methods review. That will earn you some Brownie points! Note that the experiments are numbered consecutively so that experiment numbers are not repeated. Do not repeat comments about analysis or problems that recur. Keep it short.

Title

Give each experiment a title. It should be descriptive and brief. Titles help the reviewers keep track of what is planned for the project and how its different parts interrelate. It helps them communicate with the other reviewers and makes the task of critiquing several experiments easier. A typical title for a project involving the effect of deafferentation of the lateral hypothalamus on the arcuate nucleus might be, "Hypothalamic deafferentation: Arcuate nucleus effect."

Hypothesis Corollary

Experiments are done to gather data that will test hypotheses or answer questions. Unless the purpose of an experiment is explicitly stated, the reviewers may not understand why it is being done. Avoid this by providing an explanation. If use of the term "hypothesis" is not appropriate, call the statement "purpose." Do not assume that the reviewers will understand what you fail to say!

Rationale

In our modern world the task of gathering data is very easy indeed. Modern instruments abound in every laboratory. Commercial test kits enable the investigator to accurately test for the presence of innumerable compounds; computer programs provide incredible statistical power to complicated calculations. The problem of the investigator is to select the best experimental approach among a myriad of possibilities. For instance, in a study of cell proliferation in wound healing, it may be desired to evaluate the effects of a cytokine. But which cytokine? There are far too many available to be able to test them all. This Rationale section can be used to justify the selection made and must be persuasive. Data are collected to describe a process ("look-see" research is not very interesting) or, preferably, to test a hypothesis. The rationale for an approach is that it will in fact test a prediction. But a common failing of proposals is summed up by the negative comments, "no new data will be obtained," "the data will not be definitive," "the data will not answer the important question," or "the hypothesis will not be tested." In these instances the reviewers were not persuaded of the validity of the experimental rationale.

The strength of a proposal is based on the hypotheses to be tested and the probability that data can be acquired that will prove or disprove them. Each Specific Aim should encompass one or more experiments designed to test a particular hypothesis or its corollaries, or to distinguish between crisply stated alternative hypotheses. The relation of hypothesis to Specific Aim should have been presented in Background and Significance, but space limitations often prevent adequate exposition in that section. In addition, the logic of a particular experiment may have been lost by the reviewer as the intervening Preliminary Studies forest was penetrated. The Rationale section may include references to the literature, but must present the logic of the approach clearly and forcefully. After reading this paragraph the reviewer should understand why a particular experiment will be done and how the data gathered will relate to the Specific Aim.

Design

Every attempt should be made to keep this section brief. A short list of procedures is best. The reviewer should be able to scan this section and determine what will be done, how many of what type of animal will be used, what interventions or manipulations will be done, and how many observations will be made. Complicated protocols may be best shown with a table or a flow chart.

Tables are an effective method with which to indicate what will be done in an experiment involving several manipulations or procedures. Tables should indicate the number of animals (or cultures, etc.) used, time to sacrifice, and timing of procedures. If an indication of the time required for each procedure is added, these tables become an effective statistic in the Budget Justification of nonmodular proposals in support of a request for technical help. The more detailed the table, the more impressive the proposal from the standpoint of careful preparation, providing that the numbers add up and correspond to those of the text. It is difficult for a reviewer to argue that a project needs only a half-time technician when the PI has provided tabular data that show a requirement for 1800 hours of labor per year. Of course the allocation of time for a particular procedure must be realistic and in accordance with general experience or the table will be counterproductive and may be used to support a contention that "the PI seems unfamiliar with the requirements of this procedure."

Tables from the Design can be used as the basis for justifying the use of a certain number of animals (see Table 8.1). For instance, such a table might show the need for 5 animals for each of six drug doses to be sacrificed at 1, 2, 4, and 8 days after administration, justifying a request for 120 animals. Tables can also be used as justification for a particular piece of equipment; they provide a convincing argument that the need has been identified through a thoughtful study of experimental requirements. It is much more persuasive to be able to state that "the fluorescence microscope will be used to examine 5 slides from each of 136 specimens every 2 months (see Table 3)" than to state simply, "the fluorescence microscope will be heavily used."

Table 8.1 *Experimental Design for Specific Aims 1 and 2*

Gp	Rabbits[1]	P. acnes Inoculum[2]	Serum[3]	Aqueous[4]	Vitreous[5]	IOL[6]	PLC[7]
Natural History Studies (Experiment 1)							
A	32 pseudo-phakic	Live	224	64	32	16 BC 16 FITC	16 BC 16 FITC
B	32 aphakic	Live	224	64	32		16 BC 16 FITC
C	16 pseudo-phakic	Saline (control)	112	32	16	8 BC 8 FITC	8 BC 8 FITC
D	16 aphakic	Saline (control)	112	32	16		8 BC 8 FITC
Nonviable P. acnes Studies (Experiment 2)							
E	16 pseudo-phakic	Heat killed	112	32	16	8 BC 8 FITC	8 BC 8 FITC
F	16 pseudo-phakic	Lysed	112	32	16	8 BC 8 FITC	8 BC 8 FITC

[1]Number of rabbits receiving unilateral ECCE surgery with (pseudophakic) or without (aphakic) IOL implantation, and followed clinically for 6 months (Specific Aim 1).

[2]Inoculum preparation injected into anterior chambers post-ECCE surgery (Specific Aim 1).

[3]Number of serum samples (7/rabbit) collected during 6-month follow-up period for the ELISA determination of antibody used for P. acnes and/or lens protein (Specific Aim 2).

[4]Number of aqueous specimens, collected at time of surgery and enucleation, for bacterial culture (Specific Aim 1) and ELISA determination of antibody titers to P. acnes and/or lens protein (Specific Aim 2).

[5]Number of vitreous specimens, collected at time of enucleation, for bacterial culture (Specific Aim 1) and ELISA determination of antibody titers to P. acnes and/or lens protein (Specific Aim 2).

[6]Number of IOLs collected at the time of enucleation for bacterial culture (BC) and immunofluorescent (FITC) identification of P. acnes (Specific Aim 1).

[7]Number of posterior lens capsules (PLC) collected at the time of enucleation for bacterial culture (BC) and immunofluorescent (FITC) identification of P. acnes (Specific Aim 1). The remainder of the enucleated eye will be submitted for histopathologic studies.

Timetable for Specific Aim 1: Experiment 1 will be performed over the first 17 months of the proposal period. We will complete the Group A and B animals in a series of four trials using 16 rabbits at a time (8 each, pseudophakic and aphakic). The Group C and D animals will be completed similarly in two trials. Experiment 2 will be performed over months 13 through 21 of the proposal period. We will complete Group E and F animals in two consecutive trials beginning at 2-month intervals as described for Groups A–D. There will be some overlap of time with the viable P. acnes long-term natural history studies described above. We will begin a trial every 2 months to provide for the appropriate use of space in the animal housing facilities and to optimize the scheduling and completion of the research week.

Table 8.1 nicely illustrates the above points. It describes the design for two experiments relating to Specific Aims 1 and 2 of a successful proposal concerning endophthalmitis.

Diagrams and flow charts are useful for indicating complicated relationships and particularly paths to be taken depending on a variety of different experimental results. The diagram in Figure 8.1 illustrates and relates a series of experiments composing Specific Aim 1 of a proposal to study an animal model of uveitis. The chart indicates that three stages of the condition will be studied. The right eye of each animal will be tested for the lipid peroxidation products specified and the left eye will be used for histopathology involving morphometry.

The flow chart in Figure 8.2 was used in a proposal to present a complicated series of electrophysiological tests; which test would be used depended on the nature of the response recorded when a cell was penetrated with an electrode. The proposal received an excellent priority score and was funded. This flow chart saved nearly two pages of text and probably eased the task of review.

Data Interpretation

Far too many applicants pay a high price for skipping this section of the proposal, leaving the reviewers to their own biases as to how the outcomes of the studies will support or refute the hypotheses. We are amazed at how frequently Summary Statements (the reviewers' evaluation reports) criticize the PI for failing to discuss his or her plans for reducing

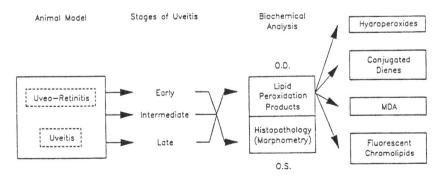

Figure 8.1

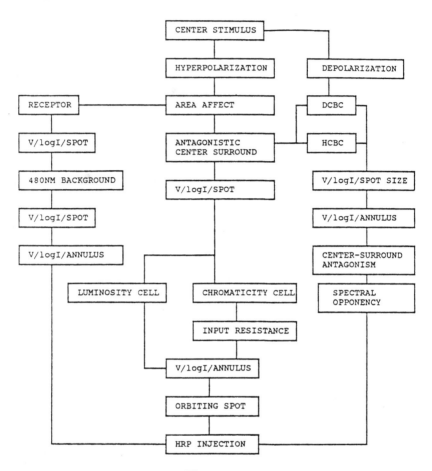

Figure 8.2

the data to an interpretable form and making an interpretation. Thus, a Data Analysis subsection is vital to all projects. Depending on the nature and number of experiments, it may be better to discuss the form the data will take as part of each experimental protocol; alternatively, the results of individual experiments can be discussed together in a subsection following the design subsection. Data analysis is sometimes presented as the last part of Methods, but it logically belongs with the Research Design. The goal of this subsection is to tell the reviewer what the data will look like, how they will be analyzed, and what they will mean in terms of the hypotheses. Alternative outcomes must also be discussed if appropriate.

Quantitative data that can be subjected to statistical analysis are always stronger than qualitative or phenomenological data. It is almost always possible to design experiments so that they can be evaluated statistically. Many biomedical researchers have little or no background in statistics and may fail to appreciate how relatively minor alterations of their experimental protocols will give them a statistical basis. Medical schools and universities have many faculty who are trained in statistical methods; they are excellent collaborators and should be sought out. Unless you are a competent statistician, it is highly likely that your research proposals can be strengthened by input from or collaboration with such a person.

Do not assume that the reviewers are familiar with your methods of data reduction. If the techniques are complicated or involve mathematics, their basis must be described in detail. If this is too lengthy for the Methods, as a mathematical proof would probably be, it should be included as an appendix section. It is sometimes necessary to include in the appendix a fundamental paper published by another author in order to provide the basis for an analysis. If the reviewer is familiar with the procedure, no harm is done. If help is needed, you have provided it and saved the reviewer a trip to the library. This is not a strictly correct maneuver but will be much appreciated by the reviewer.

Problems and Solutions

Problems anticipated or that the reviewers might anticipate should be discussed in this section. This is a very sensitive part of the design. An inexperienced PI will probably reveal naiveté by a lack of appreciation of the difficulty involved in the interpretation of data obtained by certain procedures. This will not only be very apparent to the reviewer but will probably cause a good deal of irritation. To a scientist who has spent years perfecting a technique such as intracellular recording, it is very distressing to encounter a cavalier attitude about its problems. Even though the problems may be well known in the industry, they must be reiterated and dealt with in this section by the young investigator. If there are already publications by the investigator based on a procedure, it is enough to state that the same approach will be used, providing the paper is appended. It is not enough to refer to publications of other authors with a casual statement: "Concentration of interleukin-1 in the culture supernatant will be assayed as described by Jones."

Problems appropriate to this section include those of interpretation. In the case of intracellular recording, procedural problems like electrode manufacture and use are best handled in Preliminary Studies, where it can be shown that the procedures work in the hands of the PI. A typical interpretation problem with intracellular recording is the tendency for electrodes to select structures of larger size, causing a sampling bias that must somehow be handled. To ignore the problem would be to invite criticism of a very damaging sort: "The validity of the data will be questionable due to electrode bias."

A strong proposal includes few if any experiments whose outcome is totally unknown. Enough preliminary work should have been done so that at least the nature of the data produced will be known. Occasionally it is necessary to include unpredictable experiments. If any part of the project is dependent on the results of such experiments, it is necessary to discuss possible results and the alternative research paths to be followed in each instance. It is of the utmost importance that no experiment be so pivotal to the rest of the project that failure of the experiment would destroy the project. For example, a proposal to develop an animal model of a disease and then carry out a number of experiments on the model amounts to nothing if the model does not work. There must always be clearly defined alternate research paths so the project will be productive regardless of the outcome of any particular experiment.

It is very bad practice to incorporate into a proposal any procedure with which the PI or a collaborator is not familiar. But science marches on and it is sometimes tempting to include procedures discussed at the latest scientific meeting. If this will really help a proposal, every attempt should be made to enlist the support of someone familiar with the procedure. In the case of the above interleukin-1 assay, an investigator who has developed the procedure would very likely welcome the opportunity to use it, particularly if the use is supported financially. A proposal that is ludicrous because it involves procedures that are clearly beyond the expertise of the PI becomes very strong with the addition of a few thousand dollars in the budget for a contract with an acknowledged expert who will do the procedures.

The following is an example of the Design section for one experiment from a successful NIH R01 proposal.

Experiment 9
Title: The effects of Ang1 and Ang2 over-expression in RPE and CEC in a 3D co-culture system.

Hypothesis: When Ang2 > Ang1, VEGF-induced 3D networks continue to grow and are sensitive to growth factor withdrawal. When Ang1 > Ang2, VEGF-induced 3D networks show slower growth and are less sensitive to growth factor withdrawal.

Rationale: RPE and CEC can each be transduced using retroviruses to over-express genes of interest and can be selected to provide pure overexpressing cultures. Cells over-expressing Ang1 or Ang2 will be used in 3D co-cultures to see effects on CEC tubular networks.

Hypothesis Corollaries: Over-expression of Ang2 relative to Ang1, in CEC and possibly RPE, should destabilize CEC and, in the presence of VEGF, promote angiogenesis. The vessels should remain immature and should be sensitive to growth factor withdrawal. Over-expression of Ang1 relative to Ang2 in RPE and possibly CEC should mature vascular networks and provide resistance against effects of growth factor withdrawal.

Design:

1. Produce early passage bovine CEC and human RPE
2. Produce retroviral vectors for Ang1 and Ang2 (METHOD # 18)
3. Transduction with retroviral vectors; selection with G418; production of high titer viral supernatants (Ocular Gene Therapy Labs)
4. Produce 3D RPE/CEC co-culture overlay system (METHOD # 19)
5. Observe Ang2 CEC + Ang1 RPE co-cultures. Measure area of tubes formed as criterion of effect.

Analysis and Potential Problems: Vector production and concentration are routinely performed in our Ocular Gene Therapy Lab (see Appendix 4 and ref #57). Cells will be carefully examined for toxicity, although none is expected. Control experiments will use "empty vector retrovirus and B-gal retrovirus." Specimens will be processed as previously described by our laboratory. Images will be digitized and measured using Image ProPlus software.

The following is a part of the Design and Methods for a proposal that was not successful. It demonstrates the evils of mixing design with method. This particular part was three pages long. Only part of the first page is shown.

Experiments are grouped in sections 1–4, corresponding to the Specific Aims above. Unless otherwise stated, infection with MHV-4 refers to inoculation of 6-week-old C57BL/6J mice with 1000 plaque forming units of MHV-4, given intracerebrally, as previously described (14).

Identification of critical immunological components of pathogenesis.

During MHV-4 infection. Histological studies show a characteristic generation of multi-focal plaque-like lesions in CNS white matter.

Definition of the phenotype of inflammatory cells in these lesions will yield insights as to their origin, nature, and role in pathogenesis.

Representative mice will be bled on arrival, to assure they are seronegative for MHV (3). Mice will be infected with MHV-4, killed by CO_2 narcosis and the brain and spinal cord removed. Standard histological examination of MHV-4 induced demyelination in these and the following experiments will consist of paraffin embedded sections stained with hematoxylin-eosin, luxol-fast blue (for myelin) and Bodian silver (for axons), and immunohistochemical demonstration of viral antigen (avidin-biotin; monoclonal to MHV-4 Protein), performed as previously described (27). In selected animals, tissues will be embedded in epon and stained with toluidine blue or examined by transmission electron microscopy, as previously described (13, 27) (please see letter of support from Dr. John Jones).

For the specialized studies of this section, designed to evaluate cell phenotypes and cytokines, tissues will be snap frozen and stored at $-80°C$. Cryostat sections of the brain and spinal cord, 8μm thick, will be used for immunohistochemical examination. The immunoperoxidase method will be used. Monoclonal antibodies reactive with all T-lymphocytes, L3T4+ T cells, Lyt2+ T cells, MHC Class I and Class II(1a) expressing cells, B cells, and macrophage-monocytic cells are available from ATCC and are routinely used in Jones' laboratory (see letter of support). In collaboration with Dr. White, sections will also be examined with antibodies to IL-1, IL-2, prostaglandin E, and tumor necrosis factor (see letter of support from Dr. Green).

Groups of mice will be sacrificed at days 3, 6, 9, 12 and 60 after infection. Corresponding to the stages of early viral replication, initial cellular infiltration, marked cellular infiltration, subacute demyelination and chronic demyelination, respectively.

And so on for three pages! If the editorials and methods are eliminated, the Design part of this is as follows:

Design

1. Infect 75 seronegative C57BL/6Jmice with MHV-4
2. Sacrifice, 15 each, at days 3,6,9,12, and 60.
3. Routine light and electron microscopy, 2 mice per period
4. Immunohistochemistry to determine cell phenotypes (L3T4+ T-cells, T-lymphocytes, Lyt+ T-cells, MHCI, MHCII(1a) expressing cells, B-cells, IL-1, 2, prostaglandin E, and TNF macrophages)

Analysis: Bystander hypothesis supported if there are prominent L3T4+ T-cells early, Mac 1+ cells subacutely, and TNF+ macrophages late. **Immune Regulated Oligo Cytolysis hypothesis** supported if Lyt2+ (DC8+) cells and MHCI cells are prominent.

This is the information the reviewers want. It is enough to reveal the thinking of the PI, and what will be done. It takes up a third of a page instead of three pages.

Time

Time is an important consideration in a proposal. The use of time should be logical. The PI who proposes 12 experiments and simply partitions them over the life of a 4-year grant period makes a serious mistake. Experiments take varying lengths of time; some must follow others. Sometimes all of the proposed experiments can be run simultaneously. If this is reasonable and actually is what will be done, it should be so indicated. It is common, albeit poor practice, to allocate a few left field types of experiments to the 4th or 5th years of a grant period. This is an open invitation for these experiments to be cut out by the Study Section. This action must be justified by negative comment, and any negative comment may impair the priority score.

Grant Length

Grant length is an important consideration in proposal preparation. A request for 3 years of support will not be shortened by the Study Section and will almost always be stronger than a request for 4 or 5 years. It is very difficult, particularly for first-time applicants, to propose serious studies to be done 4 and 5 years into the future. Most such proposals can be reduced to strong programs for 3 years and "more of the same" for years 4 and 5. The Study Sections will accept this from a proven investigator. Until recently the Institutes actively encouraged applications for the full 5 years, but it has now been mandated by the Congress that the average of all the NIH grants shall be 4 years. For every 5-year grant awarded, a 3-year grant must be made.

The authors disagree, mildly, about grant length requests. Ogden, being older (but not necessarily wiser), is more conservative; he advises that every proposal be as strong as possible, and that only the strongest should request 5 years. The downside of this approach is the proposal for 3 years that gets into the second percentile and could easily have been awarded 5 years of support. Goldberg, being more aggressive (but not necessarily wiser), suggests that most proposals should be for 5 years, based on the belief that reduction in time by the Study Section does not damage the priority score that much. The downside of this approach is the proposal that almost, but not quite, gets funded.

The new investigator perches uncomfortably on the horns of a dilemma. A 3-year request will be stronger than a 5-year request. But if this first proposal involves setting up a new laboratory in a new university, the poor investigator will be submitting a renewal application after only about 12–18 months of productivity. However, to ask for 5 years is to ask for a critical discussion of what is proposed in the 4th and 5th years. This is to practically solicit negative comments, requests for additional pilot data, and a suggestion that the proposal should be cut to 3 or 4 years. This is hardly fair, and most Study Sections try to give the new scientist the benefit of the doubt. As a compromise, it is probably best that the first-time applicant, with a strong proposal, requests 4 years of support and later regrets not asking for 5. In the final analysis, what duration to request is a judgment call that should be based on a realistic appraisal, hopefully influenced by an external knowledgeable evaluation, of the strength of the proposal.

The primary argument used by the NIH in promoting requests for 5 years of support was not that the research requires it, but that such grants provide a more stable base of support and reduce the number of proposals that an investigator must write. This actually may be detrimental to some researchers. Proposals should be part of the research business in much the same way that the publication of papers is part of the research business. Proposals reflect thoughtful preparation and planning that should be a continuous part of every researcher's academic life. There is an unfortunate tendency for many of us to immerse ourselves in experimental work until a project is completed and then put on our academic robes, dust off our word processors, run some literature searches, and write up the results for publication. We approach proposal writing the same way, except that during this time neither research nor publishing is accomplished and the time is considered wasted, albeit with grudging acknowledgment that it is a necessary waste.

This modus vivendi is counterproductive from both a scientific and a psychological viewpoint. It is very common with this lifestyle to discover, while writing up the experiments, a defect or oversight in the research that requires correction. This necessitates (or excuses) a return to the laboratory and a halt in writing. In the case of proposal preparation where everything else is stopped, typically 2 months before the deadline, problems have to be handled with imaginative prose since there is not enough time to gather necessary supporting data.

METHODS

The goal of the Methods section is to convey a maximum of information about the procedures to be used. It should provide at least as much detail as a publication, and for difficult procedures a great deal more. Too much detail cannot be given since the reviewers will simply breeze through the part with which they are familiar, but they will definitely pick on anything that is missing. Experienced investigators have no real problem with the methods because they simply tell it the way it is. Investigators who have not actually done a procedure reveal themselves very quickly by including trivia and omitting essentials.

Take, for example, a proposal from an experienced biochemist that wants to include some electron microscopy (EM) of cultured cells in his project. He is not an electron microscopist and will have the work done by a service laboratory. He calls the laboratory and a technician assures him that they will be glad to process the tissue if it is fixed in Karnovsky's solution. In his Methods he states that "cultured cells will be fixed in Karnovsky's solution and examined with the electron microscope." The omission of details of processing, embedding, cutting, and staining would make most reviewers highly skeptical that usable EM would be obtained. This perception would be reflected in negative comments, perhaps a recommendation to eliminate funds for the EM studies from the budget, and most certainly an impaired priority score.

The methods listed should work and should be state-of-the-art. They do not need to be recent discoveries. For instance, the Golgi procedure has been used in neuroanatomic research since the 1890s. Its practitioners, although few, are highly skilled and use their own state-of-the-art tricks to gain the results they want. The decision to use a particular procedure, old or new, should be handled in Design or Preliminary Data. In the Methods only the instructions for its performance are given. If the methods are not the latest, a statement should be added to indicate that the PI is aware of newer ways to do the procedure but prefers those listed. In making things easy for the reviewer, avoid the excessive use of abbreviations. Remember that those most familiar with the procedures will probably only glance at the text, while those with questions or who do not understand the procedures will read the section more carefully. Their attempts to understand may be thwarted by abbreviations that may be your stock-in-trade, but with which they are unfamiliar.

Hazardous procedures should be described in a special section of Methods. List only those procedures considered hazardous by the Safety Office of your university. A statement should be made that standard procedure for safely dealing with the hazardous material will be followed. If the hazardous procedure has been reviewed by a special committee of the institution, this should also be stated. For instance, some institutions require a special review of all proposed AIDS-related research involving live HIV, and it would be appropriate to mention the committee approval in this section.

Modern molecular studies involve a large number of different procedures that are standard in the industry, but very complicated. PCR, oligonucleotide synthesis, amino acid sequencing, fluorescein activated cell sorting, HPLC, immunoblots, and a myriad of bioassays are just a few of the commercially available tools used. Expertise in their use must be established by training, Preliminary Data, and publications. There is simply not enough room in a proposal to provide any detail concerning their use. Care must be taken, however, to specify the source of reagents (a new probe, for instance) that are not commercially available. A common failing of Methods is to state something will be done that requires support that is not obviously available. For instance, a study of genetics

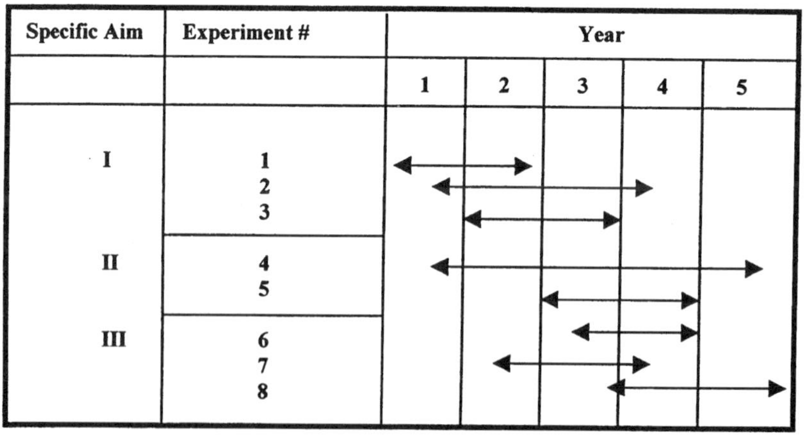

Specific Aim	Experiment #	Year				
		1	2	3	4	5
I	1 2 3					
II	4 5					
III	6 7 8					

Figure 8.3. The project timetable.

of 100 Hispanic multiplex families with insulin-dependent diabetes mellitus would be certain to fail in review unless it were clearly proven that the families were available for study.

Timetable

A timetable (Figure 8.3) is required and should be at the end of Methods. It is important in most proposals to provide an explicit accounting of priorities. A timetable is a useful way to relate the sequence of experiments and to show the estimated time for each. This can take many forms, but a Gant chart is convenient and concise. The estimates of the time required for each experiment must be realistic, and correspond to the available manpower. Ideally one or more experiments will require the entire grant period. This may protect you from reductions in time.

9

The Budget

Today, more than 80% of NIH R01 grant proposals are submitted with "modular" budgets. Before budgets became modular they were scrutinized by every member of a Study Section, probably with the negative intent of discovering an impropriety. Members of sections who have laboratory or clinical experience in the area of proposed research know what the going rate is for the goods and services requested, and have a good sense of levels of effort required for different types of research. If they saw anything that seemed out of the bounds of their experience, they questioned it. Too much attention was paid to minor differences in experimental preferences. This sometimes had a negative impact on considered evaluation of the science. This quibbling over pennies has been stopped by removing most detail from the budget presentation. The modular budget greatly simplifies the burden of the PI, and this is good. If the Study Section feels the budget is too large, it imposes cuts in increments of $25,000, and this is bad.

Detailed instructions for filling out the budget are given in the PHS 398 application packet (<http://grants.nih.gov/grants/forms.htm>), and are supplemented by instructions and sample forms presented at the "NIH Modular Research Grant Applications" web site (<http://grants.nih.gov/grants/funding/modular/modular.htm>). These should be carefully followed. In many institutions, this is the responsibility of the business office or the Office of Contracts and Grants. The PI, who gets the credit for any errors, should check it carefully.

MODULAR BUDGETS

The modular budget system is used for projects with direct costs of $250,000 per year or less. No itemization is required and the budget is allocated in modules of $25,000. The amounts requested should not change over the years, with the exception of the first year, which typically includes an extra module for equipment. A typical budget is shown in Figure 9.1. *The Modular Budget Format page in the PHS 398 packet must be used, instead of the standard PHS 398 budget pages* (form pages 4 and 5). The only budget numbers permitted are for those categories in Figure 9.1.

Example: Modular Budget Narrative

Robert Jones, M.D., PI, 50% effort. Dr. Jones will examine all patients in the study during a dedicated half-day clinic. The study calls for enrolling 100 subjects to be examined at 2-month intervals (600 examinations). He will also analyze the data, supervise data collection, and administer the project.

Samuel Smith, Ph.D., Co-I, 30% effort. Dr. Smith will supervise the DNA analyses and provide data interpretation of the subject genomes.

Jane Brown, M.S., Technician III, 100% effort. Ms. Brown is an experienced molecular biologist. She will conduct approximately 600 DNA analyses per year.

Edward White, M.D., Ph.D., Consultant. Dr. White will consult on the genome analysis and will provide patients for enrollment in the study.

Equipment: An additional module is requested in the first year to permit the purchase of an ABI sequencer ($30,000). The equipment used to obtain our preliminary data is already over used, and cannot support the additional demands of this study.

This short narrative is all that is required, providing that the Experimental Design is sound. Support for the percentage efforts should be implicit in the design of the project. Percentage effort is usually not stated for a consultant. A letter of collaboration should be appended to the proposal, and the consultant's Biosketch should be included.

Developing a modular budget is easy. Start with the regular budget pages of the 398 form. Use them as a guide only. Fill in the personnel section, including fringe benefits if appropriate, and all salaries, to obtain a total annual cost of personnel. Fill in the cost of consultants, equipment, supplies, travel, and other expenses for the first year. The goal is to de-

Initial Budget Period	Second Year Support	Third Year Support	Fourth Year Support	Fifth Year Support
$175,000	$150,000	150,000	$150,000	$150,000

Figure 9.1. A typical modular budget.

termine a realistic estimate of the cost of your proposed work. Add up all direct costs, less the equipment. Increase the first year budget by 4% for each additional year, to provide coverage for inflation. Add up the totals for the years requested (probably 5) to derive the total cost of the project, and round it to the nearest $25,000. Divide the total cost by 25,000 to get the total number of modules. Distribute the modules evenly over all years, with the possibility of having one additional module in the first year.

In the example of Figure 9.1, actual direct costs required for year 1 were calculated to be $170,000, including $30,000 for equipment. Increasing $140,000 ($170,000 less $30,000 for equipment) by 4% gives us $145,600 for year 2, $151,200 for year 3, $157,400 for year 4, and $163,600 for year 5. The 5-year total is $758,096. Rounding to $750,000 and dividing by 25,000 gives 30 modules total. Division by 5 years gives 6 modules per year ($150,000). The $30,000 for equipment rounds to 1 additional module for year 1, for a total first year direct cost of $175,000.

The average direct cost of different projects varies considerably among the Institutes, as shown in Table 9.1. For the estimate of modules in this table, actual direct costs awarded for the first year were averaged for each Institute. It is seen that modules varied from 7 to 11, but averaged about 8. These figures combine both new and competing proposals. New investigators should not request more than this in year 1, which can include 1 additional module for equipment. Subsequent years should not request more than 7 modules. Obviously operating costs escalate each year. It is the responsibility of the PIs and their grants administration people to distribute the funds so that there is not a shortfall in the last year. Since the budget request cannot reflect cost-of-living or anticipated inflation adjustments, the amounts cannot fluctuate unless specifically justified. The effect of requesting 7 modules each year, instead of 6, is obviously to increase the total award by $125,000. Thus, it is clearly to the advantage of the PI always to round the module request upward. This does present a dilemma because there is a threshold of concern about the total budget that cannot be exceeded without endangering the priority score.

A strong budget for a new investigator is one that is modest considering the proposed work, and features not more than one Co-Investigator and one technician. Consultants are paid less than $1000, equipment is less than $25,000, supplies, other expenses, and travel are less than one module, and patient costs (if any) are modest. No alterations or renovations are required, and no consortium arrangements are needed.

Table 9.1 *Average Modules by Institute Funded*
Competing R01 Grants in 2000
(Amounts Awarded for the First Year)

Institute	Average total award[a]	Modules
NIA	225	9
NIAAA	220	9
NIAID	205	8
NIAMS	200	8
NCI	205	8
NICHD	205	8
NCCAM	200	8
NIDA	235	9
NIDCD	205	8
NIDDK	195	8
NIDCR	170	7
NIEHS	215	9
NEI	200	8
NIGMS	180	7
NHLBI	215	9
NHGRI	240	10
NIMH	215	9
NINDS	215	9
NINR	235	9
NCRR	285	11
All competing R01s	**210**	**8.4**
New proposals	**205**	**8.2**
Renewals	**215**	**8.6**

[a]Direct costs times $1000.

This ideal budget is thus less than two modules plus salaries. Assuming a salary budget of about $100,000 (50% PI, $40,000; 30% Co-I, $30,000; 100% technician, $30,000), the bottom line is around $150,000 for the first year, or $175,000 if equipment is included. This is ideal for a beginning investigator in that it is well balanced and it will probably slide through without comment.

The average first-year award for new grants in fiscal 2000 was $205,000. This included both first-time applicants and established investigators with new proposals. The first-year budget of NCRR grants is large because most contain large purchases of equipment. Technically, these are not qualified to be modular. The trial period for introduction of the new modular system is over. The NIH now expects all proposals with annual budgets less than $250,000 to be in compliance. The following list names the common forms of noncompliance that will result in the proposal being returned to the PI *without review:*

1. Failure to state the budget in $25,000 modules
2. A detailed itemized budget is submitted in addition to the modules
3. Budget justification narrative includes comments about equipment, supplies, travel, other costs, etc., although the modules requested each year are the same.
4. The Biographical Sketch is not properly completed according to the PHS 398 instructions.

Supplies for modular budgets should not be itemized. However, if the budget is unusually large because of some aspect of the study, it is appropriate to point this out at the beginning of the budget narrative. For instance, a study involving several strains of transgenic mice may well involve as many as three modules in animal expenses. The reviewers will surely recognize this. However, you will not be faulted if you start this section with the statement, "Our transgenic mice colonies cost $.10 per mouse per day. We currently house 2000 mice. Annual costs are about $70,000."

The NIH is serious about rejecting noncompliant proposals. Certainly, it is not wise to stress the system. The main complaint seems to be a compulsion for investigators to add details to the budget justification that are no longer required. Justification is required for all personnel. The justification should focus on the percentage effort. This must be reasonable to accomplish the proposed work. For each individual, state what they will do. Do not laud the expertise of personnel; their Biosketches will be included. Technicians are considered "key personnel" (and must be listed on form page 2) only if they possess uncommon, unique skills that are required for the proposed work. Our advice is to include their Biosketches, in addition to comments in this section, if they are named on publications, and they have special training or experience.

NONMODULAR BUDGETS

The following comments are generic for proposals that are not qualified for module treatment, i.e., greater than $250,000 in direct costs per year. WARNING—An application requesting $500,000 or more in direct costs for any year must include a cover letter identifying the NIH staff member and Institute that agreed to accept assignment of the application.

Different types of research have very different budgets. These comments are directed primarily to laboratory research proposals and to small clinical studies. The budget requirements for multicenter clinical trials are very different. This advice applies to all proposals, regardless of strength, but is particularly important for those not likely to be in the highest (5–10%) percentiles. A strong investigator can survive a degree of bad grantsmanship and budgetary imbalance based on reputation alone. The investigator whose position in the field is not secure must use every available resource to improve proposal rating, and will likely pay a penalty for deviating from the ideal.

The perception of the reviewer is what counts. Budgets are not carved in stone, and the reviewers are well aware that the funding Institute may not be able to fund at the recommended level. Moreover, the PI has a great deal of latitude as to how the funds are eventually expended. Once the funds are awarded, salary money can be used for equipment or supplies, and equipment money can be used for travel or anything else, providing your institution is approved by the NIH for "extended authorities." These institutions include virtually all universities and research institutions. Permission for such budgetary changes can be granted by the university accounting office, providing that the amount is less than $25,000, and this should be easily obtained.

The primary goal of the budget exercise is to achieve funding, so you must generate a believable balanced budget that enhances the overall strength of the proposal. For example, certain equipment may be essential for a project, but to request it would dangerously inflate the budget and might suggest that the PI has no experience with it. In contrast, a commitment from your institution to purchase the equipment for you will have a beneficial effect on the reviewers. When the funds are awarded, needed equipment can be bought with a reallocation of funds from your other available sources. Of course, the reviewers must be comfortable with the feasibility of the project as proposed. That is, the budget must be reasonable within their experience. If your institution does not have the extended authority, permission for budgetary changes must be obtained from the awarding Institute. In our experience, this is always forthcoming if the request is properly justified. Such requests should always be preceded by a telephone call to the Institute Program Manager. There is no problem in transferring funds from one salary to another, particularly if specified personnel have been assigned to other projects.

The ideal proposal leaves nothing to chance. Only established procedures are proposed. Only data will be gathered. Nothing will have to be "developed" in order for success to be achieved. The budget will not include funds to "improve data collection," "perfect the computational model," or "develop an improved electrode puller," or for any other item that requires extensive justification.

Fallacy: "Give Them Something to Cut"

This is a common and major mistake in grantsmanship. Many investigators think that the Study Sections feel compelled to cut something out of the budget, so a questionable item such as a quarter-time photographer to prepare illustrations for publications is included. The hope is that this item, rather than something important, will be cut. This is bad thinking. A good budget is tight. Every item in it is fully justified and is required for the proper execution of the project. Anything less than this may weaken the proposal, and anything that weakens a proposal may impair its score. An item cannot be cut from the budget without some justification or comment, which invariably must be negative. "The requested photographer is not justified" may seem innocuous, but it carries the implication that the PI's judgment is poor, or that the project will not be sufficiently productive to require this item. Such a comment will certainly not strengthen a proposal, and any comment that does not strengthen a proposal is likely to weaken it in the minds of some of the reviewers.

Annual Direct Costs

The bottom line is, of course, the most important item of a budget. There is a threshold for concern about the bottom line or total that varies from Study Section to Study Section. It is determined by the personal experience of the individual members. If most of them have annual budgets with direct costs in excess of $250,000 for each of their grants, they will not be alarmed at such a request. Their NIH funding is a matter of public record through the NIH home page (<https://www-commons.cit.nih.gov/crisp/>) the "crisp" database of funded grants may be found there. If there is a question about the size of a budget, this information should be checked. The most important number in the budget is the annual direct cost of the first year. The budget is scrutinized for soft spots and these are discussed after the proposal has been approved. The discussion is of course negative as reasons why the budget is excessive are aired. Such statements as "the productivity of the PI does not warrant the request for four full-time technicians" not only justify the cut of a technician but also impugn the investigator's productivity when it otherwise might not have been faulted. Another common comment is along the lines that "four technicians are not warranted by the amount of work proposed." This also suggests that the PI does not fully understand what is proposed and the amount of work it will involve. Such comments from experienced scientists, although made in an offhand way, may raise serious questions in the minds of some of the other less-informed reviewers, who will adjust their scores accordingly. Above all, the impression that the budget is padded must be avoided. This is accomplished with a detailed and quantitative Budget Justification. Finally, anyone asking for in excess of $250,000 per year had better be of senior status and is certainly well aware of the above.

PERSONNEL

The following comments apply to all budgets. Percentage effort must be stated for each participant.

The *Principal Investigator* is assumed to be the author of the proposal. In this era of uncertain funding it is becoming increasingly uncommon for an investigator to fund his or her entire salary from a single grant. To have a large percentage of the PI's salary in the budget is particularly undesirable because of the inflation it causes. A credible involvement for most projects is 50%. Less involvement than this must be carefully justified with sensitivity to the feeling of the Study Section that the PI is simply turning a postdoctoral fellow loose on the problem without adequate supervision. An involvement of 5% is meaningless and is a very large red flag. Involvement of 10–20% is not that uncommon among senior investigators with established productive laboratories and several funded grants. It is accepted that these scientists are skilled research administrators and that they will guarantee the quality of the work. However, 20% involvement by a young PI who will spend the remainder of available time teaching or conducting a clinical practice would be viewed very critically, and such proposals do not do well. There is a counterproductive feeling that the PI lacks commitment to research. Section members are all professional researchers. They have very little sympathy for amateurs. A few institutions allow a PI to request a smaller percent salary than appropriate for the percent-time commitment. This is an excellent arrangement from the standpoint of grantsmanship since the commitment is large but the budget is kept under control. Be sure to state that the institution will support the research effort proposed, including fringe benefits.

Time commitment is limited to 100% of the total professional effort of the PI. This limitation used to refer only to regular academic duties and particularly to federally funded activity. In recent years the funding agencies have been tightening the reporting criteria, but there are some superstars with a total of 100% involvement among several grants who still manage to have a busy clinical practice, teach, and attend meetings around the world.

A *Co-Investigator* at 20% time is perfectly acceptable. Note that the NIH does not recognize the title Co-PI or Co-Principal Investigator. There must be balance between PI and Co-I involvement. The PI is the leader of the team. If less experienced than the Co-Investigator, the involvement of the Principal Investigator should be proportionately greater. Co-Investigators without salary can be construed as window dressing and their inclusion may actually weaken a proposal. Such individuals are more properly listed as unpaid consultants. Multidisciplinary proposals of necessity include a number of Co-Investigators. These proposals are much more convincing if the Co-Investigators are salaried. Of course, this does bad things to the budget, which quickly gets out of hand. If possible, limit the Co-Investigators to one or two. They will need to be fully justified and their Biosketches should be as strong as possible, with current publications pertinent to the proposed research.

Postdoctoral fellows are often called Research Associates. The first proposal of a new investigator should not include any Research Associates. To include a postdoctoral fellow in the budget will inevitably lead to discussions concerning the qualifications and experience of the PI. Unless the PI is exceptionally strong, the proposal rating will suffer. Research Associates are easily accepted in proposals by more experienced investigators. Do not use "TBA" (to be announced) to identify the fellow. This is asking for the position to be deleted. The reviewers know how hard it is to recruit an outstanding postdoctoral fellow. They need to evaluate the credentials of scientists who will benefit from grant funds. There is no accountability in the naming of Research Associates since the actual hiring may postdate the proposal by as much as 1 year and the proposed fellow could elect to work in some other laboratory. The stronger the Biosketch of the fellow the better. The ideal is a fellow with expertise needed in the work of the project, who wishes to acquire a broader knowledge base in the field of the study. If it later turns out that this stellar fellow elected to train elsewhere, it is not the fault of the PI. Obviously, discretion should be used in selecting such fellows, who must be contacted and permission to submit their name secured. We recall several instances where Study Section members had personal knowledge that a proposed fellow had accepted a fellowship at another institution. This obviously puts the application in a bad light. However, to simply put "TBA" in the budget provides no support and may weaken the proposal.

Two Research Associates in a budget is one too many. It is a liability for even the strongest proposals. Requests for less than full-time personnel should be explained; for example, an outstanding collaborator might assign a well-trained fellow to spend 50% of effort to bring a much-needed technique to the laboratory.

Technicians usually are accepted without question. A request for two full-time technicians will probably give rise to special scrutiny and requires solid justification. As with the Research Associates, the use of "TBA" should be avoided. Always list the name of the proposed staff member. Qualifications can be presented in the budget justification or Biosketch if appropriate. The listing of a technician's name indicates progress toward accomplishing the goals of the proposal. It shows that qualified personnel are already at work on the problem and start-up delays will be minimal, and instills a good feeling about the prospects for success of the work. As with the Research Associates, there is no subsequent accountability for the listing of a specific staff member. First-time proposals from new investigators should not request more than one technician.

Part-time technicians are often listed. In practice it is hardly ever possible to hire a part-time technician with high qualifications. For the listing of a half-time electron microscopy technician, for instance, to have credence, the technician must be identified and a discussion presented describing how the technician allocates time.

It is preferable to use a service facility rather than hire a technician part-time if this is feasible. For instance, a project may require histopathology on 200 specimens. Average time required per specimen might be 2 hours. A suitable technician for the work would be a 25% effort histotechnologist. This requires a great deal of justification. It is much simpler if your institutional histopathology laboratory offers the service for, say, $25.00 per specimen. The funds will be awarded without comment, providing there is actually a need for histopathology. The funds can be used to hire the technician if desired, but the proposal will be strengthened by the alternate approach. It is common to see glowing claims about technicians' abilities in the budget justification. These are taken with skepticism unless the technician has publications, in which case include the technician's Biosketch and refer to it in the Justification. The technician's expertise can also be established by reference to data presented in the Preliminary Data section. If the Biosketch of a technician is not particularly strong, it probably should not be included.

Secretaries are rarely funded at more than 25%. It is best not to include secretarial assistance in a new proposal unless it is absolutely required by the university. Be sure to state this requirement if it pertains, as it will shift the onus of justification away from the proposal. A required secretary can probably be cut without doing much damage to the priority score. Clinical proposals that require substantial telephone time in contacting or following patients can justify clerical help, whereas laboratory research proposals cannot.

Virtually every other type of personnel in the budget carries a substantial burden of justification and a great potential for weakening the proposal. Computer programmers, electrical engineers, and machinists may well be needed to carry out the proposed experiments, but to request funding for such personnel causes inflation and establishes that the means to do the research are not in hand. These staff help develop research tools, but everyone knows that research tools have a habit of not working. To request this type of technical support is to admit the possibility of failure for technical reasons. This is a weakness that an established program can overcome but that can destroy the prospects of a young investigator or a marginal proposal. Obviously the development work must be done. Good grantsmanship suggests that the costs for the development not be displayed as line items in the budget!

Biostatisticians and/or *epidemiologists* are virtually mandatory as part of the research team of most clinical projects. For an R01 proposal, their percentage involvement should ordinarily be small.

Consultants and *collaborators* strengthen most proposals. However, if there is not a perceivable weakness, there is no need to list a consultant, although one may actually be involved informally in the project. The name and affiliation of a consultant should be listed if a formal arrangement is to be used and the consultant paid for services. If there is an area of weakness in the proposal, for instance, a procedure with which the PI is not qualified is featured, then a consultant with expertise in the area may be listed. This must be accompanied by a letter from the consultant stating willingness to participate. This letter should be as specific as possible, listing the services to be provided. A consultant adds much more strength to a proposal if payment for services is included and the relationship is specified in enough detail to make it plausible. Unfortunately, many proposals list several unpaid consultants, often with letters stating simply, "I am happy to participate in your study. . . ." These may actually detract from, rather than strengthen, the application. To be certain that a proper letter is forthcoming, the PI should write exactly what the letter should say and give this to the consultant with the request that it be modified if necessary, typed on the consultant's stationery, and signed. Consultants often are not coauthors on papers. Collaborators usually are coauthors. Collaborators usually contribute more to the general conduct of a proposal than consultants do. Collaborators, unless providing a service, generally do not receive funds. Funded collaborators are really Co-Investigators. If they are in a different institution, they may have their own budget as part of a consortium grant.

Judicious use of one or at the most two consultants is good grantsmanship. The listing of more than two is problematic, is probably window dressing, and may have an effect on the reviewers quite different from that intended. The rationale for the use of consultants and a brief summary of their qualifications should be included in the Budget Justification whether they are to be paid or not. The Biosketches of consultants and collaborators should be included with those of the regular personnel. All collaborators and consultants, paid or not, should be listed, and their letters of intent should be included in Section i of the Research Plan entitled "Consultants" (not in the appendix).

EQUIPMENT

Equipment is the dilemma of grantsmanship. Research cannot be done without equipment. Study Section members know this as well as anyone. However, most members have well-established laboratories that are quite productive, without the latest bells and whistles. It is psychologically difficult to award something you wish you had yourself to a competitor you may feel is less deserving. Young investigators have a particularly difficult time of it. A molecular biologist, for instance, who has accepted a first appointment, may need to equip an entire laboratory at a cost of over $250,000. Unless the PI is clearly destined for a Nobel prize, such an equipment budget will not survive review. Worse still, without the equipment, the research cannot be done. Someone will point this out and the section will vote approval with some or all of the equipment, but with very low enthusiasm. The study will not be funded although, had the equipment already been available to the PI and not been added, a fundable priority might have been received.

Young investigators in equipment-intensive research should negotiate the purchase of necessary items with their new institution. It is unrealistic to believe that the R01 mechanism will supply a large equipment budget.

As indicated above, the threshold for equipment cost scrutiny is one module for most types of proposal. As with the other items of the budget, there is no real accountability in equipment purchases. It is now standard to request some equipment in the first-year budget of new and competing renewal proposals, but rarely in future years. This needs to be properly justified and it will usually be awarded. If the requirements of the project change, or the equipment becomes available from other sources, the money can be used for other purposes. The same piece of equipment must not be requested on succeeding budgets!

To reiterate an important philosophy of grantsmanship, it takes a strong proposal to get funds; every part of a proposal should be as strong as possible. Once funds are received, the PI is not constrained to use them in exactly the way specified in the application. Even if the Cadillac is desired, ask for the Ford, and when the funds are available, pool other resources to permit purchase of the Cadillac. This is not only good grantsmanship, it makes good sense.

Some equipment items in each specialty are sensitive by virtue of the fact that there are too many requests for them. Personal computers, HPLCs, and PCRs have gone through such episodes. Other equipment, such as a confocal microscope that is shared in most universities, is difficult to obtain for a single investigator. Such items require extensive justification. Inclusion in a proposal will probably weaken it. Replacement of outdated equipment also weakens a proposal if more than a module is requested. This is not a serious problem for established projects that are likely to have the old equipment, but such requests are hazardous for new projects of young investigators using borrowed or cast-off equipment. The NIH will permit lease and lease-purchase of equipment. These arrangements help deflate an oversized first-year budget. However, deferral of equipment purchases to later years of the grant in order to reduce the first-year direct cost is counterproductive. The use of special grant mechanisms for equipment is discussed in Chapter 25. Remember that requests for equipment never strengthen a proposal and may actually weaken it.

Supplies for nonmodular budgets should be listed in detail by categories where the amount of each category is greater than $1000. The usual categories are animals, histology, electron microscopy, tissue culture, chemicals, radioisotopes, oligonucleotides, biologicals, photography, surgery, computer, glassware, etc. Details of each category, including unit costs, should be provided in the Budget Justification. Some large items such as diamond knives are considered supplies, and diamond knife resharpening is usually included in the supply budget. The threshold of budgetary impropriety differs greatly in different disciplines. A feeling for this line should be acquired from discussions with experienced colleagues. Supply budgets of $20,000 or less are probably not questioned. The largest items in many budgets now are related to the purchase and maintenance of animals. These are generally accepted without great discussion if the project is considered strong, and if the numbers and types of animals are appropriate. The costs of animals are usually set by the university and are out of the investigator's control. The numbers of animals requested are scrutinized very carefully and, if justified statistically, are not usually an item of contention in the budget exercise. We often hear that certain Study Sections have established informal rules of thumb for supply budgets, based on the number of personnel. It is very important that you ascertain the threshold of concern from knowledgeable colleagues in your field and limit your supplies request to that amount. In addition, details for each category should be provided in this section; it is easier for reviewers to reduce estimates than precisely defined and justified amounts. A budget that lists five general categories of expense, each at a ballpark figure of $5000, is in big trouble, even if some justification is provided.

TRAVEL

For nonmodular budgets, requests for travel funds are accepted without question if they are reasonable: $2000–$3500 for one investigator.

Requests for travel funds for several investigators or for staff are likely to run into trouble, and foreign travel requests are a no-no. The amount of requested money above $1500 is probably small, but the discussion it engenders is large and damaging. It is not worth it for a few hundred dollars. Other budgeted funds can be used for travel at the discretion of your institution. You can even use your grant for foreign travel without NIH approval. It is far wiser to avoid negative discussion in the Study Section meeting and make the necessary adjustments later.

Much larger travel budgets can be tolerated by a proposal if travel is absolutely necessary for completion of a study. For instance, a collaborative study involving a virologist in California and monkeys in a primate center in Louisiana may entail bimonthly cross-country round trips, which are easily justified as a requisite of the proposal. In this case the logistics will be considered along with the science.

PATIENT CARE COSTS

Patient care costs are fully explained in the proposal packet. As in all proposal categories, these costs must be reasonable and appropriate according to community practices. Only inpatient and outpatient charges and laboratory fees are listed in this category. The university will usually set these costs according to a regular schedule that has been negotiated with the NIH. It is common practice to reimburse volunteers and patients seen as outpatients for their travel and other expenses. This should be placed in Other Expenses.

ALTERATION AND RENOVATION COSTS

These are theoretically possible, although new construction is not supported by the R01 mechanism. Small renovation projects are best submerged in the supply budget. Larger projects can be funded but are unusual and require extensive justification. Convenience is not an adequate justification. Conversion of a large laboratory into a smaller room and a darkroom to permit autoradiography would be a good justification. But only if the PI had not previously done autoradiography within the institution, had no other facilities in which to do it, and proposed a strong study that was dependent on the procedure. The argument that a darkroom previously used for autoradiography was taken away from the PI is weak. Another reasonable request would be for a coldroom to house experimental amphibia. But, again, the request is strong only if the PI had not previously used such a facility at that institution. To be appropriate for the R01, the renovation should benefit primarily the PI, and be required for this project. If it provides a shared facility, other grant mechanisms are more appropriate. Other weak requests would be for division of an office into two smaller offices, division of a lab into two smaller labs, and alteration of a room into a surgery. In the last case, vivaria facilities are usually considered the responsibility of the university. It is best not to request funds in this category; however, do include a statement that much-needed renovations for the project are being funded by the university if this should be the case.

CONSORTIUM GRANTS

Consortium grants involve more than one institution. In a common situation the PI is at the primary institution and the Co-Investigator is at another university or, perhaps, in an industrial laboratory. Unless modular in form, application pages 4 and 5 should be completed with all details of funds required by the PI. The full budget request for the Co-Investigator (Direct Costs *and* Facilities and Administration Costs) is listed on the line "Consortium/Contractual Costs." Copies of budget form pages 4 and 5, with complete details of the breakdown of the Co-Investigator's budget, are inserted after the PI's pages 4 and 5. A letter from the financial officer of the Co-Investigator's institution must also be included, stating that the budget is appropriate. Overhead costs, calculated at the rate of the consortium institution, are included in this budget as part of the consortium costs. In practice, the award is issued to the primary institution, which is billed for costs by the consortium institution. All of the usual costs are acceptable.

A consortium arrangement can strengthen a proposal if the collaboration is plausible, necessary, and carefully thought out. Cross-town consortiums are more plausible than cross-country ones. There must be no duplication of effort or personnel in the consortium laboratories. Consortium arrangements do not ring true if there is an obvious mismatch between the PI and Co-Investigator(s), or if there is reason to doubt the commitment of the collaborator to the project, perhaps because of a well-deserved reputation for overextension. Basic science R01 proposals involving more than two universities are difficult to justify; a mathematical guess is that the difficulty is proportional to the number of institutions cubed. Multicenter clinical projects are, of course, common.

A consortium proposal is strongest when the principals are, in themselves, strong, and their collaboration is logical and should produce results above and beyond those which either could be expected to produce alone. Consortiums that are contrived to circumvent university politics are rarely very strong. To generate a collaboration with a distant molecular biologist, for instance, when there is a prominent equivalent in your own group lacks credibility. It may be necessary for political reasons, but it will be necessary to use some imaginative grantsmanship to justify the arrangement. The argument that the distant collaborator will provide something unavailable in the local environment must be persuasive.

Contractual or fee-for-service arrangements are appropriate when services, rather than collaboration, that are unavailable in the local institution are required. A typical contract might involve the breeding and housing of a special strain of laboratory animal. Most universities not equipped to handle cattle, goats, and pigs contract with an outlying farm to house the animals. Large breeding colonies of dogs may be too noisy for academia, but can be cared for by contract in an approved commercial kennel. Such requirements can be handled on a fee-for-service basis, but are more conveniently and less expensively provided as contracts.

Histopathology, electron microscopy, blood tests, photography, oligonucleotide synthesis, and hybridoma generation are a few examples of services that are often handled through contracts with outside vendors or fee-for-service arrangements with investigators at other institutions. Contracting for such services is often far less expensive than providing the service within a department, given that the use of the service is limited, which is often the case. Services available within the university are generally not budgeted as contracts, but rather as Supplies or Other Expenses.

Contracting important services to professional laboratories may strengthen a proposal since it is assumed that the contractors are experts and will deliver a superior, often state-regulated, service. The credentials of the contractor should be clearly established. In the case of commercial laboratories, certification is probably all that is needed to establish credibility, although internal blind controls should be included in the experimental protocol. If nonstandard tests or services are required, it is essential that the ability of the contractor to deliver the services in a cost efficient, accurate, and reliable manner be established.

OTHER EXPENSES

For nonmodular budgets the threshold for Other Expenses of a nonspecific nature (copying, publication, and page costs; telephone costs; books; computer costs; service contracts; etc.) is about $5000. These will usually be accepted as reasonable with little justification other than that these costs correspond to current experience. Larger costs, such as service contracts for large equipment, are also acceptable provided that the PI uses the equipment in proportion to the requested share of the annual service contract. A proposal that includes about 100 hours of actual time on the electron microscope should not request funds for more than 10% of the service contract, even if the PI is the only user of the microscope. Some service contracts are excessively expensive. A computer system may cost $8000 for annual servicing, but it is bad grantsmanship to request this amount. Most service contracts are less than $5000. Funds for the entire contract should be requested only if the equipment will be used at least 1000 hours in the year. Since an EM technician requires about 4 hours of preparation for every hour on the microscope, one full-time technician can account only for about 400 annual hours on the microscope. Personnel time must be in balance with instrument use for a service contract to be properly justified.

Patient reimbursement, as opposed to patient care costs, is found in Other Expenses. It is unethical to pay patients or subjects to participate in research projects as this unfairly exposes the poor to possible experimental risks. It is permissible to reimburse experimental subjects for costs they have incurred due to their participation. The amount given should be the same for all subjects at the university. To pay more than the standard fee for all subjects for more risky or prolonged testing is obviously not permitted; this would be considered coercive by the IRB.

Equipment may be leased in special circumstances and listed in this section. The Program Director should be consulted prior to proposal submission if leasing is to be requested, to make sure that the items to be leased are acceptable to the NIH Institute. Nonspecific maintenance costs are usually not questioned if the amount is less than $1000 and maintenance-dependent equipment is central to the proposal; $1000 for maintenance is not reasonable if the only equipment is a personal computer and a stethoscope.

Computer programming is often found in this section, usually listed as a number of hours at an hourly rate. One thousand dollars for programming in Other Expenses will have little impact on the proposal. The same amount as a salary for a part-time programmer, listed in the personnel section, may give rise to a lively discussion and could hurt the priority score. Modest funds for construction of specific items of equipment may also be requested in this section. Alternatively, such items may be considered as contracts with an appropriate machine shop.

IN SUMMARY

The modular budget system has greatly simplified the life of most investigators, and will certainly be used by the newcomer. Budgets larger than $250,000 will present a substantial burden of justification for the basic scientist, even if a senior investigator. Such budgets are not uncommon in clinical studies, however. The secret of a good budget is balance and propriety, as perceived by the reviewers. A good budget is balanced in its distribution of funds among personnel (65–70%), equipment (4–9%), and supplies (10–15%). These proportions are what the reviewers are accustomed to seeing. Deviation from this pattern must be carefully justified by the nature of work proposed in Research Design and Methods.

10

Biographical Sketch, Research Support, and Resources

BIOGRAPHICAL SKETCH

The Biographical Sketch offers the opportunity to establish the credentials of the investigator as well trained and steadily productive of peer-reviewed papers. It is particularly important to the proposal success of a young investigator (see Chapter 19, Advice for Beginners in Academia). The critical reviewer seeks evidence that the scientist is productive of good science. If a deficiency in either area is found (quality or quantity), priority scores will suffer. The Biographical Sketch of the Principal Investigator follows the Budget Justification pages. The upper part of the first page contains educational information. This should be confined to college and graduate degrees. Internships, residencies, and fellowships are usually placed in the following *Positions* section, which should not be more than about six lines. It is not good to fill up the Biosketch with work trivia. What is impressive is a long list of solid publications in good journals, and on some of which the PI is first author.

Consider the unassigned reviewers, flipping through the proposal for the first time as the assigned reviewers read their written comments. Their first impression is a simple glimpse of the *length of the Peer-Reviewed Publication list*. If it is only a few papers long, the impression is bad and red flags go up. The things they want to learn quickly are how many papers; are the papers relevant; is the PI first author; is the Biosketch padded with abstracts; is productivity recent and steady; and (less important) what journals are listed. There is very little time to think about the Biosketch, so the impression of the PI's qualifications will be determined largely from the assigned reviewers' considered comments and a quick perusal of the Biosketch. The assigned reviewers will look carefully at the titles of the papers and will certainly consider the quality of the journals used.

The last page of this chapter includes a copy of a sample Biographical Sketch Format Page copied from the PHS 398 (Rev. 05/01) form, available at <http://grants.nih.gov/grants/forms.htm>. The Biosketch is limited to *four* pages. Use the first and second pages to list your publications. Use the remaining space to list your research projects that are ongoing or were completed in the past 3 years. The latter replaces the Other Support page of older PHS 398 instructions. All publications in the past 3 years are supposed to be included, and older pertinent papers may be added. A certain amount of self-censorship may be advisable. A clinician with 30 short case reports in the past 3 years would be foolish to list them in support of a basic science proposal. All the (even remotely) pertinent papers should be listed in chronological order. Be sure that they are actually in order. It is disconcerting for a reviewer who is trying to determine the flow of papers to find them listed out of order. If the list fills the remainder of two pages, stop there. If the second page is half empty, start inserting older papers that are highly pertinent to the research to fill up the void. Finally, if necessary, add less substantial papers of the last 3 years and unrelated older papers to fill the second page. The goal is to show good productivity during the past 3 years in the area of this research. Number the papers and at the top of the list state ". . . (from a total of *n* peer-reviewed papers)." Chapters, books, and non-peer-reviewed papers should be included only if they are pertinent to the proposal, and if there are not enough peer-reviewed papers to fill two pages. Such work should be listed in a separate section with the title, "Non-peer-reviewed Publications."

The Biosketch of a productive investigator who publishes strong papers in good journals is bound to be strong. Investigators with less solid Biosketches can offset some of the weakness by judicious selection of the better papers. Obviously, a dismal Biosketch cannot be helped. It is possible, however, to present a somewhat weak Biosketch in a manner that does not rub the reviewer's nose in its shortcomings.

Abstracts and presentations at meetings should not be listed in this section. To do so is interpreted as padding and actively weakens the proposal. An exception might be a PI who only recently completed the Ph.D. and postdoctoral training; but each abstract must be supported by a subsequent paper. The instructions unequivocally state, *"Do not include publications submitted or in preparation."* However, we would err on the side of noting "(submitted for journal publication)" at the end of each abstract for which this is true. If abstracts are listed and there are no subsequent publications of the material, there is a danger that the reviewer may conclude that the PI is generating unpublishable research. Do not provide them this ammunition for a cheap shot.

In the review of a Biosketch, there is a concern about the position of a young investigator's name among the authors of a paper. First authors get a lion's share of the credit and a Biosketch with 10 papers as first author is much stronger than one with 20 papers as the third of five authors. It is a mistake for a young investigator, who does not yet have 5–6 first authored papers, to publish papers as last author. Although your student or fellow may have done most of the work, and deserves to be first author, you, as a beginner, must be ruthless in claiming first authorship until the expected threshold of papers is reached. When a PI's Biosketch shows at least 10 recent, relevant papers, with 5–6 as first author, he or she can and should be generous in allowing fellows first authorship. This underscores why it may be disastrous for a fellow to be mentored by a beginning researcher who still needs to bolster his or her own Biosketch.

Some planning in publication is wise from the standpoint of the Biosketch. Clusters of publications in a certain year with no publications in the following year are common. These gaps may look bad to a casual reader who sees that there have been no papers published since 1998, but fails to note that there were four papers published in 1997. It may be impressive to readers to see three papers back-to-back by the same author, but it is far better for the Biosketch for the papers to come out sequentially so that the appearance of steady high-quality productivity is achieved. The ideal Biosketch will show at least one substantial paper published every year, and two, three, or more papers in scattered years, depending on the area of research.

Collaborators are important, and strong collaborators strengthen a Biosketch, providing that it is clear that the PI contributed substantially to the collaboration. This is best accomplished when the PI is first author of the paper. It can also be accomplished sometimes in the Preliminary Data section of the proposal or even in the Methods section of the paper, if wording is inserted indicating the roles played by each of the coauthors. This opportunity should not be missed if it becomes available. Papers published with weak or controversial coauthors are probably best not even listed on the Biosketch, unless the PI is the first author, or needs filler material.

The important point is that the time to strengthen a Biosketch is as the papers are published. Unfortunately, most young investigators do not have much, if any, choice. If their postdoctoral training happened to be in a productive environment with a senior scientist, they may acquire several publications as first author and be able to apply for their first R01 from a position of strength. If their postdoctoral mentor was less productive or just getting established, the fellow's Biosketch will surely suffer. Postdoctoral fellowships do more than provide technical training. This experience does much to establish research habits and traditions of productivity. Prospective fellows should choose mentors who are successful in their practice of science in terms of both productivity and funding. These established investigators are likely to be more generous in allowing fellows first authorship, their environment is conducive to production of more papers, and their fellows will emerge with a strong Biosketch. This may very well be the single most important variable in the success of a young investigator.

Honors are often listed after experience. The only honors that are impressive to reviewers are editorial positions and appointments to NIH Study Sections. Scholarships, traineeships, awards, ad hoc reviewing for journals, appointments to committees, etc., take up space and appear as padding in a short Biosketch. Individual NIH F32 or K awards are viewed by some reviewers as honors, but this is not true for appointment to a Training grant. The impressive honors usually go to the seniors whose Biosketch is strong in and of itself. If "Honors" are listed, they should really be impressive and no more than a few lines. It is important that the honors listed be pertinent to the subject matter of the proposal. Board certification is only relevant for clinical proposals. To list it may actually be a detriment to a basic science proposal.

The first two pages of Dr. Ogden's Biosketch are shown below. It is reasonably strong in that he is first author of 9 of the 64 publications listed. It is weakened by the fact that he has not been first author of a peer-reviewed paper since 1988. It is also clear that his publication style changed drastically in 1985. Before that time he first-authored most of his papers. A reviewer will correctly recognize this pattern as relative withdrawal from the laboratory. This will be interpreted in the context of his appointment as Associate Dean and it will be assumed that he now has little time for research. If Dr. Ogden were to apply for a grant now, he would need to show persuasively that he is fully capable of performing the proposed research and that he will be able to dedicate sufficient time to the project for success. Note that the PI's name is in bold (to help the reviewer find it), and the papers are numbered in sequence (so the reviewer does not have to count them).

OGDEN, THOMAS E. *Professor*

University of California, Santa Barbara	B.A.	1950	Zoology
University of California, San Francisco	M.D.	1954	
University of California, San Francisco	Internship	1955	Surgery
National Hospital at Queens Square, London, UK	Postdoc	1957–59	Physiology
University of California, San Francisco	Ph.D.	1962	Physiology

A. Positions and Honors

1962–1975	Assistant Professor to Professor, Neurology & Physiology, University of Utah
1974–1978	Member, Vis-B Study Section
1981–1984	Chairman, BNS-B Study Section
1975–2000	Professor of Physiology, University of Southern California
1975–1978	Visiting Associate, California Institute of Technology
1975–Present	Senior Investigator, Doheny Eye Institute, Los Angeles
1989–1992	Associate Dean for Scientific Affairs, University of Southern California
2001–Present	Emeritus Professor of Physiology and Biophysics, University of Southern California

B. Selected Peer-Reviewed Publications (from a total of 64 peer-reviewed publications)

17. **Ogden TE:** Nerve fiber layer astrocytes of the primate retina: Morphology, distribution, and density. Invest Ophthalmol Vis Sci 17: 499–510, 1978.
21. Larkin RM, Klein S, **Ogden TE,** and Fender D: Nonlinear kernels of the human ERG. Biol Cybern 35:145–160, 1980.
22. **Ogden TE,** Larkin RM, Fender DF, Cleary PE, and Ryan SJ: The use of non-linear analysis of the primate ERG to detect retinal dysfunction. Exp Eye Res 31:381–388, 1980.

23. Pierantoni R and **Ogden TE:** The internal horizontal cell of the frog retina: A morphometric analysis. Vision Res 20:761–766, 1980.

29. **Ogden TE:** Nerve fiber layer of the primate retina: Thickness and glial content. Vision Res 23:581–587, 1983.

30. **Ogden TE:** Nerve fiber layer of the owl monkey retina: Retinotopic organization. Invest Ophthalmol Vis Sci 24:265–269, 1983.

31. **Ogden TE:** The nerve fiber layer of the macaque retina: Retinotopic organization. Invest Ophthalmol Vis Sci 24:85–98, 1983.

32. **Ogden TE:** Nerve fiber layer of the primate retina: Morphometric analysis. Invest Ophthalmol Vis Sci 25:19–29, 1984.

33. **Ogden TE,** Mascetti GG, and Pierantoni R: The internal horizontal cell of the frog: Analysis of receptor input. Invest Ophthalmol Vis Sci 25:1382–1394, 1984.

35. **Ogden TE,** Mascetti GG, and Pierantoni R: The outer horizontal cell of the frog: Morphology, receptor input, and function. Invest Ophthalmol Vis Sci 26:643–656, 1985.

41. **Ogden TE,** Duggan J, Danley K, Wilcox M, and Minckler DS: Morphometry of nerve fiber bundle pores in the optic nerve head of the human. Exp Eye Res 46:559–568, 1988.

42. Zhu ZR, Goodnight R, Ishibashi T, Sorgente N, **Ogden TE,** and Ryan SJ: Breakdown of Bruch's membrane after subretinal injection of vitreous: Role of cellular processes. Ophthalmology 95:925–929, 1988.

43. Zhu ZR, Goodnight R, Nishimura T, Sorgente N, **Ogden TE,** and Ryan SJ: Experimental changes resembling the pathology of drusen in Bruch's membrane in the rabbit. Curr Eye Res 7:581–592, 1988.

44. Zhu ZR, Goodnight R, Sorgente N, Blanks JC, **Ogden TE,** and Ryan SJ: Cellular proliferation induced by subretinal injection of vitreous in the rabbit. Arch Ophthalmol 106:406–411, 1988.

45. Winslow RL, Miller RF, and **Ogden TE:** Functional role of spines in the retinal horizontal cell network. Proc Natl Acad Sci USA 86:387–391, 1989.

46. Zhu ZR, Goodnight R, Sorgente N, **Ogden TE,** and Ryan SJ: Experimental subretinal neovascularization in the rabbit. Graefes Arch Clin Exp Ophthalmol 227:257–262, 1989.

47. Mascetti GG and **Ogden TE.** The internal horizontal cell of the frog: Spatial summation. Acta Physiol Pharmacol Latinoam 39:165–172, 1989.

48. Vergara O, **Ogden TE,** and Ryan SJ: Posterior penetrating injury in

the rabbit eye: Effect of blood and ferrous ions. Exp Eye Res 49:1115–1126, 1989.

49. Zhu ZR, Goodnight R, Sorgente N, **Ogden TE,** and Ryan SJ: Morphologic observations of retinal pigment epithelial proliferation and neovascularization in the rabbit. Retina 9:319–327, 1989.

50. Nagy AR and **Ogden TE:** Choroidal endothelial junctions in primates. Eye 4:290–302, 1990.

51. Martini B, Wang HM, Lee MB, **Ogden TE,** Ryan SJ, and Sorgente N: Synthesis of extracellular matrix by macrophage-modulated retinal pigment epithelium. Arch Ophthalmol 109:576–580, 1991.

52. El Dirini AA, Saedy NF, **Ogden TE,** and Ryan SJ: Argon laser-induced retinal herniation. Am J Ophthalmol 112:602–603, 1991.

53. El Dirini AA, **Ogden TE,** and Ryan SJ: Subretinal endophotocoagulation: A new model of subretinal neovascularization in the rabbit. Retina 11(2):244–249, 1991.

54. El Dirini AA, Wang H, **Ogden TE,** and Ryan SJ: Retinal pigment epithelium implantation in the rabbit: Technique and morphology. Graefe's Arch Clin Exp Ophthalmol 230:292–300, 1992.

55. Gabrielian K, Wang H, **Ogden TE,** and Ryan SJ: In vitro stimulation of retinal pigment epithelium proliferation by taurine. Curr Eye Res 11(6):481–487, 1992.

56. Martini B, Pandey R, **Ogden TE,** and Ryan SJ: Cultures of human retinal pigment epithelium: Modulation of extracellular matrix. Invest. Ophthalmol Vis Sci 33:516–521, 1992.

57. Ye J, Wang H, **Ogden TE,** and Ryan SJ: Allotransplantation of rabbit retinal pigment epithelial cells double-labeled with 5-bromodeoxyuridine (BrdU) and natural pigment. Curr Eye Res 12:629–639, 1993.

58. He S, Wang HM, **Ogden TE,** and Ryan SJ: Transplantation of cultured human retinal pigment epithelium into rabbit subretina. Graefe's Arch Clin Exp Ophthalmol 231:737–742, 1993.

59. Wilcox MJ, Minckler D, and **Ogden TE:** Pathophysiology of artificial aqueous drainage in primate eyes with Molteno implants. J Glaucoma 3:140–151, 1994.

60. Gabrielian K, Wang HM, Lee M, **Ogden TE,** and Ryan SJ: Effect of leukopenia on experimental post-traumatic retinal detachment. Curr Eye Res 13:1–9, 1994.

62. He S, Wang HM, Ye J, **Ogden TE,** Ryan SJ, and Hinton DR: Dexamethasone induced proliferation of cultured retinal pigment epithelial cells. Curr Eye Res 13:257–261, 1994.

63. Sheu SJ, Sakamoto T, Osusky R, Wang HS, **Ogden TE,** Ryan SJ, Hinton DR, and Gopalakrishna R: Transforming growth factor-beta regulates human retinal pigment epithelial cell phagocytosis by influencing protein kinase-C dependent pathway. Graefe's Arch Clin Exp Ophthalmol 232:695–701, 1994.

64. Hao W, Chen D, Rife L, Wang XP, Shen D, Chen J, **Ogden TE,** van Boemel G, Wu L, Yang M, and Fong H: A photic visual cycle of rhodopsin regeneration is dependent on the RGR opsin gene. Nature Genetics 2001, in press.

Section C of the Biosketch, *Research Support,* refers to research funds and projects currently underway. In times past, the NIH required a separate detailed section for every key person in the proposal. With the advent of the modular grant and "just-in-time" procedures, this section has been replaced with the second half of the Biosketch for all grant proposals. You can expect the NIH to request more detailed information about your current funding and possible overlap with other funded projects at the time of funding (just-in-time). The PHS 398 instructions state, "List selected ongoing or completed (during the last three years) research projects (federal or non-federal support). Begin with the projects that are most relevant to the research proposed in this application. Briefly indicate the overall goals of the projects and responsibilities of principal investigator identified above." The sample information on the Biographical Sketch Format Page should suffice. Moreover, The PHS 398 instructions warn, "Information on other support beyond that required in the biographical sketch, should NOT be submitted with the application. Failure to comply with this requirement will be grounds for the PHS to return the application without peer review."

The guidelines state that neither the application under consideration nor, in the case of a renewal, the current PHS award should be listed as "Other Support." The "brief description" should be no more than three lines. The intent of this section is to help reviewers "assess each individual's qualifications for a specific role in the proposed project, as well as to evaluate the overall qualifications of the research team."

If there is more than one source of research support listed, or more than one project, there is more concern about experimental overlap than there is about budgetary overlap. A second project must be more than a simple extension of an existing study. It will hopefully involve the use of different technology requiring the addition of new personnel with expertise not already present on the first project. A good case might be made by a cell biologist who has a strong program of studies of growth factors, and who wishes to extend his or her studies to the molecular genetics of a particular factor. Although the cell biologist is PI of the second proposal, a qualified coinvestigator is added to provide the expertise in molecular studies. A second grant is not warranted in the case of a study that is simply too big for an existing grant. In this case a supplement might be requested. This is a "catch-22" situation, because supplements are rarely, if ever, funded.

A grant that provides a 50% salary for the PI or other worker does so on the assumption that the individual will devote at least 50% effort to the project and that the work of the project will require that effort if it is to be accomplished. If a second project is funded and the effort of the PI is reduced from 50% to 25%, half of the salary will be unallocated. When NIH administrators request more information, you should indicate that "a part-time fellow (or some other person) will be hired to perform the duties formerly required of the PI." If it is stated that the duties are no longer required, the unallocated salary might be deleted by the Institute staff. For the same reason, schedules should be arranged so that there is no effort overlap on the part of the PI, since funds for overlapping effort may also be deleted by NIH administrators.

There is always a suspicion that grants from private foundations and corporations overlap the submitted proposal. The absence of overlap must be clearly and forcefully explained (e.g., support for pilot studies), and the differences of the projects should be evident from the two- to three-line statement of goals.

The appearance of wealth is likely to weaken the percentile rating of a proposal. Small grants, usually for equipment, from private foundations or from the university do not impact major R01 projects, but may give such an appearance. Listing of such grants is unlikely to strengthen a proposal.

It is not uncommon for a new investigator to be funded from departmental funds for a period of time after joining a department. Listing these funds with the explanation that they are "start-up" funds will help the reviewer to appreciate that your institution has made an investment in your research. If Core resources or other university funds have been obtained by peer review, they should be listed as evidence of the collegial opinion of the scientific merit of the work. Usually such funds do not overlap the area of a new proposal because they are used for pilot studies in support of the R01 proposal, and the funds will be expended before the requested period of support begins.

This section is most convincing if there appears to be no other direct research support for the young investigator, but strong general support in terms of funded colleagues and abundant departmental facilities. The established scientist is strongest if there is only NIH support. Most investigators on soft money prefer to divide their activity between two grants in order to reduce their vulnerability in case of loss of funding. This not only presents grantsmanship problems with overlap, as noted above, but also may lead to the charge of career diffuseness. The existence of multiple grants weakens both new and competing renewal applications and imposes a requirement for greater strength to achieve funding. Three NIH grants cannot be justified by most investigators and should be attempted only by the superstars, who have no need of this book.

RESOURCES

The Resources Format Page follows the Biosketches. Under Facilities,

Specify the facilities to be used for the conduct of the proposed research. Indicate the performance sites and describe capacities, pertinent capabilities, relative proximity, and extent of availability to the project. Under "Other," identify support services such as machine shop, electronics shop, and specify the extent to which they will be available to the project. Use continuation pages if necessary.

If there are multiple performance sites, then include a Resources Format Page for each site. Truth be told, this information is generally ignored by many reviewers. This section usually does very little to strengthen or weaken a proposal unless there is a conflict between information given here and in the budget. If funds are requested for a computer in the budget, for instance, and the justification is that such equipment is not available to the PI, there had better not be a list of computer equipment given here. It is assumed that the claims of space on this page have some veracity and that the university, by submitting the proposal, guarantees the space listed. This section may be scrutinized in the case of a new investigator, as the reviewers look for clues concerning the probability of independent success.

The equipment listed and the information given should apply only to facilities needed for the proposed study. It is worthwhile to insert a statement concerning the free availability of an experienced team of investigators in the department, but do not call them consultants unless they are listed as such in the appropriate section of the proposal. The availability of shop facilities, operating rooms, vivarium, etc., should also be noted if relevant. The reason this page should be unimportant is that any facilities available that actually contribute to the project should be described in detail in the body of the proposal.

Principal Investigator/Program Director *(Last, first, middle):*

BIOGRAPHICAL SKETCH

Provide the following information for the key personnel in the order listed for Form Page 2.
Follow this format for each person. **DO NOT EXCEED FOUR PAGES.**

NAME	POSITION TITLE

EDUCATION/TRAINING *(Begin with baccalaureate or other initial professional education, such as nursing, and include postdoctoral training.)*

INSTITUTION AND LOCATION	DEGREE *(if applicable)*	YEAR(s)	FIELD OF STUDY

NOTE: The Biographical Sketch may not exceed four pages. Items A and B may not exceed two of the four-page limit.

A. Positions and Honors. List in chronological order previous positions, concluding with your present position. List any honors. Include present membership on any Federal Government public advisory committee.

B. Selected peer-reviewed publications (in chronological order). Do not include publications submitted in or in preparation.

C. Research Support. List selected ongoing or completed (during the last three years) research projects (federal and non-federal support). Begin with the projects that are most relevant to the research proposed in this application. Briefly indicate the overall goals of the projects and responsibilities of principal investigator identified above.

NAME OF INDIVIDUAL ONGOING/COMPLETED		
Project Number (Principal Investigator) Source Title of Project *(or Subproject)* The major goals of this project are…	Dates of Project (Entire Period of Support) Annual Direct Costs	Percent Effort

Sample

ANDERSON, R.R.
ONGOING

| 2 R01 HL 00000-13 Anderson (PI) NIH/NHLBI Chloride and Sodium Transport in Airway Epithelial Cells | 3/1/97 – 2/28/00 $186,529 | 30% |

The major goals of this project are to define the biochemistry of chloride and sodium transport in airway epithelial cells and clone the gene(s) involved in transport.

| 5 R01 HL 00000-07 Baker (PI) NIH/NHLBI Ion Transport in Lungs | 4/1/94 – 3/31/99 $122,717 | 10% |

The major goal of this project is to study chloride and sodium transport in normal and diseased lungs.

PHS 398/2590 (Rev. 05/01)   Page ____   **Biographical Sketch Format Page**

Number pages consecutively at the bottom throughout the application. Do *not* use suffixes such as 3a, 3b.

=====11=====

Human Subjects

Section *e* of the PHS 398 Research Plan concerns research that involves human subjects. Such research is subject to a number of federal regulations. The Office for Human Research Protections (OHRP) in the U.S. Department of Health and Human Services (DHHS) administers the procedures for Federal-wide Assurance of Protection for Human Subjects, and the rules and regulations for Institutional Human Subjects Review Boards (IRBs). As of March 2001, each separate institution must file a Federal-wide Assurance with this office. DHHS acceptance of the Federal-wide Assurance allows your institution to expend NIH or other federal grant funds on projects that involve human subjects. It is formal recognition that your institution has certified that it will follow the rules of the federal regulations. The review of protocols by your institution's IRB is an important component of its Assurance; IRB approval of your protocol allows you to conduct your grant project. The regulations are promulgated in the Code of Federal Regulations at 45 CFR 46 (<http://ohrp.osophs.dhhs.gov/humansubjects/guidance/45cfr46.htm>). Generally, any research that involves a living human individual subject, or data or material (organs, tissues, fluids) obtained from an individually identifiable human subject, carries a potential risk for the subject. Federal regulations pertain only to living humans, but most local authorities extend protection to material obtained at autopsy. Violation of confidentiality is also considered a risk.

In the prior editions of this book, this was an easy chapter to write. No longer. The rules and regulations have become more complex as the media have publicized untoward events in clinical trials. The ethics of medical research are under constant review and there is heightened sensitivity to the necessity to protect human subjects from questionable procedures. This has culminated in moving the former NIH OPRR (Office for Protection from Research Risks) to the DHHS. The governmental reaction is to increase requirements on investigators and their institutions. The institutional reaction is to increase restrictions. To its credit, the NIH has attempted to serve the public interest, to protect biomedical research, and also to minimize the impact on investigators. Even so, the burden in this area is great, and perhaps rightfully so. In its first year of existence, the OHRP temporarily shut down all clinical research at a number of institutions including Duke and Johns Hopkins. Ogden is old enough to remember what clinical research was like before the advent of the IRB. Modern multicenter clinical trials were unknown. Case reports were widespread and the use of statistics denigrated with the commonly heard comment, "you can prove anything with statistics."

IRBs are local groups, and there is little uniformity in how they behave. Some are much more bureaucratic than others, and all are susceptible to local politics. We know of investigators who refused to propose research involving human materials, even in cases where the human was the better model system. The reasons for this attitude were the onerous procedures of their IRB, delays in the review, and seemingly trivial reasons for IRB refusal to approve the project. Fortunately, the situation has improved and has become more rational at most institutions. IRB decisions are not subject to review. It is generally not productive to dispute them. Accept their advice, change your protocol, and get on with your life.

Check the "No" box in Item 4, "HUMAN SUBJECTS RESEARCH," on the face page of the PHS 398 form if there are no human subjects involved in the research. At Section e in the Research Plan, type, "e. Human Subjects—none."

If your research includes human subjects or human materials, you must become familiar with all of the rules and regulations. These are included in the latest PHS 398 Instructions. (See also Appendix E.) In addition, you must certify that you and your project staff have completed the "required education in the protection of human research participants." (A list of links to NIH guidelines as of March 12, 2001, is at "One Stop Shopping for NIH Information on Human Subjects and Financial Conflict of Interest" at <http://grants.nih.gov/grants/newsarchive_2001.htm>. Check for later updates.)

REGULATIONS

The March 2001 edition of the *NIH Grants Policy Statement* (<http://grants.nih.gov/grants/policy>) includes policies on the following topics under the heading, "Requirements Affecting the Rights and Welfare of Individuals as Research Subjects, Patients, or Recipients of Services":

- Ban on Human Embryo Research and Cloning
- Research on Human Fetal Tissue
- NIH Guidance for Research on Human Fetal Tissue
- Confidentiality
- Protection of Research Subjects' Identity
- Confidentiality of Patient Records
- Controlled Substances
- Human Subjects
- Assurance Requirements and Institutional Review Boards
- Education in the Protection of Human Research Participants
- Data and Safety Monitoring
- Investigational New Drug Applications/Investigational Device Exceptions
- Pro-Children Act of 1994
- Research on Transplantation of Fetal Tissue

Exemptions from the Regulations

Section *e* of the Research Plan must be completed if Item 4, "HUMAN SUBJECTS RESEARCH," was checked "Yes" on the face page of the PHS 398 form, whether or not exemptions from the regulations were indicated. Exemptions must be listed by number in Item 4a, as enumerated here (see details on page 21 of PHS 398 Instructions at <http://grants.nih.gov/grants/forms.htm>), and sufficient information must be provided in Section e "to allow a determination that the designated exemptions are appropriate."

1. Research in educational settings on instructional strategies
2. Research involving the use of educational tests, surveys, observation of public behavior, etc., and subjects cannot be individually identified nor placed at civil, criminal, financial, or other specified risks
3. Certain research involving individually identified subjects who are elected or appointed public officials or candidates for public office
4. Research on existing, publicly available or anonymously recorded data, documents, records, pathology specimens, or diagnostic specimens

5. Certain studies of public-benefit or public-service programs
6. Evaluation of taste and food quality or consumer satisfaction

Even exempt proposals must address the issues of gender, race, age, etc., in Section *d,* Research Design, and, when appropriate, in the Progress Report. Most exemptions on R01 proposals cite number 4.

Nonexempt Human Subjects Research

Multiple items are listed for response in Section *e* of the Research Plan, and page 19 of the PHS 398 Instructions provides a table to guide you through the level of detail required for each of a number of scenarios. This section has no page limitation. For most proposals, the material in Section e is only a summary that is largely for clerical purposes; it should not exceed one-half page in length unless there is a special issue. The reviewers usually breeze through this section unless a serious question is raised. Such questions should be discussed in depth in the Methods section. Avoid suggesting selective use of sensitive populations (prisoners, pregnant women, one ethnic group, children, or fetal material), but if such are essential to the project, the rationale for their use must be restated in this section. Typical responses for a limited study—not a clinical trial that would require much more detail—are indicated in quotes in the following:

- *Human Subjects Involvement and Characteristics.* ". . . 200 adult insulin-dependent diabetics in general good health. . . ." Be sure to state that subject selection will not be biased toward any particular race or gender, or better, that results will be generalizable across gender and racial lines, or best, that results will provide definitive data on differences between genders and races. Of course, back this up with your power analysis in the Research Design section.
- *Sources of Materials.* ". . . standard clinical and laboratory tests including. . . ."
- *Potential Risks.* This statement should consider only serious risks that would be apparent to anyone reading the Methods section of the proposal. It is only rarely necessary or justified to subject patients to serious risks, and this is appropriate only where life-threatening conditions exist. This section should not give the impression that risks exist where, in fact, there are none that are serious. Furthermore, do not include such potential but trivial risks as discomfort from minor routine procedures. This

statement should not be a repetition of the Risks section of the Informed Consent Form (ICF). Do not belabor "alternate treatments or procedures that might be advantageous to the subject" unless it is totally appropriate. In the vast majority of R01 proposals, this section requires only the statement, "This study does not involve physical or mental risks to subjects."

• *Recruitment and Informed Consent.* It is not necessary to include the ICF unless it is specifically requested. ". . . [S]ubjects will be recruited from the diabetes clinic; the study requirements, risks, and benefits will be discussed by the PI; and an IRB-approved ICF will be signed by the PI and the subject. . . ."

• *Protection against Risk.* For most proposals, this requires only the statement, "All data and patient records will be confidential and securely stored." If no serious risks are involved, state that "every effort will be made to minimize risks due to [pertinent procedure, conditions, etc.] . . . according to best medical practices (see Methods section) and procedures approved by our Institutional Review Board (IRB)." Only in those rare cases of great risk should details of preventive measures and emergency treatment be repeated. In this case it is appropriate to insert a few paragraphs from the Methods section. Do not yield to the temptation to discuss subject risk at length just because there is no page limitation in this section. Reviewers resent overly long proposals.

• *Potential Benefits and Importance of Knowledge to Be Gained.* Concise statements should be provided that the risk/benefit ratio of this study for the subjects and others is appropriate and that the likelihood is great that new and useful information will be obtained.

In summary, we are not suggesting that you should be cavalier about these requirements. Many investigators will have to provide copious details on all of the items in the PHS 398 Instructions. Every investigator involved in human research has an obligation to the subjects—the people who make the research possible. The standards for such research are very high, and must be met. Your actions, including what appears in your grant proposal, can have consequences for your institution and for the entire national research endeavor. However, do not overreact to the point of creating an unneeded burden for the reviewers of your proposal.

IRB REVIEW

All research that involves human subjects must be reviewed by an Institutional Review Board. Your proof of IRB approval is a letter from the

IRB that you send to the funding agency prior to funding. Research that involves no risk, either physical or psychological, can be approved by "expedited review"; but the IRB must be given the opportunity to make the determination that no risk is involved. Thus, even if a project clearly is in the no-risk category and no informed consent is necessary, notice of the study must be given to the IRB office and the IRB secretary must give you a letter stating that the project was approved under expedited review.

At one time, the NIH required the IRB certification at the time of grant proposal submission. This proved unmanageable and the requirement was extended to 60 days after submittal, and then to "before the Study Section meets." Today, with the emphasis on reducing the burden on the PI and institution, and on "just-in-time" procedures, the NIH does not require the IRB approval letter until you are called for additional information prior to an imminent award. Theoretically, this saves time and effort, and it reduces the need for IRBs to review nonfunded proposals. However, the turn-around time for IRB consideration in most institutions is at least 1 month. The PI must accept the responsibility for ensuring that all of the necessary documents are obtained and transmitted in a timely way, or suffer the consequences of a delay in the award. (Caution! Animal Care and Use Committee approval is still required together with the proposal. Most Study Sections will not review your proposal without a valid IACUC approval. See Chapter 12.)

In the not too distant past, review of human subject research performed was not done until the subject matter was presented for publication, too late for abuses to be corrected or for a poorly designed study to be strengthened. While it is true that some freedom has been lost, no serious researcher would suggest that the current system is not an improvement over the previous era of carte blanche human research. The IRB system is here to stay; it is functioning well in most institutions, and perhaps less well in others. The system, as developed by the DHHS, is not an impediment to any legitimate research. Admittedly, it is based on local review, and this introduces the possibility of local abuse. Any investigator whose legitimate projects are not approved by the local IRB may have a local political problem. This is occasionally seen in large multicenter clinical trials, where the IRBs of many institutions approve a project but the odd IRB may refuse to go along with it. This should probably be viewed as a local aberration rather than a fault of the system.

Although the Human Subjects regulations have imposed an enormous burden of paperwork and an unwieldy bureaucracy on the investigator, their overall effect has been beneficial. There is a heightened sensitivity to the vulnerability of the patient population and far less chance for abuse. Every IRB encounters the occasional proposal that they must disapprove on ethical grounds or, more often, on grounds of insufficient scientific merit to justify the use of humans. The IRBs are providing an essential element of self-policing for the research community, and often provide the valuable service of suggesting ways to improve proposed studies.

REQUIRED EDUCATION

Most recently, as part of the heightened sensitivity, the NIH has imposed an additional requirement on all individuals (the PI, collaborators, technicians, students) who are involved in the design and conduct of research, viz., Required Education in the Protection of Human Research Participants. (See "One Stop Shopping for NIH Information on Human Subjects" at <http://grants.nih.gov/grants/newsarchive_2001.htm>, and later updates.) Before funding, the NIH requires a letter that lists key personnel and the title (and brief description) of the specific course that each has completed. On-line computer-based courses are readily available at most biomedical research institutions. Ask at your research or grants office for access to the course that is approved at your institution. These are self-administered and include a test. When you pass, you can print your certificate. Some of these programs are fun, and the average training and testing time is about 2 hours. Repeated failure should make the examinee take notice. Perhaps a new profession?

REQUIREMENTS FOR INCLUSIVENESS IN RESEARCH DESIGN

Federally funded projects that involve human subjects are required to include minorities and both genders in study populations so that research findings can be of benefit to all persons at risk of the disease, disorder, or condition under study. If one *gender* or *minority* is to be excluded from the study, a clear, compelling rationale for the exclusion must be provided in the proposal. Similarly, all studies that involve human subjects are required to include *children* if appropriate. The requirements are explained in the **NIH Grants Policy Statement** as follows:

"NIH requires grant-supported research projects to be as inclusive in design as possible in order to extend the validity of research findings and allow for enhancement of the health status of all population groups."

Discussion of inclusiveness of your study subjects should be placed in the Research Design section of your proposal. There are also specific requirements in Section e. Moreover, the Progress Report for all applications that involve human subjects (competing or annual renewal) must include tables showing the representation of participants by gender, race, and age. Imbalances should be justified in terms of the science.

INFORMED CONSENT

Although it is rarely done, the regulations provide for waiver of the informed consent under certain circumstances. Paragraph 46.116.d. 1–4 of the regulations lists the circumstances:

(1) the research involves no more than minimal risk to the subjects; (2) the waiver or alteration will not adversely affect the rights and welfare of the subjects; (3) the research could not be practicably carried out without the waiver or alteration; and (4) whenever appropriate the subjects will be provided with additional pertinent information after participation. . . .

The IRB must agree that these conditions are met by the study and can then approve the omission of the informed consent.

An example of such an exemption would be the case of comatose patients found on the streets and brought to the emergency room of a large county hospital. It might be desired to include these patients in a study of immediate treatment with a drug compared with delayed treatment. But relatives are rarely in attendance at such times and the patient obviously cannot give an informed consent. The local IRB might be persuaded to exempt the PI from the ICF requirement. This would be legal if the risk/benefit ratio of the study were appropriate. You can be certain that this action would be scrutinized very closely by NIH reviewers and administrators and would need to be fully justified in this section, even if it took 10 pages of text to do it.

Any project that involves administration of drugs or invasive procedures to pregnant women, children, or prisoners is particularly sensitive and covered by special regulations. Such projects should be discussed with the chairperson of the local IRB as the proposal is written to ensure that IRB approval will be forthcoming. The rules for research involving human fetal material, transplantation of human fetal tissue, or human pluripotent stem cells are very complex and mired in the politics of "politics," ethics, and religion. On any day, there is more confusion than clear-cut directions. Even if you meet all of the NIH guidelines, get input from the chairperson of the local IRB well in advance of submitting your proposal. Such studies will be scrutinized very closely, particularly if the material is derived from nontherapeutic or nonspontaneous abortions.

Most of the provisions and requirements of the DHHS regulations make good sense; they are the result of substantial interchange between the research community and officers of the DHHS. Obviously, the regulations were formulated to protect human subjects, but it is now clear that these regulations represent the "standard of practice" for the scientific community. As such, IRB approval offers an element of protection from accusations of malpractice. Also, the IRBs are aware that they incur a degree of university liability when they approve a project. Many IRBs include a member of the institution's legal staff; this has the double value of providing informed legal counsel and an IRB member from the non-scientific community, as required by the regulations.

An Informed Consent Form, approved by the IRB, must be signed by every human experimental subject. The informed consent can take any form desired, but most institutions request the use of a standard form, of which the following is an example. It was developed over many years and after considerable debate by the faculty of the University of Southern California Medical School. It is perhaps more stringent than some, but this represents concern for research that involves primarily an indigent population.

Example: Informed Consent Form

Title: This should be in lay terms and not more than 10 words. Avoid industry phrases like "phase II study" or "open label evaluation." If the study is to test the relative efficacy of two drugs for the treatment of colitis, an appropriate title would be, "A study to determine which of two drugs (Drug A or Drug B) works best for the treatment of an irritated colon."

Investigator: Indicate the person responsible for the research and a telephone number where that individual can be reached.

Purpose: Explain in lay terms what the study is all about. A typical statement is, "You are asked to participate in a research project designed to find out which of two drugs is best for treatment of colon irritation (colitis), a condition that you have."

Procedure: Provide a brief description of what will be done, particularly, what will be asked of the patient. Mention all procedures of an unpleasant nature and the frequency with which the patient will be asked to return for follow-up. Example:

> If you decide to participate, you will be given either one of the two drugs or a nonactive drug called a placebo. Which you receive will be determined by chance and neither you nor your doctor will know which it is. You will take the medication three times every day for 2 weeks, and then return to the clinic for reevaluation, which will include looking at your lower colon through a tube called a flexible sigmoidoscope. If, in the opinion of your doctor, you are no better, you will stop the study medication and resume standard treatment. If you are improved, treatment will be continued for an additional month.
>
> You will be asked (1) to return to the clinic after 6 months for a final evaluation that will include the flexible sigmoidoscopy; (2) to keep a diary of your bowel movements until that time; and (3) to refrain from taking any other medication for digestion or bowels without consulting with your doctor.

Risks: List a realistic appraisal of the real risks to the patient involved in the research. These should include the possibility of infections, sensitivity reactions, danger to unborn fetuses, progression of the disease, bowel perforation, etc. If there are no real risks, so state. Irritation from eye drops or hypodermic needles are not risks and should not be listed here, unless your IRB requires it. Obviously, real risks should not be downplayed. If the study requires an extra cardiac catheterization, for instance, it should be stated that the risk of death from the procedure, although small, would be doubled if the patient participates in the study.

Benefits: State the benefits to the patients of participation in the experimental study. It is important to state "none" if in fact the patient will not directly benefit, and this is often the case. Possible benefits might be better understanding of a serious disease process, more examinations, or longer follow-up. Payment should not be listed as a benefit since it is not ethical to financially induce the poor to participate in experimental studies involving risk. What is appropriate is reimbursement for travel or other expenses, and this is not a benefit.

Alternative Treatment: The patient must be informed of what alternatives are available if participation in the study is declined. It is usually sufficient to make the general statement, "If you decide not to participate in this study you will receive the standard treatment as explained to you."

Withdrawal Statement: The patient is informed, "You are free to withdraw from this study at any time. If you decide to withdraw, your treatment will be continued in the standard manner." It is important that no aspect of the ICF be coercive. A threat to refuse treatment of the patient would certainly be coercive.

Confidentiality Statement: "The confidentiality of your medical records will be maintained by the investigators and the Institutional Review Board. In special circumstances the Food and Drug Administration may review your records after deletion of your name."

Signature: The patient is asked to sign the ICF beneath the statement, "By signing this form you indicate that you have read it and agree to participate as a subject in this research study." The signature should be witnessed by a nurse, physician, or clinical research coordinator.

Children, unconscious patients, and the incompetent are not permitted to sign an ICF. Special forms are required in these cases, indicating that the signer is a legal guardian. *It has become common practice in studies on children to have a competent child also sign a form indicating his or her agreement to participate.* This is in addition to the guardian's consent.

Hospitals and clinics commonly require the patient to sign general forms permitting routine procedures or surgery. In no case are these forms a substitute for the ICF, which must be individualized for each experiment and individually approved by the IRB within 1 year prior to the time that the procedures are done.

12

Animal Subjects

If your research involves vertebrate animals in any way, you must check "Yes" in Item 5 of PHS 398 form page 1, and indicate the assurance that your proposal was approved by your Animal Care and Use Committee (IACUC) by entering the IACUC approval date and the animal welfare assurance number in Items 5a and 5b. The NIH will not allow a Study Section to review a proposal involving animals unless IACUC certification is included with the proposal, or is received by the SRA within 60 days after the submission deadline. The use of animals in research is under increasing attack from a growing population of ethicists and antivivisectionists.

Research animal welfare was recognized formally by the NIH with a policy in 1966, revised most recently in 2000 (PHS Policy on Humane Care and Use of Laboratory Animals at <http://grants.nih.gov/grants/olaw/references/phspol.htm>). The NIH Office of Laboratory Animal Welfare (OLAW) has the responsibility for implementation of DHHS policy. The essence of this policy is that the responsibility for protection of animal welfare lies with grantee universities, which must file an OLAW assurance and establish, according to DHHS guidelines, committees to review all institutional use of animals. These bodies, responsible to a high official at the university, are called Institutional Animal Care and Use Committees (IACUCs). They must review every activity (research, research training, or biological testing) that involves the use of a live vertebrate animal. They must ascertain that the proposed use is justified in terms of benefit to mankind, is scientifically sound, and does not involve excessive numbers of animals or avoidable suffering. Animal research is reviewed and categorized by the local IACUC as

A. No potential suffering involved
B. Potential suffering, alleviated by anesthetic agents or analgesics, involved

C. Potential suffering, not alleviated by anesthetics or analgesics, involved

A report that includes this classification is kept on file at the OLAW and is available to the public. Animal activist groups now regularly compare published reports of animal experiments with the filed classification. If the published report suggests a class C experiment, but the IACUC report states the research was class B, a complaint is filed and animal abuse and/or scientific misconduct is alleged.

A case in point involved an investigation of corneal ulcers in rabbits and their treatment with a new antibiotic preparation. The IACUC classified this experiment as class B on the basis of administration of analgesics by the vivarium staff, and this was conscientiously done. The investigator neglected to mention in his subsequent publication that postoperative analgesics were used, and this caused a chain of events that culminated in a federal investigation. Although the investigator was vindicated, the entire process was avoidable. This example serves as a warning of the level of scrutiny of the scientific establishment exercised by the animal welfare movement. Investigators must be sensitive to potentially disastrous effects of even an appearance of impropriety in the use of animals.

There is substantial variation in the attitudes of the IACUCs of different universities, but increasing pressure from both the public and DHHS is tending to standardize animal use. The regulations require at least five members to constitute an IACUC, which must include a veterinarian, a scientist, and a community member. Most committees include several ethicists and members of the lay community concerned with animal welfare. The committees consider themselves more than a rubber stamp and closely examine each proposed experiment from the standpoint of numbers of animals used and potential suffering. They also often question the scientific validity of a proposed experiment.

Quality of science is of less concern in the case of proposals that will be peer reviewed (NIH, NSF, AHA, ADA, etc.), which constitute the vast majority of those reviewed by the IACUC. Research funded by private sources may receive little or no scientific review, and is scrutinized more closely by the committee.

Numbers of animals must be justified with specific reference to procedures and statistical necessity, showing that the number requested is based on more than a guess. This is difficult in some projects and requires an extra effort now demanded by many committees. It is not enough to simply state, "the number of animals requested is necessary to provide statistical validity to the data." The IACUC should be given the calculations used to determine the number.

Anesthesia must be used for all painful procedures and is advised before decapitation for sacrifice of rodents unless specifically contraindicated by the nature of the experiment. Full justification must be provided if anesthesia cannot be used. The most common exception is research involving blood levels of hormones or substances that might change with anesthesia. A list of papers that can be cited to support this contraindication is presented in Appendix F. The type of anesthesia must be appropriate to the animal species according to current veterinary standards. Some traditional anesthetics (chlorolose, chloral hydrate) are no longer considered good practice. Tranquilizers such as Sernylan cannot be used for primate procedures, since these agents have no anesthetic or analgesic properties. Ether is generally considered inappropriate by most institutions for safety reasons.

The fact that a particular procedure is traditional does not adequately justify its current use. Electrical stimulation has been used as an aversive stimulus for generations, but is in current disrepute as potentially abusive. Experiments involving stress or other aversive stimuli must be justified with care and with assurances that suffering is not caused. If it is at all possible, class C experiments should be avoided; these experiments require special monitoring, and will alert animal activists who may target the PI and institution for disruptive attack.

Certain experiments appear cruel to the public. Deafferentation may lead to self-mutilation in many different species. These animals mutilate themselves because they feel nothing from the involved area and they certainly are not in pain, but the appearance of such animals may be particularly repulsive and there is always the risk that pictures of them may become public property. Even though the disclosures may be made through illegal means, the effect of such publicity may be particularly damaging to individual careers and to the image of the university.

Concern over abuse of laboratory animals is clearly on the increase. Investigators must not only conduct their experiments so that suffering is absent or minimized, they must also be sensitive about how their work could be perceived by the public. Any faculty member who abuses animals or does procedures not condoned by the IACUC is a threat to federal support for everyone at the university. No faculty member can afford to tolerate such activity.

Section *f* of the PHS 398 Research Plan concerns vertebrate animals. The five items listed must be discussed if Item 5 on the front page of the application has been marked "Yes." The discussion should be brief, since this information is in the body of the proposal, and this section probably will not be read carefully by the reviewers, unless they detect a red flag. The instructions state,

> Under the Vertebrate Animals heading address the following five points. In addition, when research involving vertebrate animals will take place at collaborating site(s) or other performance site(s), provide this information before discussing the five points. Although no specific page limitation applies to this section of the application, be succinct.

Note that a *"failure to address the following elements will result in the application being designated as incomplete and it and will be grounds for the PHS to return the application without peer review."*

1. "Provide a detailed description of the proposed use of the animals in the work outlined in the Research Design and Methods section. Identify the species, strain, ages, sex, and numbers of animals to be used in the proposed work." Experiments should be listed by a descriptive title but need not be described further. State the species and numbers of animals to be used in general terms: "80 adult albino rabbits of both sexes will be used."

2. "Justify the use of animals, the choice of species, and the numbers to be used." The best justification for use of animals is that the particular study cannot be done *in vitro* or simulated by a computer model. Whether the number of animals requested is large or not depends on the nature of the experiment, the statistical design, and the species. More than 10 monkeys, 20 dogs, 30 cats, 80 rabbits, 200 rats, or 400 mice probably requires justification in terms of specific use: x drugs used at y doses, with n animals sacrificed at z times, equals $xyzn$ animals. Any use of primates is justifiable only on the basis that the primate system under study is unique. For example, studies of function or disease of the macula of the retina can be done only in animals with a macula, i.e., selected primates.

Choice of animal must be based on scientific, not economic, reasons. In studies involving primates, for instance, it may be desirable to use inexpensive squirrel monkeys rather than very expensive rhesus monkeys, but this should not be mentioned in the justification! The choice must be shown to be based on the desirable qualities of the squirrel monkey and its suitability for the proposed studies. The fact that it is less expensive will not escape the reviewers.

3. "Provide information on the veterinary care of the animals involved." Simply state that the animal facilities are operated according to all NIH and Department of Agriculture guidelines under the direction of a doctor of veterinary doctor (DVM). This arrangement is a requirement for approved facilities.

4. "Describe the procedures for ensuring that discomfort, distress, pain, and injury will be limited to that which is unavoidable in the conduct of scientifically sound research. Describe the use of analgesic, anesthetic, and tranquilizing drugs and/or comfortable restraining devices, where appropriate, to minimize discomfort, distress, pain, and injury." Procedures used to minimize pain and distress are anesthetics and analgesics for most experiments. The best statement is simply, "All procedures and examinations involving any possible discomfort will be conducted under general anesthesia." If the animals are to recover from the anesthetic, add the statement, "Routine postoperative analgesics will be administered under the direction of the veterinary staff."

For those relatively uncommon studies involving unrelieved stress or discomfort, it is necessary to describe carefully the duration and degree of discomfort and procedures used to minimize it. Such studies are class C and will be scrutinized carefully by the IACUC and antivivisection critics. Section *f* of the PHS 398 form will be read by activists if the proposal is funded, and must satisfy them that the investigator is seriously concerned about the welfare of the animals and sincerely regrets the necessity of causing discomfort for the greater good of mankind.

Class C experiments are no longer justifiable unless the research is clearly relevant to an important human disease. It is very unlikely, for instance, that many IACUCs would approve class C studies whose only justification was the relief of alopecia areata.

5. "Describe any method of euthanasia to be used and the reasons for its selection." Euthanasia should be by an approved method, such as pentobarbital overdose or CO_2 exposure. These methods are listed by the American Veterinary Medical Association. Appendix F contains a list of papers that can be cited to justify decapitation without initial anesthesia.

Publications must include appropriate words to indicate that animals were treated in an approved manner, were housed appropriately, were anesthetized for all painful procedures, and received postoperative analgesics as indicated by a licensed veterinary surgeon. It should also be stated in every publication that the procedures and species selections were approved by the IACUC.

Section *f* has no page limitations. It is possible to put much of the detail concerning animal use in this section, thereby providing more space in the Methods section. This should not be used to excuse excessive verbosity.

13

Consortiums, Contracts, Consultants, and Collaborators

CONSORTIUM/CONTRACTUAL AGREEMENTS (SECTION *h* OF THE RESEARCH PLAN)

The sample Table of Contents provided with the PHS 398 application indicates Section *h,* following Literature Cited, should discuss consortium arrangements and contracts. The next section, *i,* discusses consultant and collaboration arrangements. A consortium involves two or more institutions and investigators. A consortium arrangement is probably not appropriate for a consultant. The project suitable for a consortium is often multidisciplinary. The PI's university receives all of the funds and distributes them among the consortium institutions according to their individual budgets. The consortium proposal should include a separate budget page and justification for each institution. The rationale for the consortium should be stated clearly in this section. It is simply that each investigator has the expertise, the capability, and all of the necessary facilities for a part of the study to be carried out in each institution. It should be clear that the consortium arrangement satisfies a specific need and supports research otherwise impossible to complete. A typical consortium might concern the histopathology of the visual system of patients with Alzheimer's disease (AD). The PI might be a neuropathologist in a large hospital with many AD patients. The Co-Investigators might be experts on the retina, optic nerve, and visual cortex in three different institutions. The arrangement would provide the consortium with tissue and data on other parts of the system, thereby supporting a much more detailed study by a group of experts.

A clinical trial can also be conducted as a multicenter consortium. However, the preferred mechanism is for each clinical center to submit its own proposal for independent review and for a collaborating Coordinating Center to collect, monitor, and analyze the data of the Clinical Centers.

Consortium arrangements and contracts between institutions can only be established by the appropriate responsible officers. The details should be stated in letters written by the PI and signed by these individuals. The administrators want to be helpful but will not always understand the details of the arrangement. They will appreciate being given explicitly what is required of them, and, perhaps, the telephone number of the appropriate grants manager at the funding Institute. They will usually make a few changes in the letter, have it prepared on the appropriate letterhead, and sign it. This ensures that the best possible letters of support are obtained.

It is especially important that the grantee institution of a consortium justify their position as leader. This position is most obvious if the work proposed for the PI is clearly more than, and supports, the work of the consortium Co-Investigators. If this is not the case, a rationale must be provided. It must be made clear that the proposed arrangement is appropriate, one of the other institutions should not be primary, and the PI has a substantial involvement. A primary purpose of this requirement is to ensure that the applicant organization intends to perform a substantive role in the conduct of the project.

There are two common problems with proposed consortia. (1) Imbalance between the strengths of the PI and the consortium partner may suggest to the reviewer that the one is being carried by the other. This may lead to a recommendation that the work should be done by the stronger partner. (2) The first-year budget total will appear to be shockingly large to the nonassigned reviewers. This is because it contains the indirect costs (also called facilities and administrative costs) of the consortium partner(s), as well as its direct costs, added to the direct costs of the PI. The actual direct costs are really no larger, but are made to appear so because of the way the numbers are allocated on the budget proposal. These problems, as well as the problems inherent in integrating the activities of several laboratories, burden the consortium proposal. The strength that is added by the consortium partner must be sufficient to outweigh the adverse effect of a budget that appears to be much larger than other comparable proposals. The consortium should be briefly described as the last item in the Budget Justification. The "NIH Modular Research Grant Applications" web page (<http://grants.nih.gov/grants/funding/modular/modular.htm>) gives the following example:

Consortium
Approximately $15,000 total costs for all years.
Consortium with the University of Texas   {X) Domestic   { } Foreign
George Poole, PhD, (5% effort) will be responsible for production and
molecular biological characterization of transgenic mice expressing n-myc
proto-oncogene in photoreceptor cells. He will provide lines of transgenic
mice developing melanoma due to targeted expression of SV40-T antigen.

Obviously, this short statement leaves great questions about the nature
of the consortium. These can be addressed in Section *h*, but should have
been answered in the Research Design and Preliminary Studies sections.
For instance, this NIH example lacks credibility because the requested
funds ($150,000 per year) may be inadequate for the work. If this amount
is real, the work is being supported by other funds, and this must be explained, probably in Section *h*.

Contracts

The details of NIH contracts vary widely among different programs.
Your Office of Contracts and Grants is experienced in the execution of
the necessary paperwork and should be consulted as the contracts are fi-
nalized. Large contracts are often the result of a Request for Application
(RFA). The RFA instructions must be followed to the letter. Much of the
discussion in Chapters 21 and 22 on Program Project and Center grants
is appropriate for responses to an RFA. Also the budget may include
funds for contracts for specific services. Contracts may be let for board-
ing of large animals at commercial farms or kennels, for project development by a commercial firm, for engineering and fabrication of equipment, for software development, or for the leasing of expensive
equipment, etc.

CONSULTANTS AND COLLABORATORS
(SECTION *i* OF THE RESEARCH PLAN)

List all consultants and collaborators involved with this project, whether
or not salaries are requested. "Attach appropriate letters here from all individuals confirming their roles in the project. *Do not place these letters
in the Appendix.*" Include biographical sketches for each key consultant
and place them with those of the other participants.

Most research projects can be strengthened by the inclusion of one or more consultants. A project that lies wholly within the expertise of the Principal Investigator is probably narrow. It might well benefit from the different perspective of a suitably chosen consultant or collaborator. The association of consultants with a project evolves naturally during the development of the project, and the only decision to be made is whether the individual should be listed as a Co-Investigator, a Consultant, or a Collaborator. The NIH does not consider the titles Co-Investigator and Co-Principal Investigator to be different. One advisory from the NIH recommends against using the title "Collaborator" in favor of calling all such personnel "Co-Investigators."

An oncologist who wishes to establish a xenograft model of ocular melanoma would need to enlist the services of an ophthalmologist to obtain the tissue and an ophthalmologic pathologist to establish the cell type of the tumor. Having established the xenograft, a grant might be sought to support a study to test the hypothesis that primary ocular melanomas are fundamentally different from primary cutaneous melanomas. The ophthalmic surgeon and the pathologist might be listed as Co-Investigators, or consultants, or not at all in the proposal. The decision of which to do should be based on the nature of the proposal and the credentials of the PI. The perception that the PI lacks knowledge in an area in which there should be expertise must be avoided. For instance, if the PI has training in pathology, it would be unnecessary and perhaps even unwise to include a pathologist as either consultant or Co-Investigator. If the PI were a cell biologist, this addition would strengthen the proposal. However, it is not only the expertise of the PI that is important here, but also how the PI will be perceived by the reviewers. This perception will be based on the training and publications of the PI and the bias of the reviewer. Even though the PI is fully knowledgeable in ocular pathology, for instance, and can distinguish melanoma cell types with authority, if publications and training cannot be cited to support claims of this expertise, the addition of a consultant with such credentials will strengthen the proposal.

Generally, a Co-Investigator lends more support to a proposal than a consultant. However, neither a Co-Investigator nor a consultant strengthens a proposal much if he or she is unpaid. Also, to include a Co-Investigator or a consultant with a weak Biosketch is a serious mistake. It could weaken even the best of proposals. His or her Biosketch must be as strong as possible and must be current. To submit an outdated consultant Biosketch will cast doubt on the viability of the proposed relationship.

If a co-worker is to be listed as a consultant, time involvement and fee for services should be included to establish commitment to the project. Two consultants are probably one too many, and three consultants may be worse than none. To list a stable of consultants, all without pay, is simply window dressing and may actually cause concern about the ability of the PI to carry out the proposed research. Consultants should only be listed to fill an obvious need created by a defect in the PI's background, and multiple consultants suggest multiple defects, unless the project is logically and obviously multidisciplinary. Local consultants add more credibility to a proposal than remote consultants. Existing consultation relationships are more impressive than proposed future interactions. Preliminary data that reflect effective input from a proposed consultant greatly enhance the perception of strength gained by listing the consultant. If the proposed consultation is over a long distance, it is particularly important to provide some hard evidence that the proposed relationship will be productive. The best long-distance relationships are probably those that involve contract services. A project that involves quantitative determination of a difficult to assay substance like interleukin-1 might be less expensive and more credible if the assay were done in the laboratory of an acknowledged expert on a fee-for-service basis. Such individuals can properly be considered consultants. The consulting fee can cover the cost of the service. This is an effective way to convince the reviewers that the consultant is actually committed to the project.

Letters signed by each consultant or collaborator must accompany the proposal. An effective procedure by which the nature and timeliness of the letter can be ensured is for the PI to write it and then have it copied on the consultant's letterhead for the consultant to sign. The letter should be specific with regard to the services to be rendered, or the time committed to the project. It should reflect knowledge about the project and enthusiasm about its goals. It should be clear that the consultant or collaborator is considered part of the research by all concerned. A good letter is three-fourths of a page long.

Typical contract services that can involve a consultant are chemistries, monoclonal antibody generation and screening, histopathology, electron or confocal microscopy, tissue culture, clinical electrophysiology or echography, and other clinical examinations.

The distinction between a consultant and a collaborator is somewhat of a play on words, but generally a "collaborator" will coauthor any publications resulting from the work while a consultant will not always be listed as a coauthor. A collaborator may be listed as a Co-Investigator, as the PI in a consortium arrangement, or not be listed on the budget page at all. The greatest benefit is obtained when the collaborator is local and can be listed as a Co-Investigator. If this is not possible, the relationship should be described in this section and a letter of agreement appended. If funds are required for the collaborator in a separate institution, a consortium proposal will be needed or the collaborator will have to be considered a paid consultant.

14

Literature Cited
and Appendixes

Instructions for Section *g* of the PHS 398 Research Plan state,

Literature Cited. List all references. The list may include, but may not replace, the list of publications required in the Progress Report for competing continuation applications.

Each reference must include the title, names of all authors, book or journal, volume number, page numbers, and year of publication. The reference[s] should be limited to relevant and current literature. While there is not a page limitation, it is important to be concise and to select only those literature references pertinent to the proposed research.

REFERENCE CITATIONS

References are not considered part of the 25 pages allotted to the Research Plan. There must be neither too few nor too many citations. An average proposal should probably include no more than about 75 referenced papers. To submit more than this number is to risk being accused of uncritical reading of the literature. References that are cited merely to support a statement in the proposal and appear without critical comment about the citation should be kept to a minimum. Such references are generally classic and are mentioned to show that the PI is familiar with the literature. References to new areas of research are often controversial but must be cited to show familiarity with the current work in the field. Care must be taken with regard to which side of a debate is accepted, and this consideration should include, if possible, knowledge of the views of the likely reviewers. An important reason for limiting proposals to 25 pages was to force the PIs to be more discriminating in their citations. It was not uncommon 25 years ago to be asked to review a proposal with more than 300 references! Avoid listing more than 3 references to support a statement. More than this number is surely just padding. The references in the statement, "Type II diabetes is common in southwest native Americans[1–15]," are useless at best and detrimental at worst. If reviews are available, they should be cited rather than the original articles, in order to conserve space.

It is seldom necessary to cite directly any literature that is older than 10 years, since it will usually be included in recent reviews of the subject. It is more effective to limit references to highly pertinent recent papers, and to present these in more detail with thoughtful discussion of their relation to the proposed project.

Never cite a paper that has not been carefully read in its entirety. The availability of library searches and computer printouts of abstracts of papers published in selected areas of research often leads to citations based on reading only an abstract. But many abstracts are incomplete and/or misleading, or may represent shoddy work, even though the paper may originate in the laboratory of some "Eminent Investigator." A badly chosen citation can be disastrous if it happens to collide with strong reviewer bias. It is particularly damaging if it leads the reviewer to believe that the PI does not understand the content of a particular paper.

The citation format is left to the discretion of the investigator. Space limitations dictate that citations be numbered and so entered in the text. Superscripts take up the least space but make for a sloppy document if they overlap the preceding line of type. A small font should be used for superscripts; a 6- or 8-point font is preferred. A popular alternative is to include the citation numbers in parentheses.

- Best:
  Uveitis is one of the major causes of blindness in the United States,[16] accounting for 10% of legal blindness in young and middle-aged individuals.[17, 18, 19]

- Next best:
  Uveitis is one of the major causes of blindness in the United States (16), accounting for 10% of legal blindness in young and middle-aged individuals (17, 18, 19).

- Overlapping superscripts are messy:
  Uveitis is one of the major causes of blindness in the United States,[16] accounting for 10% of legal blindness in young and middle-aged individuals.[17, 18, 19]

- Wasted space is worst:
  Uveitis is one of the major causes of blindness in the United States (Henderly & O'Connor, 1982), accounting for 10% of legal blindness in young

and middle-aged individuals (O'Connor, Danfield, and Smith, 1981; Dinning, Grayson, Butterfied, and Fitzgerald, 1983; Gregerson, O'Connor, and Smith, 1984).

Naming of authors in the text is both ridiculous and a terrible waste of space. We recall with horror a proposal in which one page had 17 lines devoted to an endless list of papers by authors' names. Out of idle interest, we determined that the PI had used over 3 pages of the Research Plan naming authors. Of course, the text was so fractionated as to be virtually unreadable.

The reviewers of your proposal are chosen because they have some expertise in your field. They may have relevant publications and, being only too human, want to see if you have cited them. Some of the unassigned reviewers may also have publications relevant to your proposal. If you do not list references alphabetically, these poor souls will have to search through your entire list to find their names. Make things easy for them! List your references in alphabetical order. It makes absolutely no difference to anyone that the numbers of your citations in the text are not in order. Of course, it is a major mistake to fail to cite a relevant (or even not so relevant) paper of your reviewers. Obviously, you must know who your reviewers are likely to be to avoid this catastrophe. Do your homework. Identify the Study Section likely to review your proposal and its members. Use the NIH CRISP database (<https://www-commons.cit.nih.gov/crisp/>) to identify their research grants. Look up their recent publications. Cite them if it is at all appropriate.

The vast majority of proposals contain citation errors. This results from hurried preparation and a general erroneous perception that a proposal does not need to be prepared with the rigor of a manuscript to be submitted for publication. A few typos in the references are not a problem, but an incorrect citation may carry a heavy penalty in priority points if it is caught and if it gives the reviewer the impression that the PI is sloppy in writing. The best solution is to have a copy of every work cited in hand, so that it can be checked directly against the reference list. The way to achieve this is to make a habit of collecting copies of pertinent papers as they are read. This also provides a beneficial element of restraint on the number of papers cited. Do not be taken in by the belief that citations obtained over the Internet are always accurate.

APPENDIX

The PHS 398 Instructions state,

> Include 5 collated sets of all appendix material, in the same package with the application, following all copies of the application. Identify each item with the name of the principal investigator. . . .
>
> New, Revised, Competing Continuation and Supplemental applications may include the following materials in the appendix:
> - Up to 10 publications, manuscripts (*accepted* for publication), abstracts, patents, or other printed materials directly relevant to this project. . . . Manuscripts **submitted** *for publication should <u>not</u> be included.*
> - Surveys, questionnaires, data collection instruments, and clinical protocols. . . .
> - Original glossy photographs or color images of gels, micrographs, etc., provided that a photocopy (may be reduced in size) is also included within the 25-page limit of *Items a-d* of the research plan. *No photographs or color images may be included in the appendix that are not also represented within the Research Plan* [emphasis added].
>
> Note: Do not use the appendix to circumvent the page limitations of the research plan. Graphs, diagrams, tables, and charts that do no need to be in a glossy format to show detail must not be included in the appendix. An application that does not observe these limitations will be returned. . . .
>
> The appendix will not be duplicated with the application and will be sent only to certain members of the [Scientific Review Group] who will serve as the primary reviewers of the application.

These PHS 398 instructions apply to all R01 proposals. The materials are usually reprints of recently published papers and accepted manuscripts that are submitted in support of the Progress Report or Preliminary Data sections of the proposal. Although the reprints are generally those of the research team, this is not mandatory and it is a nice gesture to include key references, written by other authors, upon which great emphasis is placed. This is done for the convenience of the reviewers, in case they do not have the papers readily at hand. A note should be attached to each appendix item summarizing the reason for its inclusion. In the latter case, the comment should be added, ". . . for the convenience of the reviewers."

It is essential that any paper listed as "in press" be provided in the appendix. To fail to do this may give the impression that the claim of a paper is not true.

Material submitted in an appendix should be publication quality if at all possible. Do not submit graphs drawn by hand or substandard micrographs. Prospects of a proposal can be irreparably damaged by the addition of poorly chosen appendix material, even though they are clearly labeled "preliminary." Unpublished appendix material, after all, is submitted to support the PI's claim of progress or expertise in the absence of an actual publication. It will weigh heavily against the PI if it is not of the highest possible quality.

The appendix is not duplicated with the rest of the proposal. This material will be seen by only the assigned reviewers. Material that, it is hoped, will be appreciated by all of the section members must be included in the Preliminary Studies section of the Research Plan if it is to be seen by them. It used to be a common practice, because of page limitations, for figures referred to in Preliminary Studies to be included as an appendix. The effect of this was that the nonassigned reviewers saw the preliminary data without finished illustrations, a frustrating situation for those who were interested enough to read it.

It is essential that every item in the appendix be an important contribution to the proposal. This contribution must be noted in the proposal text. It adds nothing to simply submit a series of reprints because they happen to be available, and the extra bulk will not be appreciated by the reviewers.

Finally, the appendix must not be used to extend the 25-page limit of the Research Plan. Ogden was once involved with a proposal that contained nearly 10 pages of Experimental Method in addition to 5 pages of Experimental Design. This could not be accommodated in the body of the proposal so was presented as an appendix. Although not specifically criticized, this arrangement reflected a difficulty with being concise. The writing was too involved and the project was conceived as "diffuse" and did not make the cut for funding. In the revision, the extensive Methods section and a good deal of the other verbiage were severely truncated. The revised proposal benefited sufficiently to be funded.

= 15 =

Revision of an
Unfunded Proposal

It is a tough world. Few and fortunate are the senior investigators who have never had the gut-wrenching experience of having a proposal "approved but not funded." It is common and particularly threatening for first-time applicants to fail to get funded, but it happens to virtually everyone who stays in the business long enough. The old hands can usually rationalize that the unfunded proposal was really not that well written or the project was really not that important. However, the first-time applicant may lack sufficient self-confidence to be able to shrug off this reverse. But shrug it off you must, and proceed to a well-written, positive, improved revision. Prospects for funding of the revision are excellent. It is worth repeating that in 2000, among proposals that were successful in achieving funding, 42% of new proposals were "amended" (i.e., revised) and 35% of competing renewals were amended. Of about 22,000 R01 proposals reviewed by the NIH each year, over 40% are amended from a previously reviewed but not funded proposal. Since the use of the new "streamlining" procedures, the vast majority of unsuccessful proposals are triaged. The reviews are sent back without a priority score. *Most of these will be funded when revised!*

The proportion of proposals that are revised before achieving funding has risen sharply since 1993, and in some Study Sections the majority of those reviewed are amended. This has resulted in an overall improvement in the quality of proposals reviewed, since revised proposals are nearly always better than the originals, but has made it more difficult for new proposals to reach the funding percentile. A properly revised proposal is responsive to the Summary Statement comments. In a very real way, the Study Section itself coauthors the amended document! The Study Section actually has a vested interest in the success of an amended proposal, providing it was reasonably strong initially and the Summary Statement suggestions were rigorously followed. But beware—the comment from a reviewer that "this revised proposal is little changed" is a death sentence for an amended proposal! The PHS 398 Instructions state,

> Before a revised application can be submitted, the principal investigator must have received the summary statement from the previous review. There must be substantial changes in the content of the application. The application must include an Introduction of not more than three pages that summarizes the substantial additions, deletions, and changes. The Introduction must also include responses to the criticisms and issues raised in the summary statement. *The changes in the Research Plan must be clearly marked by appropriate bracketing, indenting, or changing of typography, unless the changes are so extensive as to include most of the text.* This exception should be explained in the Introduction. Do not underline or shade changes. The Preliminary Studies/Progress Report section should incorporate any work done since the prior version was submitted. Acceptance of a revised application automatically withdraws the prior version, since two versions of the same application cannot be simultaneously pending.

PLAN FOR RESUBMISSION

Since it is only good sense to anticipate failure of a new proposal on its first submission, and prospects for funding improve with revision, plan on revising. If you follow these suggestions you (very probably) will be successful the next time around:

1. Start work on a revision at the same time that the proposal is submitted for review
2. Get your submitted proposal reviewed by colleagues if, as is usually the case, you submitted it without such review
3. Identify the need for, and get to work on, collecting additional Preliminary Data

If your proposal fails, it is because it has some critical weaknesses. Appropriate preliminary data and collaborations can always strengthen areas of weakness. Chances are that the reviewers will pick up on these. Ask yourself and your colleagues what new data would strengthen your presentation, and get to work immediately to produce the additional material. Collaborations need time to develop. They are best supported with data gained through the collaboration. If you do this, you will be prepared to incorporate the Summary Statement suggestions in a timely manner and perhaps get your revision in for the next cycle of review. If you wait until the Summary Statement comes to start revising the proposal, you will either miss the next cycle or, much worse, submit a hurriedly prepared, poorly documented revision without new data. You cannot expect such a proposal to be successful.

RESUBMISSION

"Note: NIH policy limits the number of amended (revised) versions of an application to two and these must be submitted within two years of the original version of the application."

Most resubmitted proposals are sufficiently timely to be reviewed during the second cycle following their initial review, but some have been reviewed three or more cycles previously. Two years is the maximum time lapse permitted between the original submission and revised submissions. The need for funds, however, often dictates an expeditious resubmission. Summary Statements are returned to the investigator about 6 to 8 weeks (but often fewer) before the next submission deadline. This is just barely sufficient time for a careful revision if the process is started immediately, but not enough time for additional pilot studies. If the Statement suggests the need for such studies, they must be done, and the next cycle of review should not be attempted. But this is a small price to pay for successful funding. Of course, as stated above, if the need for new data was anticipated, and collection started early, it may be available for the next cycle. Resubmission of NIH proposals (both new and renewals) is according to deadlines (March 1, July 1, and November 1) that postdate new proposal submission deadlines by 1 month.

The Introduction (Summary Statement Response)

The only difference between a new and revised proposal is the Introduction, a 3-page response to the critique found in the Summary Statement for the initial submission. This section should precede the Specific Aims of the revised application. The Summary Statement must be read carefully and taken very seriously. Every critical comment should be listed and a response prepared for each comment. After this exercise, a summary of the rebuttal comments should be prepared and the proposal revised accordingly. Since the rebuttal comments are added, the page limit of a revised proposal is 25 pages, and up to 3 pages of response. Our experience is that a brief Introduction that directs the reviewers' attention to the changes in the 25-page Research Plan is more productive and less stress inducing than a full 3 pages of itemized refutations of the review.

The purpose of the Introduction is fourfold: (1) to establish that the resubmitted proposal is, indeed, revised; (2) to direct attention to the major changes; (3) to acknowledge and correct deficits in the original proposal; and (4) to correct errors of the Study Section (this one is dicey!).

It is important to keep the psychology of the Study Section in mind as the Introduction is prepared. The reviewers to whom the revised proposal will be assigned are most likely the same ones who were responsible for the previous review. It is improbable that they will welcome any suggestion that their previous review was defective. Whether or not true, reviewers operate under the assumption that their work represents their best effort. To be shown as incorrect to Study Section peers may be too much for some egos to bear. Since you probably do not know how ego-secure your reviewers are, it is best to assume they are fragile and tread lightly. (Note: How ego-secure *you* are is irrelevant to the revision process).

The Introduction, and the necessary revisions it describes, must be based on careful analysis of the Summary Statement, and, if available, the percentile ranking. Are the reviewers' comments consonant with the priority score? Comments substantially better than the score would indicate that there was a negative general discussion following the presentation of the reviews of the assigned members. If it was not triaged, it was in the gray zone for funding, and will certainly be funded next time if the critique is carefully followed. Large changes in the Experimental Design are not necessary or wise. You do not want to give the reviewers new targets for criticism.

It is impossible to generate an effective revision without a clear understanding of the shortcomings of the proposal *as perceived by the Study Section.* If there is a disparity between Summary Statement comments and score, every effort must be made to discover what happened to lower enthusiasm for the proposal. Both the Study Section Scientific Review Administrator (SRA) and the Institute Program Director should be contacted to determine if notes are available concerning the discussion. Sometimes an unassigned member may voice the observation, not noted by the assigned reviewers, that the work has already been done, or is not the best approach, or will not answer the important questions, etc. If the

SRA is unable to shed light on a discrepancy between comments and priority score, this insight may be obtained sometimes from Institute Program Administrators, who attend the meetings. A call to the appropriate Program Director of the Institute may provide the needed information. The SRA can usually tell you which Institute personnel were present during the meeting.

Clearly, the success of a revision is dependent on sensitivity to the concerns of the Study Section. The target of the Introduction is not the SRA—it is the assigned reviewers of the revised proposal. If successful, this section of the revision will assure the reviewers that their previous concerns have been properly addressed. Thus your task is to assure the reviewers that their prior concerns for your proposal no longer exist.

The Summary Statement should be scrutinized to identify the likely assigned reviewers. Since it is highly probable that the revision will be assigned to the same people, if they are still on the Study Section, it may be helpful to examine their recent publications for evidence of a bias that can be exploited in the revision. Ex-members of Study Sections make excellent reviewers. It may be profitable to contact a former member of the Study Section with appropriate expertise and solicit comments about the proposal. This is perfectly legitimate if the individual is no longer a member of the section. To be useful, you need a thoughtful, in-depth review. To get the time commitment needed, you may wish to suggest a paid consultant relationship and to offer adequate reimbursement (not from grant funds) for evaluation of the revised proposal; $500 is an appropriate reimbursement for the quality of review you need. Obviously, this action is strictly forbidden with someone who is still on the Study Section. Members of Study Sections should never be approached for information about grants or pending proposals. And beware, our experience is that advice from current members (gratuitous or otherwise) can be counterproductive.

Impartial analysis of the critique is a must. We have found that the best way to accomplish this is one line at a time. Give the Summary Statement to an unbiased reviewer and have them place a plus sign in the margin of the critique opposite every statement that can be construed as positive (e.g., "The hypothesis is innovative"; "This is a well trained young investigator"; New data will be obtained"; "This is an important problem"; "The work is within the expertise of the PI"; "Prospects for success are good"; and "This work needs to be done"). Ask them to place a negative sign opposite all negative comments. Any comment in the critique that begins with "but" or "however" is probably negative. Note every suggestion for deletion or alteration of an experiment or of a Specific Aim. Note every suggestion that your data will not accomplish what you claim or will in any way be flawed. Enumerate the negative comments and arrange in logical groups. You must respond to every negative comment.

Ogden's Axiom

Ogden's Axiom: The reviewer is always right.

Axiom Corollary 1: There is nothing to gain and everything to lose by contesting a comment.

Axiom Corollary 2: The goal of submitting a proposal is to get funds to support your research. Once funded, you can use the money as best suits your project. If the critique says to drop an experiment, *drop it* (from the proposal)! When you get the money, you are allowed to reevaluate the project. You may go ahead and do the experiment if you wish.

The Introduction should acknowledge that the initial proposal was flawed, that the review was excellent and helpful, and that the Study Section suggestions improved the revision. The Study Section, by implication, is given credit for important improvements in the revised proposal, and is put in a position of responsibility for some or all of the changes. The tone of the Introduction must be perceived as conciliatory. The opening paragraph should express gratitude for the effort, thoroughness, and helpfulness of the review. Repeat verbatim the best of the positive statements next: "We are grateful that the reviewers found the 'hypothesis innovative'; that 'the PI is productive and well capable of completing the study'; and that 'new and important information will be obtained.'" A statement that the suggestions have been followed, and as a result, the proposal is improved, should follow this.

The listed criticism groups should be identified one-by-one, discussed, and definitively resolved by an appropriate change in the proposal. Do not repeat responses to essentially the same comments from different reviewers. It is more effective to address issues by logical groups, such as conceptual issues, design issues, and areas requiring more data or detail, than to respond to each reviewer individually. Do not argue. A response that starts with restatement of a criticism may be seen as argumentative. The reviewers are very concerned that you paid attention to their own comments, so you must be thorough. Do not interpret the criticism or restate it in your own words. To do so is to risk allowing your own bias to color their critique, and this is asking for trouble. The best response is always to accept the criticism without argument, and to describe how the revised proposal has been changed in response to the criticism. If a particular experiment is said to be unnecessary, drop it, unless it is essential. If a procedure is said to be inadequate to the task, adopt the suggested alternative, even if this requires setting up a new collaboration. If the reviewers asked for additional data, tell them where in the proposal to find it. The response must show compliance with the suggested changes or show how they are wrong. But the latter way is dangerous indeed—a path strewn with damaged egos, argument, and confrontation, and very likely unnecessary. It is always possible to redirect an inappropriate criticism to suggest actual design improvement. In the response, it is essential that an attitude of grateful compliance be presented. The aim is to make the Study Section a party to the revised study design. If the Introduction runs longer than three pages, it is a failure. It certainly contains argumentative discussion and disagreement. You can agree and accept in a few sentences. If any of your response sentences begin with the words "but" or "however," you are in trouble.

In the unfortunate and actually rare circumstance that the Study Section seriously erred in a criticism, the response must never be confrontational. There is nothing to gain, and everything to lose, by confrontation. When it is necessary to correct a statement in the Summary Statement, it should be done with sensitivity to the manner in which the critiques are generated from the reviewers' comments. Their statements are often taken out of context from the written reviews. If a review statement is obviously wrong, attribute the fallacy to error; do not impugn the knowledge of the reviewers. If an item in your protocol was ignored, *do not* state that the proposal was not carefully read! Rather, apologize for not presenting it clearly, and rephrase the ignored material.

It is not wise to judge the adequacy of a review by what is written in the Resume section of the Summary Statement. This is a creation of the SRA, who has nothing to do with the actual evaluation, does not vote on priority score, and may not understand the reviewers' comments at all! Rather, the SRA simply summarizes any discussion that followed the reading of the typed reviews. Confine your response to issues raised in the Summary Statement. The Study Section members know perfectly well that your only feedback from the review process is what is in the report. They are reticent to hold you responsible for issues not covered in it, so it is not wise to open new territory for the reviewers to address in your revised proposal.

If a review is clearly defective and seriously flawed, it is a matter for Institute staff and council to review. The proposal should not be revised until a council has reviewed it, and either agreed that the review was defective or accepted the Study Section action, in which case the criticism must be accepted or the proposal abandoned.

Occasionally, however, a reviewer will simply make a mistake. If you presented a detailed statistical analysis only to get the comment that no statistics are considered in the design, this should be brought to the attention of Institute and CSR staff. They may agree that a rereview is appropriate, or the council could also call for rereview. Beware, however, since in a rereview, the original proposal, not a revision, is considered, although recent advances may be presented as an addendum if the SRA agrees. Reconsideration by council will also delay the review process a full cycle. It is wasteful of precious time unless success is virtually ensured. Follow the advice of the Institute Program Director in deciding whether or not to appeal to Council. The vast majority of appeals are unsuccessful.

Benevolent Censorship Is Mandatory

Preparation of an Introduction is always an emotional experience, and it is very easy to be borne along on the wings of righteous outrage. The result is the intrusion of adversarial language that is self-defeating. Thus, it is essential that a neutral third party review the Introduction with instructions to highlight anything thought to be stated too strongly. The objective is to bring the reviewers over to your side. You want them to be your advocates, not your adversaries. Ogden has found that a nonscientist can perform this service very well, and obtained his Introduction reviews from his most exacting critic, his wife.

PROPOSAL REVISION

Revision of a proposal should be viewed as an opportunity to improve it. The revision should be extensive, based on the Summary Statement comments, recent advances in the field and literature, and new preliminary data. At least 9 months will have elapsed since the initial proposal was written, and it is important to show that some kind of progress was made during that period, especially if the unfunded proposal was a competing renewal.

Major items to be changed will have been identified and a strategy for improvement developed for the three-page Introduction. As these are dealt with in the revision, every aspect of the proposal should be reconsidered, particularly the hypotheses. Are the questions they pose still important and timely? If there has been progress in the field, this must be reflected in the proposal goals and Background section. The reviewers must not get the impression that nothing much was changed. The assigned reviewers will be given the original proposal and Summary Statement, as well as the revision, and will probably compare them. The instructions call for some indication of the changed text. We much prefer that the altered parts be indicated by a vertical line in the margin along the left-hand side of the paragraph. We do not like bolding or italicizing of changed text, and particularly dislike underlining, which is actually prohibited. These things make the proposal more difficult to read. Confine these identifications to the Research Plan; marking up the Abstract, Budget, or Budget Justification looks bad, and is not necessary. It is only required that changes be marked. The method is left to the PI. Do not bother to mark single words or short phrases, unless absolutely crucial.

The best revision answers all comments of the Summary Statement, proposes substantial methodological improvements, and has an appendix brimming with reprints and manuscripts not available a year previously, when the initial proposal was submitted.

Additional collaborations should not be proposed unless the Summary Statement suggests the necessity, or new methods require it. Some experiments proposed the previous year might have been done even though there was no funding, and the results of these should be presented to support a claim for progress. Personnel changes should be explained, although it is best if there are no changes except those suggested by the reviewers. If the Summary Statement suggests reduction in personnel from full to part time, accept this suggestion. You can always reallocate funds to get someone full time (Ogden's axiom, corollary 2).

If the budget was reduced, it was by one or more modules. This is an area where you may defend your needs with specific information about costs, need for equipment, etc. However, do not quibble about reduction of small items such as travel. Save your arguments for defense of essential parts of the budget. The most common indefensible budget cut is in funds for animal per diem. These are not under the control of the investigator, and must be energetically rebutted with hard figures. If the requirement for a particular species is properly made, the per diem expenses are then required for the particular experiments.

Do not request personnel, equipment, supplies, travel, or other costs specifically deleted in the previous review. As a general rule, do not inflate the budget over that recommended by the reviewers. In no circumstances request more time than was in the original proposal. If the Summary Statement suggests a specific duration, follow the suggestion exactly.

The Preliminary Data/Progress Report section should be largely rewritten to show continued progress. It should be abundantly clear to the reviewers that this revised proposal is not simply "more of the same." We hope for a comment like, "this is a heavily revised proposal that satisfies completely the criticisms raised in the last review and shows substantial progress."

An unfunded proposal is, by definition, weak. The revision of such a proposal should operate under the mandate that none of the many proposal-weakening practices described in this book is committed. This is a proposal that simply does not have the luxury of perpetuating the sins of grantsmanship that were most likely committed in the original proposal. In our experience, resubmitted proposals have almost always received a better priority score than the original. Our best experience was a proposal that received a 328 on initial review and a funded 116 on resubmission. In another instance, a proposal received a 280 initially, a 200 the second time, and a funded 150 the third time. We know of another instance in which a proposal was funded after the fourth submission, and in 1993 there was one proposal at the NIH that was finally funded after its seventh revision! Perseverance can pay off! However, if your revised proposal receives a score that is worse than that of the original proposal, you probably reinforced rather than allayed the concerns of the reviewers.

The following are excerpts from poorly written Introductions:

- "The reviewers suggested the tumor necrosis factor (TNF) may correlate with, but not cause, axonal degeneration." This was the PI's interpretation of several negative comments in the review, none of which actually said this. Do not make up problems that are not actually stated as such, verbatim, in the Summary Statement.

- "We purposely used unphysiologic means to demonstrate a truncated form of prorenin in human chorion, because we were interested in demonstrating activity in a form of renin with only a partially clipped prosegment. This has little bearing on the present study, since none of the tissue is handled this way. Thus, control studies have *not* been proposed to address this issue" (emphasis added). The complaint was the absence of control studies. Instead of simply saying that such studies are now included, or the experiment has been deleted, an argument is presented and the suggestion declined. Bad form.

- "We agree that quantitative measurement of renin gene expression may have little bearing on post-translational processing to active renin. *Nevertheless,* gene expression is the key issue, important to the identification of the site of renin production. . . ." (emphasis added) This was followed by a half-page of argument with several references. To put it crudely, it is foolish to enter into a hair-pulling contest with a reviewer. You cannot win!

We have encountered a few frustrated and somewhat embittered investigators who responded to every criticism of their original proposal, but their revised proposal did poorly, and the new Summary Statement contained a whole new set of criticisms! This is certainly disheartening, and there is nothing you can do about it except roll with the punch, grit your teeth, and revise again. What probably happened is that both the original reviewers left the Study Section in the intervening time. New reviewers were assigned the proposal and they found problems not seen by the previous people. The bureaucrats will certainly be sympathetic, because they see this aberration from time to time. For all their sympathy, you will still have to revise. But your next revision will do much better. Persistence pays! Occasionally you may find out from the SRA that your revision went to the same reviewers who raised the new issues. This is a major problem. It is tantamount to the reviewers saying either "you have repaired your proposal and made it worse," or "now that you have clarified your proposal its faults are more apparent." Ask an independent, unbiased colleague to read the reviews of the original and revised proposals to determine what the reviewers are actually about. Then, with this in mind, revise it again.

16

Competing Renewal of R01 Projects (Progress Reports)

A competing renewal proposal is essentially the same as a new proposal plus a Progress Report in Section *c* of the Research Plan. We prefer to find the Progress Report presented as section *c.1,* before the Preliminary Studies *(c.2)* The report must begin with a statement of the years of the award and the years covered by the report. They will not be the same. Then the previous Specific Aims should be listed verbatim. The best evidence of progress is the statement, "This aim was completed. See references 1,2,3," or "see appendix manuscript 1." If a manuscript or reprint is not available, essential data should be presented. However, space is at a premium. New data supporting the new Specific Aims must be presented as a narrative after this section, which should probably be limited to about eight pages. If you must fill it up with data pertaining to the old grant, you are in trouble. An account must be given of progress on each of the aims. If there has been no progress, this must be explained briefly. Since the renewal precedes the end of the grant period by about a year, the best explanation is that the work is "in progress." Other acceptable reasons are that "the work was published by someone else"; "an essential reagent is no longer available"; or "completed studies render the additional work unnecessary." If the work was abandoned because of technical reasons, or a change in research direction, these must be explained fully.

A Progress Narrative should follow this brief review of progress for each Specific Aim. This will briefly summarize the important findings in publications to be found in the appendix and unpublished data. Publications and accepted manuscripts are then listed. Any publication or manuscript listed here must be included in the appendix. To fail to do this is to invite criticism of your credibility. Manuscripts must be publication quality in every respect. If you exceed the limit of 10 appended papers, list all you wish here, select the 10 strongest or most pertinent to your new aims for inclusion in the appendix, and mark them here with an asterisk to indicate they are included in the appendix.

A *strong competing renewal application* presents a research plan that is a logical extension of the current project. It is within the PI's expertise, and is likely to succeed; it breaks new ground, uses new procedures, and tests new hypotheses; it describes a productive period of research and solid publications in the Progress Report; and it proposes continued work in an area that is still of interest and important. Such a proposal has a high likelihood of funding. All the preceding comments about new R01 proposals apply to competing renewal proposals.

The ideal of a *continuing project* is often difficult to achieve. Research goals change; the title of the previous grant may no longer be appropriate. However, changes in title may be made without losing revised status. The best evidence of the success of the past project period is that the research is worth continuing at more fundamental levels. If the long-term goals of the project are unchanged, the renewal proposal should be presented as the logical next step. This is best accomplished if the theoretical model on which the previous proposal was based is essentially unchanged, or the new experiments clearly represent progress in evolution of the model. Thus, new hypotheses are essential. The progression often seen is from studies of cell biology to cell molecular biology. Some studies progress from experiments on the efficacy of a drug to effect a pathogenic process, to experiments on the mechanism of action of the drug. Others might progress from studies of prevention of stent fibrosis to experiments testing hypotheses about intracellular pathways upon which fibrosis is dependent. However, studies that only add yet another growth factor, cytokine, or drug to a long list of older agents, for no other reason than that they are new, are doomed to be weak.

EXPERTISE

Technology seems to be advancing at an ever-increasing rate. It is likely that there are new and more powerful procedures available now that were unavailable 4–5 years ago, when the original proposal was funded. Some of your competitors will be using these new experimental tools. A good example is the widespread availability of specific immunohistochemical agents. Studies using these reagents are best done by confocal microscopy. Failure to use this equipment will probably adversely affect the review. On the other hand, you may not have publications showing this new expertise. If there is a large change in the expertise required for completion of the proposed studies, it must be demonstrated with publications or with data in the Preliminary Data section that you are expert in the new area or have established a collaboration that will provide the needed expertise. The strongest and most interesting proposals will be those ably using the latest technology to test new, more fundamental hypotheses. If a renewal proposal has no need for new techniques, the research is obviously "more of the same," and this is almost the worst thing that can be said of a competing renewal.

PROBABILITY OF SUCCESS

Probability of success is evaluated largely on the basis of past productivity. Productivity of the previous research period will be judged primarily on the basis of peer review publications; the minimum is one per year per investigator. Chapters in books, review articles, and abstracts from meetings rarely provide support for a claim of progress, and may actually be detrimental if their addition appears to represent padding. In listing publications and manuscripts, explanatory notes should be added if there could be a perception that the work they represent was done before the start of the previous grant, or was supported by another grant. It is not uncommon for a new investigator to publish work done in a mentor's laboratory after assuming a new position supported by a new grant. At renewal time it is reasoned that these papers were prepared while the PI was supported by the new grant and can therefore be claimed as a product of it. This is beneficial if the subject matter and methodology are related to the grant, providing it is explained that the research was not supported by the grant. To be less open than this is to risk being considered not quite honest. Work that is done in other laboratories provides less support for a competing renewal than does work done in the PI's own laboratory.

Most investigators believe that their work is in an important area. This belief may be more reflex than considered. An independent appraisal of an area of research can be obtained from the appropriate NIH Institute Program Director with nothing more complicated than a telephone call, yet it is rarely sought. For instance, the neuroanatomist who traces brain paths with silver stains for degenerating fibers would be told very clearly that the state-of-the-art is now the use of tracers and that these should be incorporated into the experimental design. Competing renewals should make every attempt to include the newer procedures used by peers in the field. The pathologist who studies cell infiltration in an experimental model cannot get away with calling the cells a "round cell infiltrate" anymore, but must identify them with specific cell markers. A competing renewal proposal will receive a searching analysis to determine if it represents the latest in research strategies. If it does not, this is considered a weakness unless it is adequately justified. Previous successes will not overcome criticism leveled at poorly thought-out experiments. Intellectual sloth will turn off the reviewer of a competing renewal just as effectively as the reviewer of a new proposal.

It is sometimes necessary to leave a project because advances in the field have so outdistanced it that the research is no longer very interesting. It is not good grantsmanship to beat a dead project. It should be left in peace, and new horizons sought. Ogden's research in the early 1960s involved studies of the electroretinogram using extracellular, intraretinal microelectrodes. This was state-of-the-art compared with the work of the 1950s, which involved whole eye recordings, but was soon surpassed by studies that involved intracellular recording. Continued funding required use of the newer technology as it evolved. The problem is particularly pervasive in this modern age of molecular biology. Well-established investigators using older technology find it difficult to compete with peers testing hypotheses about molecular mechanisms or using tools based on genetic engineering.

Institute priorities change gradually over the years. Prospects for funding are better for those projects that are considered of high program relevance. This information is also best obtained from the appropriate Institute Program Director. Interest in the proposed new research will be based largely on the nature of the hypotheses to be tested. If these are new and imaginative, but are not excessively controversial, interest will be high and the work will be perceived as an advance of the field. If it appears that the PI's thinking about the problem has not progressed much over the years, particularly if peers are testing new hypotheses, interest in the renewal will be low.

Continued research in a field of study is certainly warranted if past research has been successful. The strongest evidence of success is impact on the field of study. Every effort should be made to cite instances in which past data have led to altered treatment, new hypotheses, better procedures, new concepts, new research by others, etc. It should be stated explicitly, if reasonable and exemplified, that the proposed research will impact the field of study.

Some of the competing renewals reviewed by a Study Section have a productivity problem. This is sometimes dealt with by creative grantsmanship, which, if obvious, can be more detrimental than the more direct approach of simply stating what the problems were, and how they will be circumvented in the future. As will be discussed below, a severe productivity problem cannot be circumvented, and should lead the PI to consider submission of a new proposal rather than a competing renewal.

To renew or not to renew is a strategy decision that should be based on past productivity and the desired direction of future research. Not many projects are dropped simply because research interests have changed. Many are dropped, and many more should be dropped because of poor productivity. It is bad grantsmanship to force new research into the rigid mold of an existing grant, just to avoid a new proposal. Only if the fit is comfortable should the existing grant be continued. A proposal made awkward by adherence to outdated hypotheses will lose priority points far in excess of the advantage it has by being a competing renewal. It is particularly unfortunate to attempt to resuscitate an unproductive project.

Accountability in research funding and productivity really only happens in the renewal process. It can be avoided to a degree by submitting a new proposal, rather than a competing renewal. The reviewers are not given detailed material relating to currently funded projects of an investigator when they review a new proposal, unless they specifically request it, and this rarely happens. Thus the reviewers have no way of evaluating the productivity of these grants except by looking at the Biosketch. Embarrassing questions are best avoided, and if a project has been unproductive, this can be achieved through submitting a new proposal. Reasons for lack of productivity are legion; none are fully adequate to overcome the stigma attached to lack of success. A new investigator who has recently moved to a new location, where it has been necessary to set up a new facility, may be forgiven some lack of progress, but the investigator will still suffer some loss of priority points because most of the competition will show good productivity. Since productivity is generally evaluated in terms of the previous Specific Aims, a substantial midstream change in research direction gives the appearance of low productivity. Unfulfilled Specific Aims must be addressed in the Progress Report. Even if the project was productive, and although this report of lack of success or changed direction will cost some points, the problem must be addressed. Unless there is confidence that the reviewers will accept the changes as beneficial, it may be cost effective to submit a new proposal rather than defend a failure to achieve the old Specific Aims.

The success rate for competing renewal R01 proposals in 2000 was almost double that for new proposals (50 and 26%, respectively). A major cause of this difference, of course, is that beginners form a large part of the latter group. Competing renewals have a definite funding advantage over new proposals with about the same percentile rank; the Institutes find it difficult to close down projects that may well be funded in a later cycle with an amended proposal. The necessity for revision is becoming very common; 42% of new R01 proposals and 35% of competing renewals actually funded in 2000 were revised. Revised proposals usually receive an improved priority score and have substantially improved success rates (see Chapter 15). All of these factors must be weighed in deciding whether to submit a competing renewal or a new grant. The stronger alternative should be chosen.

The renewal process should start at least 12 months before the deadline, which itself is nearly 12 months before the anniversary date of the grant. This long lead time is essential to permit pilot data to be gathered as the new research plan is developed. When it is decided to renew, pending manuscripts must be scheduled for completion. To send along a poorly written manuscript in the appendix, representing it as accepted for publication, could easily destroy chances for funding. Even worse, a reviewer who may have been asked by the journal to edit a manuscript will resent finding, in the appendix, a manuscript that it is known has not been accepted for publication. A complaint will appear in the review. Reviewers are more impressed by papers that have already succeeded in peer review.

New Specific Aims must be identified, although the long-term goals of a competing renewal proposal will hopefully be unchanged. *The short-term goals should not include any previous Specific Aims.* If a previous Specific Aim must be included in the renewal, there must be a detailed explanation of the delay in getting to it and a strong rationale must be given as to why the aim is still important. Care must be taken to provide an explanation that does not weaken the proposal. The previous proposal was too ambitious, the work was too difficult, unforeseen problems arose, subjects were not available, etc., are the usual reasons for lack of success, and each implies inexperience or incompetence on the part of the PI. Acceptable excuses are that certain experiments had to be dropped because of cuts in funds or that the experiments are in progress and will be completed by the end of the grant period. If an aim was dropped for scientifically sound reasons, such as an exciting new avenue of research, a detailed explanation must be provided and there must be complete confidence that it will be accepted. This is a judgment that must be unbiased, and that many investigators find difficult to make. We recall a grant for research involving a clinical study on a large number of rhesus monkeys. After funding, primate research abruptly became socially questionable and very expensive, and molecular-level research became fashionable. The competing renewal attributed the decision to drop the primate experiments (two of four Specific Aims) because of their cost and for reasons of conservation. This was accepted by the Study Section, which gave the renewal a fundable priority score.

New goals or Specific Aims represent the testing of new hypotheses. In the strongest projects, a theoretical model is presented at the outset that provides the foundation for the new hypotheses. It is more common for the new hypotheses to be suggested by recent work in the field, hopefully some of it by the PI. The identification of new testable hypotheses is critical to development of a successful competing renewal. Most investigators consider their research as their private domain and have a tendency to guard it jealously. This attitude has become even more prevalent as a result of the growing competition for funds. Research proposals, however, are strengthened by knowledgeable input from experts. The broader this input, the better the proposal is likely to be. In the best of worlds, a panel of experts should be convened to assist with this process. If it is not possible to meet in person, a conference call may serve the same purpose. The experts should be given a copy of the old proposal and a summary of progress and asked to evaluate progress and the suggested new aims.

Papers and proposals are essential elements in the life of a scientist. These should be complementary products started at the beginning of a project and virtually complete as the project nears completion. Writing is an activity that really does become easier with practice; it should be a part of every scientist's week. If this lifestyle is practiced, very little additional effort will be required to generate manuscripts and the occasional proposal on schedule.

PLAN TO REVISE

In 2000, only about half of competing renewals achieved funding with the first submission. This fact has important implications for every NIH-supported researcher. Plans for interim funding are essential, and funding from at least two staggered grants is highly desirable. When a proposal is not funded it can be resubmitted as an "amended" proposal. These resubmissions are becoming so common that they constitute the bulk of work in some Study Sections. Probability of funding is increased with resubmission, because the investigator has the advantage of past Study Section comments. The award rates for competing renewals of R01s in 2000 were as follows: initial, 51%; first revision, 48%; and second revision, 51%. Obviously it is wise to plan on resubmission and start the process of rewriting at the time of initial submission (see Chapter 15). It is also wise to start the renewal process at least one cycle early so that funding will be minimally interrupted if it becomes necessary to submit an amended proposal.

DIVERSITY

Ethnic and gender diversity have recently been added as yet another PHS 398 reporting requirement. If the prior grant involved *human subjects,* then you must also report on the enrollment of women and men, and on the race and ethnicity of research subjects. The PHS 398 form now provides a "Targeted/Planned Enrollment Format Page" to report this information for each relevant funded study (and for each relevant study that will be continued). These tables do not count toward the 25-page limitation.

17

Proposal Submission and Supplementary Materials

SUBMISSION DATES

Dates for submission are published on the Internet and in a table on page 31 in the PHS 398 packet. New R01 proposals are to be *postmarked* no later than February 1, June 1, or October 1. Competing renewal proposals are due 1 month later. Grant applications submitted in response to a Request for Application (RFA) must be *received* at the NIH by the date specified. Contract proposals in response to a Request for Proposal (RFP) must be *logged in* at the appropriate NIH desk by a specific hour on a specific day. It is suggested in the PHS 398 application directions that the submitted proposal carry a post office date no later than 1 week prior to the stated deadline. We strongly recommend use of an express delivery service with guaranteed delivery and dated receipt, even when it is not necessary from the standpoint of time. This admittedly reflects a bias based on some bad experiences with U.S. mail service.

Please do not accept these dates as your personal deadlines. Have your completed proposal ready at least 1 and preferably 2 months earlier. This will give you time for a knowledgeable review, and last minute editing, without which your proposal will simply not be your best effort.

GENERAL APPEARANCE

Neatness gets a better priority score than does godliness in grantsmanship. The standard of the finished proposals now submitted is very high. Today it is unusual to find a proposal prepared on a typewriter. The current high standard is made possible by the widespread use of word processors with spell checkers, which have virtually eliminated casual typos. Fonts of many sizes and styles are available. Laser printers may be purchased for less than $500 and letter-quality color printers are universal and much less expensive. The end product, both text and figures, should be textbook quality. Anything less will stand out from its fellows as below average in quality, and perhaps give a bad initial impression to the reviewers.

The instructions request that the "original" and six exact copies be submitted. These should be clean photocopies, printed on one side only. It is requested that the proposal is single-spaced, but we much prefer to use 1.2 spaces between lines for greater readability. This will not be questioned; it will slightly reduce the proposal content within the page limitation. But greater readability is always better than more words! *The use of italics and underlining impairs readability,* particularly if it is done to the extreme. **We prefer the use of boldface type for emphasis.** As in all things, moderation is indicated in the use of emphasis, lest the reviewer feel lectured. Inappropriate use of emphasis may give the impression of condescension. The "original" will be photocopied by the Center for Scientific Review and these two-sided copies will be given to the Study Section staff who will distribute them to the nonassigned members of the section, without appendix material. The assigned members will receive one of the six copies originally submitted along with its appendix material.

Illustrations should be line drawings if possible, since these will copy well. Halftone and color prints should be scanned into a computer and printed on single-weight 8.5 by 11-inch photographic-quality paper. Two or three of the six copies of the proposal submitted will be given to the assigned reviewers; all six, including the original, must be prepared with equal care. The advent of the color photocopy machine has revolutionized the presentation of preliminary data. These machines copy black and white, color, and halftone photographs with excellent fidelity and provide a final copy that is much superior to pasting photographs on pages, besides being more convenient. The copies are expensive, but it is a good investment and provides a very professional looking document. Electron micrographs, photomicrographs, and fluorescence micrographs reproduce very well with this method (see Appendix C).

Do not submit photocopied parts, such as Biosketches, of past proposals unless the part exactly matches the submitted proposal. It is not uncommon to see poorly copied Biosketches, particularly from Co-Investigators. This suggests a "quick-fix" of material that is probably out of date. It indicates either staff support insufficient to enter an updated Biosketch or poor communication with the collaborator. This may leave a bad impression concerning the productivity of the proposed collaboration.

The length of the proposal must comply with the page requirements, and the appendix material should add a minimum of bulk to the package. Each proposal copy should be bundled with the appropriate appendix material, using a rubber band. Do not staple it to original. Send actual reprints rather than photocopies, if they are available. This is particularly important if the reprint contains halftone photographs, such as electron micrographs. It is very wise to hold back an ample supply of reprints of every paper supported by a research grant to provide for the necessity of submitting reprints to the NIH. Their availability could make the difference between being funded and not being funded.

DEADLINES

Deadlines are taken seriously by the staff of the CSR, but can be extended. Each cycle thousands of unsolicited R01 proposals arrive at the CSR and are stored in a large room. They are moved out to the respective Study Section SRAs on a first-in, first-out basis following the deadline—a process that takes several weeks. Thus, it does not impair the system for a proposal to be a week or two late. A call to the CSR official responsible for assignment should be made to explain what has delayed completion of the application (a computer virus, a crashed hard disk, etc.). This will elicit the advice to go ahead and submit it late and that it will probably be accepted, but that no promises will be made. A covering letter to explain the delay should accompany the application. Within these limits, it will, in all probability (but without guarantees), be accepted. Ogden remembers with chagrin a Core Center competing renewal proposal he submitted without a last minute check. The printout computer became infected with a virus, unbeknown to its operator. The virus deleted every other paragraph! The proposal was wonderfully short, but useless. An appeal was made to the CSR and we were permitted to submit a whole new packet, 10 days late.

However in the case of R01 proposals submitted in response to an RFA, Center grants, and Training grants, review is by Institute, rather than by the CSR, although the proposals are still mailed to the CSR. In these cases, the PHS 398 instructions state,

Solicited applications must be received by the specified dates. However, an application received after the deadline may be acceptable if it carries a legible proof-of-mailing date, assigned by the carrier, and the proof-of-mailing date is not later than 1 week prior to the deadline date. These include request for applications (RFAs) and program announcements (PAs) with specified receipt dates. [Emphasis removed]

Any deadline extension must be negotiated with the Institute Program Director or official responsible for the review.

Last minute submissions seem to be the rule in most institutions. These always result in hurried proofing and errors. Budgetary errors can often be corrected, with permission from the SRA of the Study Section, simply by submitting a revised budget. Extensive revisions of a proposal are not usually allowed, but submission of last minute data and recently accepted manuscripts, as addenda, is permitted by most Study Sections. Some limit such addenda to a single page, but most will accept anything that is "reasonable." Some reviewers resent these additions, so it is important to keep them as brief as possible, preferably a single page plus two to three illustrations or tables containing data that are absolutely essential for the review. If a new (pertinent) manuscript has been submitted for publication in the interim, this should also be sent in with the supplement together with any acceptance letters for manuscripts that were submitted with the proposal. Note, however, that the appendix is limited to 10 items. If you submitted 10 manuscripts with the proposal, you should not use the supplementary submission to exceed the limit.

SUPPLEMENTARY MATERIAL

Supplementary material such as budget revisions and proposal addenda should be sent to the Study Section SRA, not to the CSR. The SRA should first be contacted by telephone or e-mail to determine that the proposed date of addenda submission and their character will be acceptable. This deadline is real. Generally, material arriving after the proposals are mailed to the reviewers will not be forwarded to them, although it may be presented to them at the meeting. Even if it is seen at the meeting, it will probably have little impact on the written review, which the reviewers will have previously prepared. Danger—supplementary material extends the length of the proposal beyond the specified limit of 25 pages. Be brief! On balance, we have more sympathy for the problems of the overworked reviewer who refuses to read more than one page of addendum than we have for the complaint of some applicants: "they didn't read my addendum!" The submission of supplementary material, providing it is pertinent and of high quality, probably carries no risk and often strengthens a proposal. It demonstrates continued progress and dedication to the project, which can be important, particularly for previously unfunded studies. As with all submissions to the NIH, the material submitted as addenda must be as near to publication quality as possible. There is a tendency for some to submit hand-drawn graphs and rough tables in addenda. This may be as damaging to an application as the submission of such material with the original proposal.

18

Your First Grant Award
(R, F, or K)

In Chapter 4 we noted that new investigators are often undecided about which of the several NIH grant programs is appropriate for their initial request for funds, and we concluded that the R01 should be used by virtually all qualified investigators, that is, anyone who is (1) overqualified for a postdoctoral fellowship and who also has (2) an independent academic or research position. We stand by this advice because the R01 has become the accepted gold standard by which the independence of an academic researcher is judged.

However, it is hard for a recent Ph.D. to prove that he or she is an independent scientist without first completing a period of additional postdoctoral training. Similarly, it is hard to accept as independent scientists M.D.s who had limited research exposure, even if they have completed a research fellowship in their clinical specialty. Fortunately, the NIH has grant award mechanisms to assist such individuals as they make the transition to independence under the guidance of a research mentor. These are listed in Table 18.2. All of these awards are available only to U.S. citizens or foreign nationals with permanent resident status.

For the Ph.D.s, there are individual postdoctoral fellowship (F32) awards. For the M.D.s and other individuals with clinical professional degrees, there are two types of special awards, the Mentored Clinical Scientist Research Award (K08) and the Mentored Patient-Oriented Research Development Award (K23). People who have clinical degrees may also apply for the F32 awards, but the allowable "salaries" of the K awards are based directly on institutional pay scales and may be more than double the F32 "stipends" (see Table 18.1). The other K awards listed in Table 18.2 are for more senior investigators. An exception is the K01 Mentored Research Scientist Development Award, which is used by

Table 18.1 *National Research Service Awards (NRSAs) Stipends—Fiscal Year 2001*

Level	Stipend ($)
All predoctoral	16,500
Years of postdoctoral experience	
<1	28,260
1	29,832
2	35,196
3	36,996
4	38,772
5	40,560
6	42,348
7+	44,412

some NIH Institutes to attract young Ph.D.s from specific, desired disciplines to work on research topics of special interest that require new approaches. For example, the NIMH has used K01 awards to attract young scientists to bring new methods from other fields to the study of child and adolescent neuropsychiatric disorders.

Table 18.2 *NIH Postdoctoral Training and Career Development Programs*

National Research Service Awards (NRSAs)
- T32, Institutional Research Training Grants
- F32, Individual Fellowships

Career Development Awards (K series)
- Mentored Research Scientist Development Award (K01)
- Independent Scientist Award (K02)
- Senior Scientist Award (K05)
- Academic Career Award (K07)
- Mentored Clinical Scientist Development Award (K08)
- Mentored Clinical Scientist Development Program Award (K12)
- Mentored Patient-Oriented Research Development Award (K23)
- Mid-Career Investigator Award in Patient-Oriented Research (K24)

Administrative supplements to R01 and other research grants
- Individuals from underrepresented minority groups
- Individuals with disabilities
- Individuals reentering science after a career hiatus

POSTDOCTORAL TRAINING

There are, actually, two types of NIH postdoctoral training awards: the T32 grants to institutions and the F32 awards to individual trainees. Both types of awards are offered by all NIH Institutes except the National Library of Medicine. They are both called National Research Service Awards (NRSAs) because, during the early years of the program, the fellows had to repay the award by working in research in the health sciences profession for an equal period after completion of training. The rules changed in 1993; now payback pertains only to the first year of postdoctoral training and may be accomplished during the second year of the award (some very clever NIH administrators are to be congratulated for easing this burden on young scientists). T32 Training grants are made to universities or departments in universities that, in turn, select suitable candidates for the awards. The T32 proposal is discussed in greater detail in Chapter 24.

Securing an F32 individual postdoctoral fellowship award is much more desirable than appointment to a T32 program for establishing your independence; you must write a full grant proposal and successfully compete against your colleagues in a review that is conducted by one of the Fellowship Study Sections in the Center for Scientific Review. The F32 award provides a stipend ($28,260 in FY 2001) that increases with the number of years of postdoctoral research experience. The award also includes limited funds for tuition, health insurance, and research supplies. Fortunately, it can be supplemented with funds from other sources, as long as there are no strings attached that would interfere with full-time research training.

Awards to fellows for postdoctoral support are limited to a total of 3 years. Longer periods of training can be obtained with permission from the awarding Institute. In FY 2000, the NIH supported 773 Ph.D.s and 77 M.D.s with F32 awards. The success rate for M.D. applicants was 47.5%, and for Ph.D.s, 45.4%.

The Mentored Career Development Awards, in contrast, are limited to 5 years (but may be funded for only 3 or 4). At least 75% of your full-time effort (80%, 90%, or more is preferred) must be devoted to research and research training during this entire period. You must have full-time faculty status and the award reimburses your salary and fringe benefits. A K award typically includes $25,000 or more for research and training expenses.

There is some confusion as to who should apply for each type of award. In general, we advise clinician-scientists who desire to conduct fundamental bench research under the mentoring of a basic scientist to apply for the K08, and clinician-scientists who desire to conduct patient-oriented research under the mentoring of a clinician, epidemiologist, or biostatistician to apply for the K23. However, some of the Institutes have more specific guidelines, so it is wise to check with the appropriate Institute Program Director before applying. The bottom line is that both types of proposals are reviewed by the same Institute-based Study Sections and compete against each other. In FY 2000, the success rates were 50% for both programs.

FORMS

The mentored K proposal uses the PHS 398 application form with special attention to the Additional Instructions under Section IV of the PHS 398 booklet. In addition to the usual requirements of an R01 proposal, these require letters of reference and specialized information about your research background, scientific career goals, and proposed career development and training activities during the award period. Statements and letters from the sponsor, other mentors, and collaborators are a crucial component of these applications (see Table 18.3). The proposal must in-

Table 18.3 *Tips on Preparing a Postdoctoral Training or Career Development Proposal*

More of the same does not work
- You have to go someplace else
- You must propose to learn, and to do, something more

Identify potential preceptors
- Do this early
- Meet with and discuss *your* goals
- Write and submit your proposal before you move (even if you are still writing your thesis)—do not wait until you get to your new institution

The success of your proposal depends on *all* of the following four major components (listed in order of importance):
1. Your preceptor (training experience, research)
2. You (scientific career plans, accomplishments, transcripts, reference letters)
3. Your training plan
4. Your research plan

clude a letter of agreement and institutional commitment from the Dean or Department Chair which certifies that you will be released from all other duties, explains how that will be accomplished, and attests to the institution's commitment to you and to the development of your research career. These proposals are reviewed by Institute-based Study Sections.

The F32 proposal uses the PHS 416-1 application packet. This can be obtained from the Office of Contracts and Grants of your university, or from the NIH web site (<http://grants.nih.gov/grants/forms.htm>).

Space limitations are severe and enforced. You must keep your responses to many of the items within the spaces allotted. It is not uncommon to see F32 proposals that almost certainly were written largely by the sponsor, despite the remonstration that the application is to be written by the applicant. These generally are professional and do well in review, if the sponsor's addition is not too flagrant. They show an active interest of the sponsor in the candidate, and bode well for successful training. It is also common to see proposals from candidates who apparently have talked with their preceptor only very briefly, and really understand very little about the project or the laboratory in which they hope to work. This is probably not the candidate's fault, but it is a bad sign and the result is a loss of priority points. Some sponsors have too many fellows and provide very little assistance to them. If they are good enough to get the fellowship, they are accepted into the laboratory.

Section 30b is the Research Training Plan. *It is limited to 10 pages.* This part of the F32 proposal is a short version of an R01. To be successful, it needs a clearly stated Specific Aims section that identifies an important hypothesis (1 page maximum), a succinct Background section that is rather more of a review than is usually seen in an R01 (3 pages maximum), and a brief Design and Methods section (5 pages maximum). The 10th page is enough for the essential references. There is a tendency to propose far more work than is possible. Keep it sharply focused. Test a single hypothesis, but make the test definitive. The work should include technology or aspects that are new to you, in which you will be trained.

Section 30d concerns selection of your sponsor. You make this selection because your career goals require training and experience in a new area that extends your doctoral training. Your proposed sponsor is a recognized, respected senior investigator in this new area. You have a problem if this Great Person is in your own institution, or if you have had a previous association. The fellowship is designed to broaden your training. It is unlikely that this broadening will be successful if you stay at home. You must be very persuasive if that is what you propose, for you must overcome this weakness. This is a common problem of fellowship proposals, usually dictated by family obligations and a tendency we all have to be more comfortable with the familiar. However, it is far better to transfer to an institution across town if this is at all possible and there is a suitable sponsor. It may be possible to develop a relationship with the Great Person as a collaboration. Just do not mention it in the proposal.

SUCCESSFUL PROPOSALS

The success of a proposal for an F32 or K award is based largely on the background of the candidate and the past success of the preceptor. Previous papers or at least some experience in a laboratory in addition to the graduate training is helpful to the candidate. Applicants are probably turned down more often on the basis of an inappropriate sponsor than because they themselves are poorly prepared.

The immediate postdoctoral research years are far and away the most important part of the training of most young investigators and in preparing the way for a successful career. The sponsor must be selected with great care; a mistake can literally ruin a promising career. A candidate should never go into a laboratory without first talking to past fellows and reviewing their publications. A laboratory without successful past fellows should be avoided (see Chapter 19). The experience of the sponsor is a vital criterion for selection. The sponsor should have stable research support in the form of an R01 that was recently successful in competitive review. Young sponsors, probably assistant professors, should be avoided, unless they have a very strong Biosketch. Make sure that their recent papers do not list them as first author. This is a position you want for yourself. The sponsor should be sufficiently established that first authorship of papers is routinely given to fellows. *If you do not complete your fellowship with at least two papers as FIRST AUTHOR, or your K award with at least four or five, you probably will have trouble getting your own grant support.*

Since your relationship with your mentor will determine the success of your fellowship, every effort should be made to meet and talk with this person before you make the commitment. A visit to the laboratory will provide insight as to the technical help that will be available and provide the opportunity to talk with other fellows. Find out who actually runs the laboratory, what services you will be expected to provide, and how productive the group is. Think twice about joining a laboratory where you will be the only fellow.

An F32, K08, or K23 application requires a *statement from the mentor* about plans for your training. This must be carefully written to indicate actual training in new procedures. It must be obvious that you will be more than a technician working on the mentor's projects. Details of training in the ethics of use of animals, human subjects, hazardous agents, etc., must be included.

SUBMISSION DEADLINES

Submission deadlines for the mentored K proposals are the same as for R01s. F32 proposal deadlines are different: April 5, August 5, and December 5 are the submission dates, with prospective funding the following September, January, and May. Like the R01, you can submit supplementary material after the submission date, providing you receive permission from the Study Section SRA. You will be notified which Study Section will review the proposal and which Institute might fund it.

=====19=====
Advice for Beginners in Academia

This chapter is written for the young investigator finishing postdoctoral fellowship training and about to seek a first appointment, quite possibly involving a change of university. It is amazing that in an age of communication, so many young scientists should be so naive about the hard facts of life of their chosen careers. Serious mistakes are common, and these can blight a promising research career.

PUBLISH OR PERISH

Researchers, for whom this book was written, are judged by their peers on the basis of the quantity and quality of their publications. An unproductive scientist will fail just as quickly at Harvard as at a small state college. A productive scientist will be just as successful at both places. But if the small state college offers better conditions than does the Ivy League school, it should be the preferred choice. The better conditions might translate into more rapid, higher productivity, and more rapid success in obtaining grant funds. Very often, eminent universities trade on their established names to attract young talent, which they promptly abandon to sink or swim. Those who sink due to lack of seed funds, laboratory space, equipment, or staff support may have their careers severely damaged by the experience. Be assured that the eminent university name will be of precious little help in securing grant support. It may actually be a detriment if their cavalier attitudes about young faculty are well known.

The *ideal university job* is one in an established department comprising some well-known investigators, most of whom currently hold NIH grants. There should be an obvious place for your particular contribution to the function of the department. It is essential that there be kindred spirits in the group, either scientifically or socially, and hopefully both. The department should be willing to provide whatever is necessary to quickly bring your research to productivity. Your new colleagues should be sufficiently ego-secure that they will not be threatened by your success. Your start-up requirements will certainly involve substantial seed money for equipment, supplies, and a technician for at least 2 and hopefully for 3 years. Your first NIH grant may be able to provide some equipment purchases, but any equipment request larger than about one module ($25,000) will initiate discussion and may weaken your proposal; it certainly will not strengthen it. This ideal job will also provide a minimum but adequate amount of space—not shared, but assigned to you—and a promise of more space if you get funded. Finally, there should be a minimum of teaching or clinical responsibility in your first year.

Move if You Possibly Can

Most young graduates tend to hold on to their alma mater. But unless highly sought-after superstars, their careers will surely suffer if they do not move. It is true in science, as elsewhere, that familiarity breeds contempt. Homegrown scientists often lack the clout to negotiate adequate salaries, seed money, or space in their own institution. Their desire to stay where they are weakens their bargaining position. They hover for a few years in the shadows of their mentors, existing on crumbs of collaboration. They may eventually be forced to leave to gain real independence. These arrangements may actually lengthen the curriculum vitae (CV), but unless there is the opportunity for mostly first-authored papers, this may not compensate for inadequate support. A tragedy follows when the young scientist's first NIH grant application, based on the mentor's collaboration, fails to be funded. A greater tragedy occurs when the first renewal comes due, but the mentor no longer feels responsible, and the investigator simply does not have the wherewithal to be productive.

Clout is the name of the game. When you change universities, it should be to your advantage. As they attempt to recruit you, they must meet your demands or you will go elsewhere. If you do not have that kind of clout, you have chosen the wrong institution.

A Research Scientist Requires Funds

To get funds, there must be a reasonable promise of success. For a new investigator, this is provided by pilot data. Your new laboratory must produce such data of high quality as quickly as possible to support your first independent proposal. Time is of the essence! Acquire (begging or borrowing as necessary) what you need to get into production quickly. If it is at all possible, produce some good pilot data during the last year of your fellowship training, so that you are in a position to immediately submit your first proposal. If it takes 6 months to get your laboratory running (an optimistic estimate) and 3 months to collect pilot data, the earliest you might expect NIH funding is 18 months along the time line, so you will need seed money for 2 years of research support in these circumstances. Since most proposals are simply not funded on the first submission, 3 years of seed support from the institution is not unrealistic if they really are committed to fostering your success.

A note from the chapter on Biosketches is worth repeating. It is bad planning to allow gaps to occur in your Biosketch. Fellowships often end with incomplete projects. They must be written up and submitted for publication without delay. If additional experiments are required and the work is not part of your major goals, it may be best to shelve it. Do not spend time completing a project if it will delay setting up your lab for your own work. If productivity in your own laboratory is delayed, your CV will reflect this unless you actively collaborate with your new peers. As long as it does not interfere with your own work, collaboration is a wonderful way to make friends and bolster the CV. It may be both informative and helpful to seek these collaborations outside your new department, taking advantage of what temporary freedom you may have from departmental politics.

The Job Offer

Scientists are usually not good business people. They are more comfortable concluding agreements with a handshake. But jobs are business. You must get a written offer listing everything you require from the university and what that institution requires from you. These offers always state academic rank and salary, but may otherwise be brief. Be sure that the words "tenure-track" appear in the offer, if appropriate. Terms like "research" and "clinical" are pejorative at some institutions; be sure you understand the connotations of their use at yours. Also, get a statement concerning how long you will be supported in the event that you fail to get, or lose, research funding.

If teaching is involved, have specific course numbers listed and a statement that you will not be required to teach more than x contact hours per semester or year. You should also get a commitment for complete freedom to do research x months of the year if this is appropriate. Beware! It is not realistic to think you can do research only during the summer months and remain competitive with full-time investigators for funds.

The job offer should also include statements concerning space. "Four hundred square feet in the Jones Building" is acceptable, but "room 303 in the Jones Building" is better. During the job interview, you must ask to see the space you will occupy. If that is impossible, you better look somewhere else. A minimum of 100 square feet for an office and 400 square feet of lab space is required for most basic science projects, and an average beginner generally gets about 600 square feet. Clinicians who expect to do some laboratory research absolutely must have a technician committed to their projects, on at least a part-time basis. They must also hold out for dedicated laboratory space, and some operating funds. The beginning clinician-researcher has a particularly difficult problem in obtaining research funds from the NIH, and needs at least 3 years of secure funding from the institution.

Temporary space in someone's laboratory is a very poor offer unless you are shown your own space under construction. These arrangements are common in older departments. They require setting up labs twice, and at best may cause delayed productivity. At worst, the "temporary" arrangement may turn out to be permanent.

Salary is often not very negotiable unless you are a clinical superstar. Levels are set by university standards and can usually be shifted only a few thousand dollars. Salary overlap and moving funds are a different matter, and should be sought. It should be possible to have your salary start 1 to 2 months before you arrive at your new location. Some universities will also pay for moving expenses. If you are moving into an impacted area like Los Angeles, where housing expenses are very high, low-interest loans may also be available from the university.

Certain equipment is essential to every kind of research. Do not be greedy, but be firm. If the standard of your new department is to use a shared scintillation counter in a Core facility, do not demand your own, even if it would be more convenient. Ask for those items used daily in your current laboratory. List them by name, model, make, and price. Then insist that your offer letter include the items on your list. If you can use equipment in a colleague's laboratory, and you know that it is available from personal conversation with that colleague, have a statement to that effect included in the job offer. Do not neglect small items like disposable glassware, magnetic stirrers, hot plates, balances, distilled water filters if necessary, fume hoods, incubators, computers (both scientific and word processing), printers (demand a laser printer), software, laboratory and office furniture and file cabinets, dark room equipment, microscopes, histology equipment, etc.

In order to provide a proper list of equipment that will not outrage your less fortunate future colleagues who quite likely have trouble getting light bulbs, you must be familiar with how they operate. If they share a communal darkroom, you should use it also unless your use will clearly exceed its capacity. Sometimes you can cement a new relationship by finding what new equipment your colleagues need and then requesting it as if you required it. This obviously must be handled with circumspection. It is inevitable that the "have-nots" among the existing faculty will be envious and perhaps resentful of your temporary clout, and a certain amount of sensitivity to their feelings may help smooth your settling in.

The written job offer is your only hope of recompense in the case of massive malfeasance on the part of the department or university. This is a serious matter. We know of a young scientist hired shortly before his new department chairman was fired. The replacement chairman restructured the department, taking most of the young man's space. Because he had specifics in his written job offer, he was able to force the institution into a substantial financial settlement as compensation for the clear damage to his finances, his career, and the cross-country displacement of his family.

The pitfalls to be avoided are the opposites of the above requirements:

- Inadequate space
- Inadequate equipment
- Inadequate seed money
- Inadequate staff support
- Excessive teaching or clinic load
- Improper balance of salary and expenses

- An unstable department
- An unhappy department
- A poorly funded department
- Unreal expectations of the department

A final word of caution about university research funds, sometimes suggested as a source of seed money. They are usually limited in amount and dispersed under heavy competition. The promise of such funds should not be accepted as a possible source of seed money; they are inadequate for more than small pilot studies, and are jealously guarded. Thus your commitments for seed money must be negotiated and written agreements obtained, signed by a responsible institution official, preferably the Dean.

Unfortunately, not all department heads are scrupulous. Some rise to their high position despite (or perhaps because of) a rather ruthless nature. The value of your job offer will be much greater if the spirit of the offer will be honored, and this depends on the character of the chairperson. Evaluate the chairperson in terms of department turnover. Talk to the newest faculty members and assess their reaction to their new positions; they may, however, not feel free to be forthright, or their standards may differ from yours. The best source of information about the department may be an ex-faculty member, or fellows who have recently moved to new positions. Ask to see a list of faculty, their Biosketches, and their funding. Try to find out if there are any second-class citizens in the group, i.e., those without funds, space, or support. Talk to them if you can. Most departments have a few such members carried for services, such as teaching, that they provide. Your new department will be your new home, and you will want it to be a happy one. Avoid departments that have a callous attitude about those who are not superstars and are, consequently, unhappy members.

Be suspicious of a department where everyone is fully funded. While it is possible that every member of the faculty, including recent appointments, is fundable, it is more likely that the absence of anyone without funds reflects merciless removal of those who are not successful. Think carefully about who does the teaching in a department of such successful researchers! Also be suspicious if there are more than a few members without funds (suggesting low standards in the group).

A good department chairperson provides strong guidance, steady support, and continuous concern for the success of young faculty. This is probably the single most important nurturing feature of many successful research careers.

ON BEING A PROFESSIONAL WRITER

The following thoughts are addressed to those of you for whom writing is not a pleasure, but hard work—for those who put it off until the last, and who are always hard against a deadline. You have no problem with the conception and the gestation of your masterwork but struggle with a painful delivery—a process in which you find no denouement, yet without which you have nothing. We sympathize with your plight, for we have experienced it ourselves, as have most of our colleagues. There is a solution. Read on.

Most scientific papers are poorly written. Even in this age of computer assistance to correct spelling and grammar, communication is impaired by inadequate organization, too many words and what has been called "pompous prose" (see Appendix F). Writing is as important a research tool as any other skill. It is a pity that most scientists have never received adequate training in English composition.

We occasionally give workshops on grantsmanship. The audience is usually a group of researchers, graduate students, and fellows. We like to start with a few "get acquainted" questions. A particularly revealing question is, "How many professional writers are here today?" Usually no hands are raised. This leads to the comment, "Well, I guess if your are not professionals, you must be amateurs!" The definition of a professional is someone who does something for money. Obviously there is a problem of attitude among the audience. They attend a workshop to improve their writing skills at requesting money, but do not consider themselves professionals. Researchers, of course. But writers? No. There is a very real competition for research funds. When you enter that competition, you must meet or beat the standards of your competitors to be successful. Since the standards of writing are actually rather low, your proposal will be outstanding if it is well written. This requires effort, but it is an effort that pays big dividends.

That research proposals are generally poorly written is probably more an indictment of American education than anything is. Most research beginners are steeped in the technology and importance of their fellowship projects and consider writing as the downside of their line of work. For many, writing is hard work. It is something of which they have done little. Writing gets in the way of what is fun: real research. Writing is done under pressure to meet deadlines, hurriedly, and generally poorly. However, those who are successful eventually come to appreciate that, in the end, *what is written is all that counts!* Publish or perish is a fact of life for the university researcher. Research that is never published, no matter how great, is a useless waste of time and resources. Also our experience is that the grant proposal that is not written almost never gets funded!

The researcher who comes to enjoy writing has the best of all worlds. The pleasure of collecting good, clean data is augmented by the process that results in dissemination of the results, the support of new ideas, discovery, and the acknowledgment and appreciation of one's peers. But how is this celestial modus vivendi achieved? Simply by doing it. Writing is an art that really does come easier with practice.

Good research training leads the student to develop good research habits. Unfortunately, most programs concentrate on the technology and ignore scholarship. We expect scholars to read something every day, and most manage this religiously. They should also write something every day, but this requires a discipline few beginners seem to have, perhaps because university life tends to fill up the hours with trivia and interruptions. Now, here is the *secret to success:* pick an hour out of your day that can be absolutely inviolate. Set it aside and spend that hour writing every day, 7 days a week, 52 weeks a year. Over the course of a year, you will be devoting a total of about 45 eight-hour days to writing! Since proficiency is directly proportional to practice, your skills will develop rapidly. Most importantly, you will be continuously productive in the only way that will be remembered and appreciated: your writing. Deadlines will cease to threaten and cause fear. Your next proposal will be gradually assembled over months or even years with ample time for thoughtful review and addition of supportive preliminary data.

What should you write? Research is always done for a purpose. The purpose is the gist of the introduction to any paper describing the project. Ergo if you are doing research, you are in a position to write the introduction of the relevant paper—the purpose of your research. Your computer should always contain one or more fetal papers and at least one grant proposal. Your papers will be part of the Preliminary Data for the proposal. Your accompanying literature reviews will be appropriate to both. So, before you start a new project, write the introduction for the relevant paper, and list the pertinent literature.

As the research progresses, you use the procedures that will constitute the Methods section of the paper. This is the best time to write the methods, since they are fresh in your mind. Sometimes papers are written months after procedures are done and the details are long lost. Avoid this by writing up the methods in publication form, as they happen.

What do the data mean? This is the discussion part of a paper. It should be written in approximate terms as the data come in, a time at which you should be thinking deeply about interpretation and significance. A common failing of beginners is to concentrate so intensely on collecting the data that the significance is ignored. When the results are finally considered seriously, perhaps months later, deficits are seen and more experiments needed. A poor way to do business.

As they begin to accumulate, collate the data from an experiment immediately and generate several publication-quality figures to describe them. Write legends for the figures. By the time the last data are in, usually months after the project was started, the paper will be essentially written. All that remains is to edit it, select the best figures, and write a discussion that is appropriate for the results actually obtained. You will never be in the position of rushing a paper out with inadequate preparation, because you will have spent months writing and rewriting and thinking about it while the research was in progress. There is a possible downside to this lifestyle, and it must be avoided. There are some that develop productivity constipation as a result of an obsessive-compulsive drive for perfection. They are never quite satisfied with their product, and rework it to destruction. This is a behavioral problem. An effective solution is to develop collaboration with someone who is productive and will push the papers out.

University life requires periodic reports. These also should be continuously massaged and kept up to date. You should always have your Biosketch current in two forms. The first is your curriculum vitae for the university. Include all teaching, presentations, invited talks, review articles, book chapters, papers, etc. Also include committee service, graduate students, and fellows. When promotion time comes, your promotions packet will be all but written. The second should be the NIH R01 proposal four-page Biosketch. Thus it will always be up-to-date. When you are asked to be a Co-Investigator or collaborator on a colleague's proposal, and your Biosketch is requested, it will be immediately available and a credit instead of a liability. If your institution subscribes to "Community of Science," be sure to keep your listing in their database up-to-date as well.

How should you write? Obviously you must use a good word processor. We prefer Microsoft Word. As you use it, add your specialized words to its dictionary, spelled correctly, of course. Use the grammar checker to help you write short sentences that will more effectively communicate your ideas. We have a love for sentences with many convoluted phrases. This is anathema to our word processor, which uses green underlines to shut us off. Our ideal is a paragraph sans green. Identify the journal to which you will send each paper. Write papers in compliance with the "Instructions for Authors" of the journal. Most journals follow the recommendations of the International Committee of Medical Journal Editors (ICMJE), or the *American Psychological Association Style Book* (also see Appendix F). If you start out with the appropriate style, you will avoid tiresome revision when it comes to publication. Write proposals strictly in accordance with the R01 grant instructions for the same reasons.

Style is less important for a proposal than for a paper. The minimum requirements for each section are described in the relevant chapters. Style of published papers has a lot to do with their acceptance. The comments in Browner's *Publishing and Presenting Clinical Research* (Appendix F) are well worth reading and apply equally to basic research papers. Of course the standard reference for biomedical scientific writing style is the *American Medical Association Manual of Style* (Appendix F).

Stephen King, the best-selling author of more than 30 books, has written an excellent little book, *On Writing* (Appendix F). He offers some very good advice: "The second draft = the first draft less 10%." I prefer to work with somewhat looser restrictions. Try to limit your first draft of a 25-page proposal to 30 pages (Specific Aims, 2 pages; Background, 4 pages; Preliminary Studies, 10 pages; Research Design and Methods, 14 pages). Then be merciless with the second draft.

Start with the Specific Aims. The two-page draft must be reduced to no more than one page with lots of spaces. Reduce the actual Specific Aims to one sentence per Aim plus a title. Eliminate all of the background comments not directly related to the hypotheses. If you do not have specific hypotheses, this may explain excessive length! Reduce or eliminate descriptions of methods to be used. Delete all editorial comments (e.g., "These studies will open new avenues of therapy for whatever"). Delete all references. If the reviewer has to look up a reference to get your message, you have failed. In the best of all worlds, and if you do your editing properly, you will have room for a self-explanatory diagram that presents your hypotheses in the context of a larger model and reveals the logic of your Aims. Of course, all this must be on one page, and be readable in 3 minutes.

The Background and Significance must not be longer than three pages. If you did not write it from an outline, make one now, complete with titles for the paragraphs. If your diagram successfully represents your proposed work, use it as a guide for the logic of this section. Ruthlessly eliminate all statements of the obvious (e.g., "Alzheimer's disease is a serious dementia-producing illness of the elderly"). Trim out excessive, intrusive, unnecessary, and, to the reader, aggravating adjectives. Scientists have a specialized vocabulary, and tend to be overly fond of it. Excessive, unnecessary, and, to the reader, aggravating employment of technical terminology tends to burden otherwise erudite, incisive, epistemic compositions. Such writing is, in fact, "pompous prose" (see Appendix F). It leads to excessive, unnecessary, and, to the reader, aggravating verbosity (as hopefully proven here). But we do love our special words. Here is where an uninvolved reader can be a big help. Give them carte blanche to cut. Remember the *Scientific American* principle: keep it simple. Rewrite any sentence longer than two lines. If possible, use tables and diagrams to reduce words. When referring to preliminary data, do not go into detail that belongs in Preliminary Studies. Concentrate on the relevance of the data in support of the proposal. Methods belong in Methods, not in Background. Sometimes an animal model is central to a study, and it is appropriate to extol its virtues, briefly, referring to supportive preliminary data in the Preliminary Studies section. Do not clutter up the Background with such data; only refer to it. If the significance of your work is not obvious to the reviewers, you are in big trouble anyway. So do not waste much space stating the obvious. It is, however, customary to either open or conclude this section with a short paragraph concerning significance (impact on the field) and future directions of your research.

The Preliminary Studies section can usually be limited to eight pages without difficulty. If it is longer than this, it probably contains too much method description. As stated above, methods belong in the Methods part of Research Design and Methods. The legends here should be similar to those found in publications—just the facts. A picture is really worth a thousand words, and it is not helpful to belabor, with words, the obvious. Delete anything that is included in appendix material, unless it is going to get you the Nobel prize. Do not repeat descriptions that are in the preceding Background section. Repetition is the bane of good writing. That is, if you present an idea succinctly, with incisive brevity, the first time, you should not have to repeat it repetitiously, again and again.

You should have 13 pages left for Research Design and Methods, after editing. If there are many experiments to be described in Design, there may be a squeeze in Methods. This can be avoided by being brief and limiting design as described in Chapter 8. Do not mix Design with Method. In Methods, refer to published papers (hopefully of your own) if possible. Do not repeat methods described in papers (not necessarily your own) included in the appendix; rather, refer to them, noting modifications. Be careful in what you delete from Methods. Nothing essential can be left out. In this section more than any, a knowledgeable review will keep you out of trouble. Each Study Section has its own set of expectations for the inclusiveness of this section. If you leave something expected out, you will pay a price. Only someone familiar with your Study Section can help you avoid this. Often that someone is your fellowship mentor, if you are lucky.

If English is not your first language, you may never write at the level of your America-born competitors. Accept this as a truism and do something about it. Have your papers and proposals edited for English grammar. Every university has an English Department filled with students well qualified to edit the writing of those for whom English is not the primary language. The more common errors are in the use of articles, plurals, and phrasing. The cost is minimal, but the process requires time and some effort. If your school has a student-work program, it may actually pay for this service. Professional writing does not contain grammatical errors (very often), and you decided to become a professional writer when you chose a career in science. If you do not already have them, now is the time to start developing these skills. They are every bit as important to your success as any technical expertise you have acquired.

Part Two: Advanced Grantsmanship

Chapters 20 to 25 cover the Small Business grant programs and institutional grants for Program Projects, Centers, Construction, Training, and Instrumentation. These are not programs for beginners, but even experienced researchers will have to get their feet wet for a first time and may benefit from reading of our experience with these more complex programs.

20

Small Business Grants

The Small Business Innovation Research (SBIR) and Small Business Technology Transfer (STTR) programs were designed to facilitate the transfer of newly developed technology from the university to industry and ultimately to the public. The programs were inspired by the explosive development of the biotechnology industry exemplified by numerous small companies involving university-based scientists. Congress decided that practical application of new developments derived from federally funded research were slow to enter the marketplace and thus were of small benefit to mankind. The NIH, NSF, and DOD, and most federal components that have budgets for extramural research, must use a proportion of their funds for SBIR and STTR grants and contracts.

The SBIR grant program (R43, R44) was initiated in 1985. Its stated goals are: (1) stimulation of technological development; (2) to involve small businesses to meet federal research and development needs; (3) to increase private sector commercialization of innovations derived from federal research and development; and (4) to foster and encourage participation by minority and disadvantaged persons in technological development.

The NIH and other federal research agencies are required to expend 2.5% of their current extramural research budgets for small companies to conduct research and development programs funded by SBIR grants. They must also devote 0.15% of their budgets to support STTR grants.

The program guidelines define a small business as being independently owned and operated with fewer than 500 employees. An individual or a private medical practice can qualify. The PI of an SBIR grant is required to be primarily (more than 50%) in the employ of the business before the starting date of an award. This requirement does not apply to STTR grants, providing that the PI has some kind of formal appointment with the company. Advice on eligibility of a business can be obtained by calling the NIH Special Programs Office (301-496-1968), or the program staff at any of the Institutes.

These grants are awarded in two phases: Phase I ($100,000 total costs) lasts 6 months (SBIR) or 12 months (STTR) and establishes feasibility. Phase II (SBIR, $750,000; STTR, $500,000 total costs) lasts 2 years and continues research and development to the point where final development can be financed with nonfederal dollars (Phase III). Application submission deadlines for both grants are April 1, August 1, and December 1. At least 67% of SBIR Phase I work and 50% of SBIR Phase II work must be carried out by the small business, which is the prime grantee for the SBIR award. The remainder of the budget may be used for consultants and subcontracts, such as with a university. The STTR award generally is to a research institution, where the PI may have a primary appointment. It is not possible to get a Phase II award unless Phase I has been completed—Phase II applications are only given to successful Phase I investigators. "Fast-track" review of these grants is possible in select cases. When this is chosen, proposals for both Phase I and Phase II are reviewed together.

The SBIR program had some success in supporting university spin-off companies (a great many of which have failed), but had limited success in achieving its goal of encouraging university grantees to transfer their discoveries into the public sector. This was perceived to be the result of the restriction of the SBIR program that the PI must be primarily an employee of the industry. A university entrepreneur was required to relinquish university status in order to participate as PI, and many were unwilling to do this.

The STTR (R41, R42) program is the result of the Small Business Research and Development Act of 1992, which requires the NIH and NSF to reserve a specific amount of their budget for extramural research for small business technology transfer. The goals of this program are more specific: (1) stimulate and foster scientific and technological innovation through cooperative research and development carried out between small business concerns and research institutions (universities); (2) foster technology transfer between small business concerns and research institutions; (3) increase private sector commercialization of innovations derived from federal research and development; and (4) foster and encourage participation of socially and economically disadvantaged small business concerns and women-owned small business concerns in technological development.

The STTR program differs from the SBIR program in an important way: the PI can be a full-time employee of the university. The business still submits the proposal and is the grantee, but more of the research can be done off-premises, i.e., at the university. Only 40% must be done by the business; at least 30% must be done by the university. The university must certify that dedicated space is available for the proposed work. All aspects of the work must be done in the United States.

The relationship of the PI to the business can be much less formal in the STTR program; the PI need not receive any remuneration from the company as long as some kind of official relationship exists. However, care must be taken to provide assurance that a university-employed PI will be able to devote sufficient time to the proposed project to achieve success.

THE PROPOSAL

There is no real difference between SBIR and STTR proposals. These proposals are funded by NIH Institutes and are reviewed by ad hoc NIH Study Sections that are convened by the CSR. These committees usually consist of scientists who are used to R01 proposals plus scientists from small businesses who have competed successfully for their own SBIR grants. All the criteria of a good R01 proposal apply here, except those remarks concerning development. A project to develop a commercial product makes for a weak R01 proposal, but is the essential basis for the SBIR and STTR projects. Applied research is not very competitive among R01s but is entirely appropriate to these programs. This is the basis for a problem faced by the SBIR/STTR applicants: reviewers are asked to apply different criteria to these proposals, which are assigned priority scores like R01s. This is difficult to do and some scientists, chafing at the low award rates of R01s, are not particularly sympathetic to the goals of the program ("to make money for someone"). Thus SBIR/STTR proposals probably have a competitive disadvantage in review, but not in funding, since funds for this program are set aside and cannot be used for support of R01 applications.

Application forms for SBIR/STTR proposals may be found on the Internet. Section VI ("Small Business Research Grant Programs") of the PHS 398 form is used (<http://grants.nih.gov/grants/forms.htm>). Additional information about these programs can be seen at <www.grants.nih.

gov/grants/funding/sbir.htm>. The Research Plan is essentially the same as that of an R01, with the exception that Preliminary Data is not required and a business plan is. For Phase I proposals, the entire application may not exceed 25 pages (including form pages 1–4, Budget, Research Plan, and Literature Cited, but excluding letters of support and Biographical Sketches), and Items *a–d* of the Research Plan are limited to a total of 15 pages. For Phase II applications, the Research Plan is limited to a total of 25 pages, with no other limitations on size.

No appendix material may be submitted with Phase I applications.

The Budget and Budget Justification are similar to those of modular R01 proposals. Funds transferred to other investigators should be in the form of a subcontract and should be itemized and justified. Additional information will be requested by NIH "just-in-time" to make an award.

A small business, before receiving its first SBIR/STTR award, is faced with the necessity of completing an indirect cost agreement, and certain business-related assurances, with the NIH. This complicated process is beyond the scope of this book.

The requirements to provide assurances concerning human subjects, animals, minorities, women, etc., that apply to the R01 also apply to these proposals. Small businesses do not have the necessary Institutional Review Boards (IRBs) and Institutional Animal Care and Use Committees (IACUCs) required for these assurances, but can use those of the collaborating institution, providing there is in place an appropriate agreement.

Proposal review is by ad hoc Study Sections of the CSR. They are given somewhat different criteria by which to evaluate a proposal (see pp. 96ff of PHS 398 guidelines). The emphasis is on both scientific and technical merit *and* potential for commercialization. Standard NIH priority scores are used (1.0 to 5.0) with "triage."

1. *Significance.* Commercial potential to lead to a marketable product or process, societal benefit, advancement of knowledge, and development of new technology that is better than existing technology.
2. *Approach.* Good design, feasible studies, problems are dealt with, and definite testable milestones.
3. *Innovation.* State-of-the-art technology, and original aims and ideas.
4. *Investigators.* Well trained, capable, productive, and experienced.
5. *Environment.* Resources, existing equipment, facilities, collaborations, and supportive atmosphere.

The Study Section SRA will provide a Summary Statement as with an

R01. Unsuccessful proposals may be revised and are more likely to make the funding cutoff when amended. Revised proposals should have an additional page (26 pages total), an Introduction of 1 (not 3) page that responds to the criticisms of the original proposal found in the Summary Statement.

A MODEL PROPOSAL

This section presents an example of a successful SBIR proposal. Submitted by a small biotechnology company, it addressed the problem presented when cell proliferation associated with normal wound healing causes pathology, in this case intraocular scarring, retinal detachment, and blindness. It was suggested that the proliferation of a particular type of cell, the fibroblast, is excessive, and prevention or control of this proliferation would prevent the complication. The company had patented a process in which a cytotoxin is conjugated to a monoclonal antibody (mAb). The combination of the mAb with its target cell results in death of the cell.

Based on the reasonable assumption that control of fibroblast proliferation would prevent intraocular scarring, the company proposed to develop a fibroblast-specific mAb to test its ability to destroy fibroblasts *in vitro* when conjugated with ricin and to test the conjugate against an *in vitro* model of cell proliferation. The Background and Significance was 2 pages, followed by 1 page describing the experience of the PI and colleagues (this could have been in the Budget Justification). One page of preliminary data was provided to establish their ability to make the cytotoxic conjugates in pure form, without ricin contamination, and the Methods section was quite detailed, covering 10 pages.

This successful proposal was a revision. The original version also included development of an animal model of intraocular scarring. The critique noted that the PI had no experience with such models and offered no preliminary data pertinent to the model; this part of the proposal lacked credibility. In the revision, the animal model was deleted, but the rest of the proposal was essentially unchanged. The *in vitro* studies were supported.

The SBIR/STTR instructions suggest that preliminary data are not required for these proposals. However, there is no better way to demonstrate the probability of success than good preliminary data. It is not likely that a strong proposal can be written without it. The whole nature of the Phase I project is to demonstrate that a particular idea for some application is feasible. The more preliminary data available to support this contention, the better the proposal. As the example above demonstrates, failure to provide pertinent supporting data can sink an SBIR proposal as quickly as an R01.

INSTITUTE INTEREST IN THE SBIR/STTR PROGRAM

The Omnibus Solicitation for SBIR/STTR grants is available at the above web sites. It contains sections for each NIH Institute that list the specific areas of the programs for which they desire SBIR/STTR grants. These lists are not necessarily the same as the Institute programs, since they represent areas their Advisory Councils feel need applied rather than fundamental development.

A WORD OF CAUTION

These grants are not suitable for the long-term support of an academic career. They may be very helpful as an adjunct, but they are no substitute for R01 support. Investigators who get involved in applied projects must consider carefully the complications of conflict of interest that arise when scientists derive financial gain from the success of their research.

21

Program Project Grants (P01)

Program Project, or P01, grants are large integrated, usually multidisciplinary projects involving three or more investigators who, in most cases, would benefit from sharing some type of core facility. Successful P01 projects convince the reviewers that "the whole is greater than the sum of the parts." The interaction and/or core facilities made possible by the P01 strengthen the individual projects of each of the members. The quality and quantity of their data are improved, and collaboration among the members is enhanced. In fiscal year 2000, the NIH reviewed 410 P01 proposals and funded 215. This is a success rate of 52%. In contrast, the success rate of all R01s was 31%. The difference is the result of the senior status of most investigators involved with Program Project grants. Program Project proposals are considered in this chapter, and Center grant proposals in the next.

P01 grants are awarded to institutions on behalf of a principal investigator for the support of a broadly based, often multidisciplinary, long-term research program with a particular major objective or theme. A program project involves the organized efforts of groups of investigators who conduct research projects related to the overall program objective. The grant can provide support for the projects and for certain shared resources needed for the total research effort. Each project supported under a program project grant is expected to contribute to the overall program objective.

Center grants, awarded to institutions on behalf of a program director and a group of collaborating investigators, provide support for long-term, multidisciplinary programs of research and development. The distinction between Program Project and Center grants is that the latter are more likely to have a clinical orientation and are usually developed in response to announcements of the specific needs and requirements of an Institute. Center grants support programs in critical health problem areas including research and development; demonstration of advanced techniques for the diagnosis, treatment, prevention, or control of disease; education; and other related nonresearch components.

235

Funding for P01 grants varies greatly among the Institutes, from no funding (NEI) to 23% of the total Institute budget for investigator-initiated research projects (NHLBI). The NIH funding of P01 grants for 2000 is shown in Table 21.1. P01 awards are the equivalent of three to seven or more R01s. The size of the awards varies greatly among Institutes. The success shown is in terms of ratios because the numbers are small. Again, the variation is great among Institutes. Six did not make P01 awards in 2000.

P01 and R01 grants are funded from the same dollars so Institutes with large numbers of P01 grants can fund fewer R01s. This explains, at least in part, the higher R01 success rate of the NEI and lower R01 success rates of the NIA, NCI, NIEHS, NINDS, and NHLBI (see Table 1.3). The essence of a strong Program Project is a group of productive researchers, each successful in obtaining R01 funds; all share a common broad research goal, but use widely different experimental approaches that, nevertheless, require common resources and can benefit from group interaction. Projects suitable for P01 support are broad, and are often specifically identified by the granting Institute. Such projects might be obesity and hypertension, atherosclerosis, diabetes, breast cancer, immunotherapy for cancer, or a portion of the human genome. Projects are also often oriented

Table 21.1 *Institute P01 Awards in 2000*

Institute	Average direct costs × $1000		Success rate	
	New	Renewal	New	Renewal
NIA	1165	1559	18/54	24/45
NIAID	903	1001	11/31	5/10
NIAMS	886	1318	1/3	1/1
NCI	1521	1559	18/54	24/45
NICHD	804	1136	7/13	13/17
NIDA	1198	884	11/31	5/10
NIDCD	600	1120	1/1	4/4
NIDDK	948	1150	15/28	7/9
NIDCR	899	928	5/8	2/3
NIEHS	832	1019	3/6	2/2
NIGMS	1136	1307	6/13	2/2
NHLBI	1421	1673	10/15	23/26
NIMH		1282	0/4	2/2
NINDS	1074	1310	11/21	7/17

Note: No awards were made by the NCRR, NIAAA, NHGRI, NEI, NCCAM, and NINR.

toward a common research theme such as molecular genetics, transport processes, or transplantation biology.

P01 proposals that are in response to an RFA or Program Announcement must adhere rigidly to the requirements of the Institute. Investigator-initiated P01 awards are probably less common. Before such a P01 proposal is submitted, the appropriate Institute staff should be consulted to determine the specific interests of the Institute and to obtain the Institute's guidelines for multiproject proposals. If they will agree, give them a preproposal to critique. It is particularly important to identify prospective reviewers and to structure the proposal goals to support the Institute goals and reviewers' biases. The NIH has ruled that a proposal requesting more than $500,000 direct costs for any year must be accompanied by a letter that identifies a Program Director who has agreed to accept the proposal. Since P01 proposals always exceed this amount, they require such a covering letter.

PROGRAM LOGIC

The best Program Projects feature a group of investigators whose work logically interconnects. A typical program might involve collaboration of a clinician whose patients are diabetic, a basic scientist with a colony of atherosclerotic rats, a molecular biologist with an interest in the intracellular pathways activated by insulin, and a scientist studying the dependency of atherosclerosis on MAP kinase pathways in endothelial cells. Their interactions are best represented by a diagram that also includes Core Modules, perhaps for a vivarium, tissue culture and biostatistical support, etc. (Figure 21.1). The functional model might feature hypertension, diabetes, and obesity as these relate to each project. Thus, this is generally a model for the pathogenesis of a disease involving a number of related hypotheses, each of which is central to one of the projects.

Unfortunately, this is an ideal seldom achieved in the real world. Most P01s are the result of Institute announcements or initiatives. These identify the focus desired and set limits on the nature of the research. They often set deadlines a few months after publication of the announcement. Typically, a successful PI with a class-A personality and a need for a core facility starts organizing a program 2 or 3 months before the deadline. He or she casts about for likely collaborators and tries to persuade them to make the effort to join the group. All too often, the ones willing to join

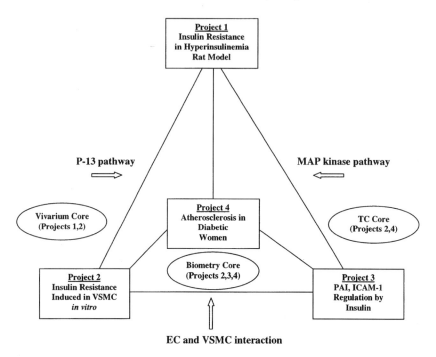

Figure 21.1. Example diagram of a multiproject proposal on insulin resistance and atherosclerosis.

are unfunded, or at least have a recent proposal that failed. They have already done the writing and are all too happy to give it another try. The group is a polyglot of dissimilar interests. The challenge is to get them to interact enough to generate a coherent proposal featuring some sort of logical interaction. The silver lining to this dismal cloud is that this is a disability that afflicts most P01 proposals. If you can do better than this, you will probably succeed.

There is a solution. The nucleus of the group should be formed long before the submission of the P01 is contemplated. In the above example, a "Hypertension Study Group" might be formed. It should meet on a regular basis, with refreshments, to hear members of the group describe and discuss their research. This will lead to new collaborations and awareness of who is doing what. Cross-town membership should be encouraged. Minutes of the meetings should be kept as important support for a later P01. When a critical mass of interested parties has been gathered, perhaps after a year or two, it is ready to develop a proposal. Meetings should focus on the integrating model and the hypotheses. If this is done correctly, and the faculty is strong, the resulting proposal will succeed. The secret is a combination of organization and time. You must have both. Some diplomacy is required when proposal time comes. Some members of the group will lack funds. They must not be assigned to be Project PIs. Make it a hard and fast rule that all Project PIs must have a funded R01, or at least some NIH support. Your unfunded colleagues can probably be Core Module Directors without harming the review.

Investigator strength explains the success of most funded P01 proposals. Each Program Project has a Program Director in whose name the award is made, and who must have a funded R01 grant. There must be at least three projects in the program: the Program Director is the PI of one, and two or more additional projects each have a PI. In the strongest projects every PI has an R01 grant. Thus the strongest group is one in which every member has at least one funded R01 grant, and several of their second R01s will be "rolled over" into the P01 if it is funded. The advantage for these investigators is that the P01 will provide important core support they would not otherwise have. In the past, Program Projects had a well-deserved reputation for supporting one or more investigators who were unfundable by the R01 mechanism. This is one reason why some Institutes spurn such grants. However, in the present era of intense competition, it is very unlikely that a weak PI will survive P01 review. Thus, it is a mistake to include such investigators in the proposal; most Study Sections simply delete weak projects, but the discussion justifying such action is always negative, and is likely to depress the overall priority score. Obviously Program Projects are not for beginners. They are designed to encourage interaction among senior investigators. They are a way for the rich to get richer.

CORE RESOURCES

A Program Project is a collection of R01 projects with a common theme and sharing one or more core resources, called Core Modules. If there is no real need for a core resource, there is little to be gained from a P01 grant. Such a proposal would be weak and unlikely to be funded anyway.

Typical Core Modules are:

1. Vivarium (providing animal models of hypertension or neuronal degeneration, or a colony of transgenic mice; supporting a colony of miniature pigs or breeding monkeys, etc.)

2. Laboratory (providing special methods, tissues, or tests such as blood catecholamine or renin levels, cytokine levels, fluorescein-activated cell sorting, hybridoma generation, or confocal or electron microscopy)

3. Analytical (providing statistical support or mathematical modeling; such modules usually provide a salary for a biostatistician or other professional)

4. Computer (providing networked programs for sharing software and data, telemedicine units, special programming, etc.)

5. Shop (supporting construction of specialized instruments or electronics)

6. Administrative (providing staff support or internal review, or facilitating communication or use of core facilities)

7. Epidemiology or biostatistics (usually providing salary support for a professional)

8. Clinical (inpatient or outpatient, providing service, diagnostic or laboratory testing, treatment, or supervision not available through regular hospital services, or a NIH-supported General Clinical Research Center)

9. Research support (reviewing and awarding small grants for pilot projects)

These and other modules are described in more detail in Chapter 22 on Center grants. The advantage of the P01 mechanism is that it provides larger budgets than do most Center grants. However, this varies among the Institutes.

It is essential that the Director of any Core Module is obviously qualified by experience and publications, and be capable of devoting an appropriate amount of time to the project. This last is sometimes a problem because Module Directors are often Project PIs, and tend already to be heavily committed. The reviewers must be convinced that real direction will be provided. This is best handled by providing a schedule of meetings and times during which the Module Director will interact with module personnel. The primary duties of the Director, besides overall supervision, are to monitor the Core Module product to ensure good quantity and quality of data, and to collaborate with nonexpert core users.

A case should be made that each Core Module will foster collaboration among the users and will be extensively used by the P01 participants and by PIs with related R01s. A good way to do this is to include in the Research Plan for each project a section called "Collaboration." This paragraph should supply details of how each of the other projects and Core Modules will interact with the project. This description must agree with the information shown on a diagram that illustrates these relationships.

ADMINISTRATIVE CORE

Although the nature of Core Modules is determined by the circumstances of the program, every P01 should have an Administrative Core Module headed by the proposal Program Director, and with a Co-Director from among the other PIs. It is primarily the Administrative Core that extends the strength of a P01 beyond the sum of its parts. Its role is to monitor the activities of all P01 projects, facilitate communication among project members, facilitate the intellectual activities and methodological capabilities of the Study Group, arrange for seminars, visiting speakers, external reviewers, and consultants, and handle the paperwork generated by the program as a whole. The description of the Administrative Core should include agreed-upon rules of data handling and sharing, and authorship. This core will arbitrate differences and initiate policy changes as required. Provide a diagram to illustrate administrative relationships. The arrows in Figure 21.2 represent lines of communication and collaboration.

Administrative staff could handle some paperwork of project members, but it will be questioned if more than minimal assistance is suggested. Generally, it is felt that staff support is warranted only insofar as

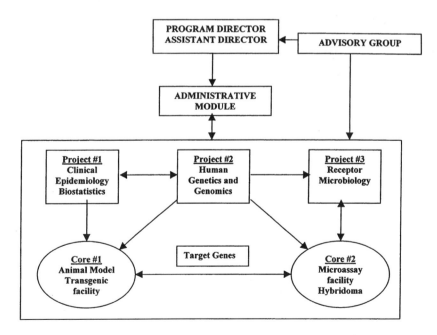

Figure 21.2. Diagram of administrative organization.

it is appropriate to the productivity of an individual project. The location of the Administrative Core staff should be specified and should be in close proximity to as many researchers as possible. The Administrative Core should be a shared resource. If it appears to be just another secretary for a superstar PI, the proposal will be weakened. Since the best Program Projects involve more than one department, it is good strategy to represent the Administrative Core staff in a different location than that of the PI. This will help allay the suspicion that the P01 PI might monopolize the services of the unit. This is a valid concern because it commonly happens and is a root cause of the failure of these large projects to achieve their full potential.

APPEARANCE IS IMPORTANT

The best evidence of a strong Administrative Core is a tightly organized, logical, integrated, attractive, well-written proposal. In addition to supplying a budget for its own activities, the Administrative Core can be used to summarize, with a table, the use of each additional Core Module. Appropriate tabulated module usage should be about 85% of capacity, leaving room for expansion but justifying the budgeted items. Of course, each individual Core Module should provide a more detailed table of projected use by each of the P01 or related R01 projects, and separate itemized budgets.

Most P01 proposals appear poorly written because a committee in which the members do not communicate writes them. The sections lack uniformity, each of the Biosketches is different, different fonts are intermingled, and the numbering on the figures is not consecutive. In short, they look like they were written by a committee. This can be avoided by producing an outline of the projects and insisting that it be followed, and that the format for each project and module be the same. The Biosketches must be redone to be uniform. Figure labeling and legends must conform. The same section titles should appear throughout the proposal. These are simply the requirements of good grantsmanship.

Repetition is the bane of P01 proposals. The proposal starts with a review of the rationale for the project. The background of the general problem and the overall model and hypotheses are presented with rave reviews of the sterling qualities of the faculty. The need and great benefits of the Core Modules are described, along with the administrative arrangements.

Then the individual research projects are presented, followed by the Core Modules. There is a boring tendency for each of these sections to rehash the background presented up front. Rather, each should take up where the Introduction left off. This requires organization and communication because each section will have a different author. Start with a detailed, paragraph-by-paragraph outline, and then stick to it. If necessary, freely rewrite sections to ensure their conformance. Usually the Introduction and Modules are written at the same time, but by different authors. Someone, usually the PI, should rewrite each project and Core Module to delete these vain repetitions and to unify the proposal. If this is not done, the best the proposal can be as a document is average.

Facilities are crucial to an effective P01 proposal. Usually, each PI has existing facilities as required for his R01 projects. The P01 usually represents some expansion of research and the reviewers must judge whether adequate additional space will be available. To be credible, this requires an institutional commitment, described in a letter of support, of additional usable space.

INDIVIDUAL RESEARCH PROJECTS

The Program Project proposal is, in the final analysis, rated on the basis of its constituent projects, each of which should be written up like any R01 proposal. In addition, each project should include sections explaining in detail exactly how the project will be strengthened by the Program Project and by use of the Core Modules. If, for instance, use of a Vivarium Core is part of a proposal, the number and types of animal models should be specified, with discussion of why these require the core facility. Convenience alone is not an adequate justification for a Core Module, which should provide services beyond the practical reach of an individual project. Similar sections should be provided for each Core Module, including the Administrative Core. Ideally, animals, reagents, patient materials, etc., will be shared and correlated among the projects.

The page limit of an R01 applies to these individual projects, but the proposal will be vastly easier on the reviewers if a 20-page limit, rather than 25, is imposed. The individual budgets must be reasonable and should err on the side of too little. Many PA or RFA Program Projects have a budget limit under which everything must fit. This cannot be exceeded. Unsolicited proposals may have no such limit, but in a practical sense, all have a threshold above which there is certain failure. Contact the Institute Program Manager for a review of the budget and follow his or her advice. There is no prohibition on requests for equipment, but such should be kept to an absolute minimum. The budgets for individual projects of a Program are usually somewhat smaller than those of R01s. If a funded R01 is to be rolled into a P01, the budget should remain the same or be only slightly increased. While equipment can be requested for Core Modules, the request should be strengthened by the specific needs of individual projects with the same caveats that apply to an R01. Personnel and supplies also should correspond to a typical R01. The budgets of each project should be well balanced and approximately the same in size to achieve overall balance in the program.

Although every project should be dependent on the core facilities, the individual projects should be relatively independent of each other, so that elimination of a project by the Study Section does not threaten the integrity of the entire program. Care must be exercised to avoid duplication of activities of any project with that of a Core Module. Thus, if the Morphometry Module contains a histology technician, this position should not be requested for an individual project unless the scientific requirements are clearly different and explained.

Review of Program Project proposals is usually by site visit, often by an ad hoc committee of a CSR or Institute Study Section. Recently "reverse site visits" have become common. In these, the applicants either come to the NIH or are contacted by telephone for the review. The ad hoc committee reports its findings to the parent Study Section at its next meeting. A typical site visiting team might contain two members of the parent Study Section, two to four ad hoc reviewers chosen for expertise in the science of the individual projects, and a NIH administrator. For large, complex proposals a research administrator may be included among the reviewers. The site visitors prepare the usual critique of each part of the proposal and provide answers to a long list of specific questions. These questions are published in the Institute guidelines and should be specifically addressed in the proposal. The site visitors generally vote a priority score for each part of the proposal and for the proposal as a whole. The parent committee then reviews the entire program, possibly deleting some projects, and votes a priority for the remainder. This final priority may be much improved through elimination of weak sections, and is the basis of funding. In most Institutes, P01 proposals are inserted into the appropriate R01 list on the basis of priority score rather than percentile, and are funded from the same funds, in competition with the R01s.

SUPPLEMENTARY DATA

Program Project proposals are notoriously difficult to coordinate and usually are submitted at the last minute, with inadequate internal review and incomplete pilot data for some projects. In some Institutes, they are reviewed only once a year and many months may elapse between the submission deadline and the site visit. Other Institutes may have P01 competitions on a regular cycle. Supplementary data, which are listed below, should be submitted about 4 weeks prior to site visit review, so that the reviewers can see it at their leisure. Additional supplementary material can be provided at the time of the visit, but will add to the burden of reading of the reviewers, so must be kept to a minimum.

1. List alphabetically all professional personnel (include consultants, external and internal advisory committee members, and institutional officials) who are included in your application. Indicate their roles in respective projects or cores, their institutional titles, their departments, and their organizations.

2. List all of each investigator's grants and contracts (federal, foundations, associations, industrial, pharmaceutical, etc.), both active and pending, including project(s) or core(s) in this application. Provide the grant number and the individual's percent effort in each of the above. Describe all areas in which the grants or contracts overlap with this application, and how such overlaps will be negotiated. Compile information for all professional personnel, and list them alphabetically.

3. Copy the entire budget section of each project and core if these have been changed.

4. Compile supplemental information for each project and core, but only that not already included in the proposal.

a. Curriculum vitae of all professional personnel associated with the project or core, if not included in the application.

b. Selected reprints or manuscripts, representing work related to the scientific content of the project or core.

c. Further description, procedures, materials, hypotheses to be tested, timetable for completion of different studies within the projects, and any other information, if incompletely described in the original application.

d. New data demonstrating feasibility of proposed studies within the projects (figures, tables, photomicrographs, etc.). This information should be presented during the Project or Core Director's presentation at the site visit. Hard copies of slides should be made available to the reviewers at the site visit.

e. Informed consent forms for use of human subjects in research in any of the projects or cores.

f. IRB approval for use of human subjects in each project or core if such was pending during submission of the application.

g. IACUC approval for use of animal subjects in each project or core, if such was pending during submission of the application. (Some Institutes may permit submission of items e, f, and g "just-in-time" when funding is awarded.)

h. Line drawings, detailed cost estimate, and justification of any requested renovation or alteration.

A supplement should not seem to revise a submitted proposal. This is not permitted. But a supplement can correct errors and provide additional data.

The Institutes, Centers, and Divisions of the National Institutes of Health accept a variety of large unsolicited grant applications, such as those for Program Projects and other large, complex coordinated research grants. However, guidelines and policies governing preparation, review, and funding of these applications are not uniform across the NIH and may differ because of a variety of factors such as legislative mandates, fiscal constraints, and programmatic management. Therefore, in order to serve the extramural community better, the NIH advises that prior to submission of any application for an unsolicited, multifaceted grant, applicants communicate with appropriate Institute staff. This action will allow the applicant to be apprised of the guidelines and policies that govern the preparation, review, and funding of such applications for a particular Institute. Of special concern is the fact that the different Institutes have different dollar limits for those multifaceted programs, and applications that exceed these limits will be returned without review.

The assignment of an application to a potential funding source within the NIH is based on scientific guidelines developed for each Institute in conjunction with the CSR and is the responsibility of the CSR, not of the individual Institute. Although the proposal is developed with the help of an Institute Program Manager, it is submitted to the CSR, and then assigned to the Institute the CSR prefers. Thus, when the potential applicant discusses plans for a complex program grant application with the initial Institute contact, he or she is strongly advised to inquire whether other Institutes might be interested. Dual assignment is advantageous.

Since Program Project grants are Institute-specific, the appropriate Institute officer should be contacted to obtain up-to-date information. These individuals change regularly so the best way to start such contacts is to visit the web site of a specific Institute. At <www.nih.gov/icd>, follow the links to the desired Institute, then go to "Funding" or "Grants," and then search for "program awards" and links to program staff.

22

Center Grants

There are several classes of Center grants: Core Center (P30), Specialized Center (P50), Comprehensive Center (P60), and Planning Center (P20).

• *Specialized Center grants* (P50), also called Specialized Centers of Research (SCOR) grants, are designed to provide shared facilities and resources to support multidisciplinary programs of research on specific diseases or biomedical problems. This program is very similar to the Program Project grant (P01) with the exception that each P50 program is usually instigated by an NIH Institute with an RFA and is tracked very closely by the Institute staff. A typical SCOR program (with which Ogden was associated) concerned hypertension and was initiated by the NHLBI. The important thing about SCOR grants is that they are designed by the NIH Institutes with very specific goals in mind. They are awarded on the basis of slavish adherence to the guidelines, which are very specific, the innovative nature of the research program, and the strength of the research team.

• *Comprehensive Center grants* (P60) are designed to bring together into a common focus divergent but related facilities within a given community. P60 grants are usually based within a university, but may involve other related resources such as hospitals, clinics, regional centers, primate colonies, or computer centers. P60 grants may include R01, P01, or P30 grants as integral components. Comprehensive Centers, also solicited by RFAs, usually include community outreach and educational programs. These types of activities are usually not supported by other NIH research awards.

• *Planning Center grants* (P20) are limited grants to support development of larger Center grants. They provide funds for strategic planning and preliminary administrative activities needed to be successful. Very few Institutes use this award mechanism.

- *Core Center grants* (P30) are designed to provide infrastructure support. They are similar to P01 or P50 awards consisting solely of Core Modules.

We have only limited experience with the P60 grant, and there is no real difference between the P50 and Program Project (P01) grants discussed in depth in Chapter 20. Thus, we have elected to concentrate in this chapter on the Core Center grant (Core grant for short). Core grants are receiving more emphasis by many NIH Institutes, and are the only type of Center grant awarded by the NEI. They have a good record for success in fostering the productivity and building up of research groups.

The Core grant is designed to support an independent group of NIH-funded investigators with facilities or services beyond the scope of the usual R01 program. These grants do not support specific research projects, but should enhance the institution's scientific environment and capability for conducting research, facilitate collaborative studies, and support the recruitment of new faculty in a specific NIH program area. From the institutional viewpoint, Core facilities reduce duplication of equipment and staff, and thus save space and effort—precious commodities.

Eligibility of an institution to apply for an NEI Core grant is based on the needs of at least eight R01-type projects that must be funded at the time of proposal submission. Each module or functional unit of the Center Cores must have at least three R01-funded users. The users should be productive, and the larger the participating faculty, the stronger the proposal. The Core faculty should be of excellent quality and should demonstrate a high probability of even greater productivity and excellence as a direct result of the availability of the proposed Core facilities and services. Eligibility requirements vary with different Institutes. The faculty does not need to be in a single department, or even in a single institution. However, the faculty must be focused on an integrated area of research targeted by an Institute, and must interact. The Vision Science Core grant to the Doheny Eye Foundation at the University of Southern California (USC) has a faculty with appointments in ophthalmology, physiology and biophysics, molecular and cell biology, pathology, and pediatrics. The laboratories of these investigators are in separate buildings at USC and across town at the Children's Hospital of Los Angeles. Their proposal was strong because the 18 faculty were well funded and productive. There was widespread collaboration among them involving many areas of research considered important by the NEI. The group produced well over 100 publications each year, all of which involved the use of at least one of the five Core Modules.

Center grants (P30, P50, and others) are currently available from most of the Institutes in a multitude of programmatic areas. These are easily viewed on the NIH web site (<www.nih.gov/icd>). The appropriate application form for these proposals is the PHS 398, the same form used for the R01. *It is essential that applicants contact the appropriate Institute staff for advice and additional information about specific programs before applying.*

Core grant proposals describe facilities or services that are needed by existing funded faculty. They present a plan by which the needs will be provided, and they describe in detail how the research of each user will be enhanced in quantity and in quality by the Core Center. The criteria of Core grant review are based on these expectations. Foremost is the quality of the faculty. A strong research faculty is probably growing, productive, independent, and publishing important papers in the best journals. An older established faculty is unlikely to be very persuasive that their research needs the facilities of a P30 if they have managed very well without it for 15 years!

Collaboration enhancement is an important review criterion. The facilities and services of Cores are usually arranged in modules, each headed by a Director. Use of the module by other investigators forms a natural pathway for collaboration among them. This is less persuasive if each Core Module Director has already been collaborating with all of the users. The proposal must demonstrate "added value." It is useful to recruit from other departments for the proposed new Core facilities, as this should lead to interdisciplinary collaborations.

Increased productivity should be soundly argued. This may result from better equipment, better access to a facility, or availability of a technology not previously at hand. For instance, an Ultrastructure Core with automated tissue processing equipment might greatly increase tissue throughput since the processing would be done on a 24-hour basis. Such an argument should be supported with detailed discussions of the time required to process a single block and justification of the assertion that a specific number of blocks will be processed. This, however, is not enough. The new equipment will reduce the required technician time, and the use of this free time must be accounted for in terms of more rapid advancement of the participating R01 projects. Productivity may also be improved if a facility is close at hand. If a DNA synthesizer at a neighboring institution was used previously, its availability down the hall would clearly improve productivity. Again, if time is saved, it is important to provide details of how it will be used to advance the goals of the R01 projects.

Quality of research should also be enhanced by the proposed facility. This is usually based on the availability of new technology that will take a given study to a deeper level. Quality improvement may also result from the availability of a module supervisor who will oversee an instrument, such as a confocal microscope, to ensure its continued good function and servicing, and to provide training and supervision of users. Improved quality may result from collaboration of experts; hence the importance of collaboration in the Core guidelines.

Core facilities benefit everyone in a research group, particularly those who are not funded. Such facilities are commonly used to collect pilot data that are later used to support a research proposal. Although this type of benefit is obvious, very desirable, and applicable to practically all groups, it is not worth much in the review. *What counts is the number of NIH-supported faculty who will benefit* and how compelling the presentation is that the quality and quantity of their research on a topic of interest to the Institute will be enhanced.

Recruitment of new faculty is also a benefit derived from a Core Center grant. The new faculty should be identified as fully as possible. The best case is based on a Biosketch from the anticipated new member and a letter indicating why the proposed facility is important. Such claims should be credible. They are counterproductive if, for instance, someone on the Study Section knows that the proposed new member has accepted a job elsewhere.

Faculty strength is very important. Every member should be publishing regularly in good journals. Participation in Study Sections is a strong plus. The strongest proposal lists only funded faculty, but some faculty members are invariably weaker in funding than others. Heavy use of a module by unfunded faculty is not very persuasive unless they are highly productive and do excellent work. Unfortunately, some Study Sections concentrate on faculty weakness rather than strength, but this can be minimized by deleting the weak members. It is far better to have a small strong group than a larger one containing some obviously weak members.

A *focused program of research* is stronger than a broad program. Most departmental groups applying for Center Core grants are reasonably focused. If focus is not real, and the faculty is large enough to permit it, selection of participating faculty should be made to enhance the perception that the faculty share research interests and are therefore likely to collaborate. Thus, a group from several different departments interested in the interrelationship of diabetes, obesity, and hypertension, for instance, would be stronger than a group from the same department interested in retinal degeneration, cataracts, and dry eye syndrome, three totally unrelated conditions. The research of the group should also show evidence of continuity and provide promise, based on past performances, of continued steady progress toward the same or similar goals. The best evidence of this kind of continuity is research grants in their 6th or more year of funding. The best evidence of collaboration is multiauthored publications.

Budgets of Core Centers vary among Institutes, but generally are capped at about $500,000 per year or less. Thus the smallest Core grants of two or three service modules might provide direct costs approximating an R01. Most Core grants have more than three Core Modules and proportionately less support for each. In developing a Core proposal, consultation with the Institute manager is essential. This should be done early on to avoid unproductive effort. Center direction and administration are key review considerations for all P-type proposals. The Director must be a successful scientist who is also known for his or her administrative skills and ability to bring the group of participating "independent scientists" together.

Core Modules provide scientific expertise in the form of a skilled specialist or specialized shared equipment, or both. The module personnel typically perform services for occasional users who lack their own technicians or supervise the use of the equipment by the technicians of heavy users. Thus the module technician often functions as a Core Supervisor and is responsible for maintenance of equipment, quality control, and training of users. A strong justification for these module supervisors is that they will enhance both the quantity and the quality of the work done in the module, and will demonstrably facilitate the work of specific Institute-funded investigators.

TYPES OF MODULES

There are many different kinds of modules that can compose Cores. These modules may be found in any of the different types of Center grants and in Program Project grants. Below, 13 are briefly discussed. These are common, but are by no means the only possibilities.

1. *Administrative Module.* This module is not allowed by some Institutes. Unlike the Program Project, it is a difficult module to justify for a Core grant since it is generally accepted that the university is responsible

for providing administrative support to funded investigators. If a group is sufficiently large, however, it may be possible to justify provision of an editorial assistant to assist with editing manuscripts. This person should not be a word processor and should handle at least 30 manuscripts per year. Services can include reference verification and literature searches. A strong argument for such a position is a current practice of obtaining such services on a freelance basis at a considerably higher cost than the salary of a part-time or full-time editor.

The justification for the editorial assistant must be NIH-supported work. Book chapter and review editing must not be proposed unless directly supported and required by an NIH grant. The cost of an editor varies across the country; an average wage in southern California in 2001 was $45,000–55,000 per year plus benefits. The total cost of an Administrative Module featuring only an editorial assistant might include $2000–3000 in supplies, but no equipment, and would be approximately $50,000–60,000 per year.

Some Cores include purchasing agents, grants managers, statisticians, secretaries, etc. These positions are exceedingly difficult to justify. Generally, the Administrative Core is the most difficult of all modules to justify, even without positions such as secretaries to burden it, and you are well advised to request scientific rather than administrative modules.

2. *Biometry Module.* This is a popular and easily justified Core Module for a group of eight or more investigators who conduct clinical research, human genetics studies, or research heavily dependent on statistical analysis. Justification is facilitated if many of those involved are directly engaged in clinical research. There is widespread recognition that the quality of clinical research is enhanced if experimental design, data management, and data analysis are handled by a biometrist. This has led to new programs of support for Biometry Modules.

Use by basic science investigators strengthens a Biometry Module but is insufficient by itself to justify a proposal. The strongest Biometry Module is headed by an experienced biometrist with at least 2 years involvement in clinical trials after the Ph.D. and 10 or more publications in the field. The group of users should be composed primarily of clinicians, with a good funding history and experience in clinical research. Unlike the other modules, R01 support is usually not a prerequisite for this module.

A strong justification for a Biometry Module is that it will facilitate development of new projects by experienced faculty who are simply too busy to develop the protocols and necessary "Manual of Procedures." The latter task is often handled by an experienced clinical coordinator working under the supervision of the biometrist. Most Biometry Cores also assist with data analysis, and so feature some computer equipment and a data entry specialist. In the latter case, it may only be necessary to have a half-time biometrist.

In a typical Biometry Core, the biometrist meets with the faculty to develop the experimental design and protocol. Working with a clinical research coordinator, the biometrist guides the development of the Manual of Procedures, often a lengthy document describing all procedures, and the data entry forms. The research coordinator trains those who gather data, if necessary, in the acceptable procedures for the tests and supervises data acquisition with random inspections to determine that correct procedures are followed and data are correctly entered. The data entry person works from the data entry forms and, under the supervision of the biometrist, provides the computer analysis of the data and necessary reports, graphs, histograms, etc.

The budget for such a module will be at least $60,000 per year and could include some computer equipment (not more than $10,000) in the first year.

Recall that a half-time position requires about 900 hours of identified work. A clinical protocol could reasonably require about 90 hours of effort. On this basis, a half-time biometrist should work on 10 projects in a year, one each from a faculty of 10 clinicians. A manual of procedures will take 2 to 4 weeks of preparation—a maximum of 20 projects in a year for a full-time person. Data entry requires perhaps 10 minutes per patient per visit and data analysis about 2 weeks per study. Whether the data entry clerk is full or part-time will depend on the numbers of patients and visits, and the types of analyses.

The important point is that the justification for these positions should be based on calculated hours of involvement, and this should be supportable on the basis of the publication records and research experience of the faculty.

3. *Clinical Research Center (CRC) Module.* These are similar to Biometry Modules, with which they may be combined. They are not a substitute for the General Clinical Research Centers (GCRCs) supported by the NCRR, but serve a similar function on a much-reduced scale. The CRC Module provides the physical facilities to conduct clinical trials. A Clinical Research Center could justify a substantial equipment budget in the first year, and space for patient examination and data storage.

Personnel could include nursing staff, technicians, and a clinical coordinator. These must be justified in terms of the services performed, the time each service requires, and the number of times a service will be performed. It is rather unlikely that a CRC Module would be awarded to a group that was not already heavily engaged in clinical research, i.e., already participating in a number of funded clinical trials. It is also very unlikely that a CRC Module would be awarded if a GCRC were available.

4. *Computer Modules.* These are among the most difficult to justify, yet are often very useful. The Core consists of a single individual, in most cases, with programming experience and a broad knowledge of modern personal computers, hardware, and software. These individuals are extremely helpful in large groups but are difficult to justify from the standpoint of research. In most large groups, those using computers extensively either are themselves experts or employ their own specialized computer people. The needs of users vary so much that it is difficult to assemble a large enough group of moderate users to justify a professional. Development of research software is often too time-consuming for a Core to handle. Finally, identified projects may require computer programming at a high level initially, but this is usually not sustained and complicates justification.

To be successful, a Computer Module must provide convincing evidence that the requested support will enhance the quality and quantity of research now and in the future for at least four to six funded investigators. The cost of such a Core should be $50,000–60,000 per year, and could include some equipment.

There are other types of Cores that use computers and may need programming (Morphometry, Imaging, and Biometry). These are considered separately.

5. *Histology-Histopathology Module.* This is one of the most common and easily supported Core Modules, providing it supports modern procedures such as *in situ* hybridization. Histology requires a trained technician and certain equipment that occupies substantial space. Many different types of research require some histology. It is wasteful of space and equipment if these routine studies are done in each laboratory. A shared facility makes good sense and is easy to justify if the faculty have NIH-funded projects requiring histology. Histology Modules typically charge a fee per slide or tissue block. These charges are easily justified and simplify budget preparation for R01 grants. To justify a full-time supervisor/

technician for a Histology Module, approximately 1000 tissue blocks should be processed per year.

It is not reasonable for one investigator who produces 1000 tissue blocks per year to propose to do this in a Core Histology Module. That investigator obviously needs a full-time histologist. The module equipment could be used, however, and the use supervised by the Module Supervisor, with training provided to the technicians of the users as needed.

6. *Instrumentation Module.* Large research groups often share equipment such as ultracentrifuges, freezers, DNA synthesizers, amino acid synthesizers and sequencers, scintillation and Coulter counters, flow cytometers, liquid nitrogen storage tanks, and some PCR units. Someone must have the responsibility for maintenance and supply for each instrument. A strong argument for an Instrumentation Module can be made if the instruments can be located in one area and are actually shared, and the users are funded. Most investigators usually prefer to have frequently used instruments in their own laboratories. However, as space becomes scarce, removal of large equipment to a central location where it can be shared becomes attractive. The reclaimed space compensates for the inconvenience. This is especially true if someone else takes responsibility for maintenance and supervision of the instruments.

Instrument Modules usually operate by sign-up sheet with a supervisor who trains users and maintains the equipment and necessary supplies. Such a module might have several faculty codirectors, each expert in the use of different instruments and each responsible for the proper training of the Core Module Supervisor, who in turn trains the technicians if necessary. The sign-up sheets are particularly helpful at renewal time to verify the level of usage. They should be carefully maintained and saved for this purpose. The Core Supervisor may also collect data for unfunded pilot projects of new investigators, and should maintain lists of Core-supported pilot projects that developed into successful R01 proposals or publications.

The reviewers must determine several things: (1) that the equipment is used by NIH-funded users; (2) that the Supervisor and/or Core Module Directors are expert with each of the instruments; and (3) that use of the module will improve both the quantity and the quality of work.

The module budget is generally for the supervisor's salary, some supplies, and maintenance contracts for the instruments, usually $5,000–10,000 per instrument. The total budget should probably be about $50,000–60,000.

Equipment can be requested as a part of any Core Module but this is not usually done. It is certainly unwise to request an expensive instrument as part of an Instrumentation Module, except with especially strong justification. The instruments should be at hand and in use, and hopefully available to move into the new space dedicated to the Core Center. The module facilitates shared use and improves the quality of data obtained through better supervision and training of the users.

7. *Media Services Module.* This module usually includes shared facilities for photography for publications, artwork, preparation of slides and presentation materials, and occasionally even word processing. This is a difficult module to justify by any but the largest research groups. The justification must rest on use by NIH-supported investigators to produce material related to NIH-supported research. The amount of artwork involved in most kinds of research is insufficient to provide the demand needed. Also, it must be shown that the university facilities cannot accommodate the special needs or demands of the funded research projects. Convenience is not a sufficient justification, and preparation of teaching materials should not be mentioned. Activities associated with teaching and production of books, treatises, and review articles are not supportable by research funds and cannot be used to justify a Media Module.

A Media Module justification must be based on numbers of special illustrations or services provided and a calculation of the hours required for each. Also, in this age, it is tenuous to suggest that your graphs must be drawn by an artist, when your peers are using computers.

8. *Morphometry Module.* Morphometric equipment is often included as part of an Ultrastructure or Histology Module, or may constitute a separate unit. Morphometry Modules usually feature expensive computer-based quantitative morphometric equipment such as the ACAS confocal microscope, Quantimet, or Zeiss IBAS automated microscopes with or without fluorescence. The confocal microscope particularly is new and is rapidly becoming used by most investigators. Most potential users would like to gain access to this equipment to do what they are already doing, but better, more efficiently, faster, and with quantitation. These are valid reasons, but more compelling justifications highlight new scientific abilities. The best reason to get new equipment is that it will support new research. The obvious "catch-22" is that the reviewers may not accept that a particular new application is feasible without pilot data, but without the instrument, how can one collect pilot data? It can and must be done! If the instrument is not available, use one in another department or

institution, or the manufacturer may be enlisted to provide the data. This is usually a successful approach. The pilot data are essential for a strong application.

As with other module types, the strength of the proposal is ultimately based on the credibility and credentials of the users. With a module based on a new instrument, it is difficult to establish the likelihood that the proposed users will actually use it. It is common practice to enlist the aid of as many funded scientists as possible in support of a module. If none of them have ever used the new equipment, there will be considerable doubt that they ever will use it. This can be allayed with pilot data from every user. If this is not possible, divide the presentation of users into those with pilot data (primary users) and those without pilot data (secondary users). The major support will come from the primary users.

It is actually difficult to justify morphometric equipment. Examination of the justifications from many of the prospective users will usually reveal that they could accomplish what they propose with a much less expensive instrument. These users should not be listed as primary. To do so will certainly weaken the proposal. It is also common for a prospective user to propose uses for which the instrument is not designed. These must be eliminated entirely to avoid the accusation that "the users do not understand the uses and limitations of the instrument."

The request for a Quantimet to perform automated counts of autoradiographic grains is a good case in point. The instrument works very well on thin specimens with only moderate labeling, but accuracy drops off drastically as grains become confluent. If the emulsion is not perfectly planar, automatic focusing must be provided. However, given the right materials, the instrument performs very well. Unfortunately, there are usually only one or two users whose material is perfectly suited to the instrument, and many others for whom the uses are questionable at best. The Quantimet cannot be easily adapted to automatically count and measure nerve fibers, corneal endothelial cells, muscle fibers, or Betz cells, or to a host of other applications. To suggest such uses is to invite criticism of why it will not work, and rejection of the proposal. The dilemma of proposing a Morphometric Module is that many users are needed, and yet their individual applications must be valid.

9. *Photography–Darkroom Module.* Growth of research groups is often attended by proliferation of small darkrooms and photographic facilities. Those researchers using histology, autoradiography, morphometry, and electron microscopy particularly need darkroom facilities. From the

institutional standpoint, this proliferation wastes space. A central facility with an experienced photographic technician to maintain fresh solutions is easily justified. If it contains enlargers and automatic print processing equipment, it can relieve the usual congestion around the EM darkrooms as well as serve as a general-purpose facility for preparation of prints for publication, slides for presentations, and photography of specimens. This type of module may overlap with, but is different from, the Media Services Module described above.

Review criteria include the number of NIH-funded users and careful evaluation of overlap in the funding of individual grants, many of which include funds for photographic chemicals and other supplies. These must not duplicate supplies requested for the module. While each of the users might supply their own film and paper, it would be unrealistic for each to supply his or her own chemicals. As with each type of module, it is important that the competing proposals of the users reflect the availability of module services and not request duplicating funds. On the other hand, a morphologist doing a lot of autoradiography and photomicrography might have such heavy darkroom requirements that use of a shared facility would be impractical. Such an investigator needs to be self-sufficient and should not be listed as a module user.

It is appropriate to request funds to renovate existing space into a Core darkroom and to purchase some equipment such as developing tanks, print processors, and enlargers. A better approach, however, is to request the space renovation without equipment, if the latter can be moved into the space from individual laboratories. It should be established that the facilities will be used to at least 80% capacity. Since much of the work will be done by user technicians, the supervisor should not be at more than 25% effort. With reasonable supplies, the budget should be about $40,000 for salaries and supplies.

10. *Shop Module.* These modules are basic to research groups involved in bioengineering or physiology, but are very difficult to justify otherwise. It is not cost effective to build your own equipment if it can be obtained commercially. Electronic equipment is too complex for repair by any but professional technicians, but now such repair often can be circumvented by simply replacing a circuit board. This can be done by any investigator.

Research groups doing bioengineering development usually are based on extensive shop capability and do not require shared facilities, so the proper combination of needs to justify a Shop Module are seldom found.

There is no question that a central facility employing a "jack-of-all-trades" machinist/electrician (with a supply of plastic and metal stock, fuses, machine screws, nuts and bolts, brass tubing fittings, gas fittings, and hand tools, along with a drill press, band saw, mill, and lathe) is of great general utility to a wide variety of laboratory researchers. It is probably best to provide such a shared resource from university funds. A shop might be justified on the basis of specific projects or instruments being developed, but this is strongest as a separate proposal in which the science can be fully presented. Also, most universities have such shops. They are usually slow, expensive, and inconvenient, but these defects are not strong justifications for duplicating a facility.

11. *Tissue Culture Module.* This is a common module in recent years due to a widespread increase in *in vitro* studies. Heavy users of tissue culture are usually independent but can benefit from a central facility for dishwashing, autoclaving, purchasing, liquid nitrogen storage, media preparation, and technician training. Occasional tissue culture users may benefit from a central source of specific cell lines, such as fibroblasts or retinal pigment epithelial cells, used in generating animal models of human diseases. For instance, the injection of fibroblasts into the eye of rabbits causes a condition similar to proliferative vitreoretinopathy in humans. This animal model has been widely studied in an attempt to develop methods of prevention or treatment. The investigations involve primarily *in vivo* studies of the pathogenesis and treatment of the condition. If an outside source of fibroblasts is available, more laboratory resources can be brought to bear on the primary problem. If several such projects are underway, provision of cell lines from a Tissue Culture Module is cost efficient and contributes directly to an improved project. Tissue Culture Modules may also provide specialized instrumentation, such as Coulter counters, scintillation counters, special facilities for work with radioactive substances, and time-lapse photography. Alternatively, such instrumentation may be included in an Instrumentation Core (see above).

Highly specialized tissue culture facilities such as those approved for HIV work are usually associated with individual investigators, although they are appropriate for a module if at least three funded projects require their use.

A Tissue Culture Module could consist simply of an expert in tissue culture who maintains some shared cell lines and trains and supervises individual technicians working in different laboratories. It is more common, however, for a Core to consist of a laboratory with the necessary support equipment, such as an autoclave or coldroom, and several separate culture rooms, each with a laminar flow hood and an incubator.

12. *Ultrastructure Module.* These modules are easily justified by most research groups with Core grants. Funds are usually provided for a facility supervisor and equipment maintenance, with a budget of about $50,000–60,000. As with the other service modules, heavy users provide their own technicians who operate the equipment [electron microscopes (EMs), microtomes, dark rooms, etc.] under the supervision of the Core person who also trains the technicians up to high performance standards. These facilities require constant maintenance with regular replacement of gas tanks, photographic chemicals, etc.

The Core Supervisor may also provide a limited EM service for occasional users who have too little work to justify the expense of a technician. Many proposals list part-time EM technicians, but it is rarely possible to hire such a person on a part-time basis. If a Core is available, the funds can be conveniently used to support a project carried out by Core personnel on what amounts to a contract basis.

Some Ultrastructure Modules offer specialized morphology support with photomicroscopes, fluorescence or confocal microscopes, cryostats, or facilities for autoradiography. The specialized equipment is maintained and supervised by the Core Supervisor and use is allocated by sign-up sheet. These sheets should be kept in a file and used to apportion maintenance costs and to verify usage at the time of the grant renewal. It may be convenient to combine ultrastructure and morphometry functions in a single module; however, it is probably better to keep the responsibilities and technology of a Core as focused as possible since the supervisor should be expert in all aspects of its work.

Maintenance contracts may also be a substantial budgetary item of an Ultrastructure Core. EM and SEM maintenance contracts are typically between $5000 and $10,000 per year, and are appropriate to include in the Core budget.

A problem faced by Core administrators concerns the fair sharing of costs by funded users. One way to ensure this is to charge them a proportion of the maintenance contracts of the instruments. Yearly use should be a matter of record and easily justified in a proposal. Those who will use an EM 10 hours per week should be encouraged to ask for 25% of the contract costs. These requests are seldom refused if use of the instrument is justified. Some Cores charge users by the hour; others levy no charges and in effect subsidize the users, who very likely have requested such funds in their R01 budgets anyway. If the funds are not allocated for the module, the users are free to use them for other purposes.

Supply items such as diamond knives are also appropriate for an EM Core, providing their use can be substantiated. A strong justification for a diamond knife is a project that requires some serial sectioning.

Quality control is particularly important for an Ultrastructure Module since the reputation of a group may be damaged by poor-quality micrographs. The Module Supervisor is in a position to critique the output of the unit and provide assistance where it is needed, which is an important function to emphasize.

13. *Vivarium Module.* These modules must provide services not provided already by the university's vivarium services. Proposed services may be trained surgical assistants or operating room personnel, technicians to perform special tests (e.g., EEG, ERG, photography, ultrasound, or radiography), production and maintenance of shared animal models, maintenance of large colonies of transgenic mice or colonies of purebred dogs with a genetic defect, etc. If the activity is sufficiently large, it may well justify existence as an individual Core, i.e., a Transgenic Mouse Core or Atherosclerosis Primate Core. Such Core Modules are possible only if the user group is sufficiently large.

The basis of such a request is the necessity for regular attention beyond that routinely afforded by institutional vivarium staff. As an example, a group of several hypertension researchers would profit from a Core colony of SHR rats maintained on special diets with daily blood pressure readings. A single technician, hired to perform the tests and keep the records of the colony for use by five or six projects, would be very cost efficient compared with each of the projects providing these functions separately. Also, the number of animals required could be reduced by the sharing of animals among different projects. Such a module request is strong if each user has a funded NIH grant, if it is demonstrated that the number of animals used will be reduced, and if it is clear that the quality of the data will be improved.

Labor-intensive projects involving animals are best staffed with full-time personnel hired by the individual project. It is only in those projects requiring limited access to highly specialized procedures that use of Core technicians makes sense. However, if a number of projects require full-time animal technicians and many specialized procedures, it may be possible to request a Vivarium Supervisor to train the technicians and supervise their use of shared facilities, such as cameras, operating microscopes, lasers, and ultrasounds. This requires solid justification based on the need for such training and supervision, and the proposition that untrained technicians can be hired for less money and adequately trained for the work required.

Vivarium procedures requiring sterile surgery involve a wide range of supplies. A Core facility can function as a central supply in a cost-effective way if there are enough users.

Justification of vivarium personnel must be based on actual hours of work accomplished by each employee. This requires that every procedure be described accurately as to preparation, execution, and clean-up time. Justification is then easy if it can be shown that the total procedures required by the funded grants of the users involve about 1800 hours per year for each full-time employee. The tabulation of procedures should be specific (anesthesia rat, anesthesia rabbit, anesthesia primate, etc,).

One method by which a Core Vivarium Module can operate is to set a charge for every procedure, from taking rat blood pressure with a tail cuff to bypass surgery in dogs. The cost of the procedures is then recovered from the users.

Review considerations for Vivarium Modules bear heavily on overlap between the services of the module and the resources of individual grants. If a number of grants provide funds for part-time animal technicians, it is very difficult to justify additional funds for vivarium personnel. This generates problems with new vivaria modules. Prior to the first competitive renewal of such modules, the users should remove overlapping personnel from their grants. A strong argument for continuation of a Vivarium Module is that five or six good projects are based on its existence and could not function without it.

There are many other types of Core Modules that can be suggested; Molecular Biology and Hybridoma modules are two that come to mind. The principles of grantsmanship discussed above will pertain to any module. Contact the appropriate Institute Program Director for help in developing the proposal and identifying supportable and unsupportable modules. A Core grant is a tremendous boon to an active research group. It will relieve individual grants of support expenses that are a real encumbrance to review. It will provide strengths in many subtle ways that are widely beneficial. Core grants are only a burden for the PI, who must be willing to expend the time for the betterment of his or her research family. It is an effort that pays great dividends when successful.

=====23=====

Construction Grants

When an outline of this book was submitted to the publisher, one of the reviewers, obviously an experienced grantsperson, voiced the opinion that the sections on Core, Program Project, Training, and Construction grants should be eliminated—no novice would attempt such projects, and anyone who did would not need tutoring. We do not agree with this attitude. Every investigator is called on, sooner or later, to develop proposals that are outside his or her areas of expertise. Also, there is a first time for everyone with each type of proposal. We believe our experience and ideas about these institutional programs will be of interest to others, and we hope they will also be helpful.

Construction awards are highly individual. Generic rules of grantsmanship are obvious for R01s, but less defined for these kinds of institutional projects. Our comments therefore are directed more to a process of grantsmanship that has been developed gradually, and with increasing effectiveness. This is a process that can be applied to any type of large project.

Construction funds for new construction or alteration/renovation of research facilities are available as C06 awards from the NIH, through the National Center for Research Resources (NCRR), as determined each year by specific congressional appropriations. Before 1994, only the NCI, NHLBI, NIA, NEI, and NCRR had construction authority. Since then, construction funds for all biomedical purposes have been available mainly through the NCRR. In fiscal year 2000, 49 construction awards were made by the NCRR (3 of these were funded by other Institutes). The availability of funds is limited, and competition is always keen. Funds available for Construction grants in the year 2001 were $75 million. One-to-one dollar matching is required, using nonfederal funds. Twenty-five percent of available construction funds are set aside for those institutions that have achieved special recognition as Centers of Excellence (COE).

COE awards are usually made to large institutions with a relatively large minority enrollment.

Political factors such as regional location may play a subtle role in fund allocation at various federal agencies. Funds are allocated for construction as a result of the congressional budgeting process. A Request for Application (RFA) or a Request for Proposal (RFP) usually announces new programs. Most RFPs reach general distribution only about 3 months or less prior to the proposal deadline. Thus, those who are aware of an upcoming RFP are in a position to begin proposal preparation well in advance of those who receive the announcement through regular channels. This can be immensely important in a construction project, which will probably require consensus faculty support, substantial planning, architectural input, development of 50% matching funds, local approvals, and a cost analysis in addition to a well-written proposal supported by hard data. It is very difficult to prepare a strong construction proposal in a short period of time.

Some construction and renovation funds are available for specific purposes. The NCRR program was originally designed to alleviate hardships caused by new federal regulations concerning vivarium facilities. For instance, vivarium construction or upgrading has been supported to permit bringing existing facilities up to changes in standards. Primates now are required to have available special exercise cages. These cost about $30,000 each. RFAs called for proposals to upgrade animal resource facilities with grants of up to $500,000 for construction costs and $200,000 for fixed equipment. As with all Construction grants, matching funds were required. From time to time, an Institute will provide Construction grants to support specific types of activity. For instance, the National Eye Institute (NEI) provided grants in the 1980s to build clinical research facilities for eye research.

Strong proposals are essential to secure funding in an intensely competitive arena. Generally, it is difficult to get Congress to approve funds for construction, and the occasion of their availability leads to extreme competition. Proposals for such funds must be well written and well justified, tightly organized, and supported by careful architectural detail to be competitive. Success is based on the number, strength, and productivity of facility users. There must be a compelling presentation that the proposed facilities will lead to expansion of research activity with an increase in both the quantity and the quality of the work performed by the group. In the case of animal facilities, upgrading to the new standards is justification enough if the facility is used by a sufficient number of investigators with R01 grants.

The nature of a strong construction/renovation proposal is defined by certain obvious principles. The proposal:

1. Must accurately meet the criteria of the funding program, for example, upgrading of a vivarium to meet new standards
2. Must come from a strong research institution
3. Must represent the efforts of a strong research group with multiple NIH grants
4. Must present a project that will clearly benefit this faculty
5. Must demonstrate strong administrative and institutional support
6. Must show the necessary matching funds

Preapplication information is crucial to a successful application. Since competition for construction dollars is keen and often involves many strong programs, grantsmanship may be the key to success. Construction programs always represent a response to a widely perceived need. Guidelines for review are prepared with this need in mind. It is essential that those responsible for preparing construction proposals be fully informed concerning the purpose of the particular program. If members of an Institute council are known, their knowledge of the Institute program should be sought. This in no way suggests a conflict of interest, if only information is requested. It is essential that the NCRR Program Director or official responsible for the program also be contacted. Every effort should be made to understand the concerns of the council or other advisory body that led to initiation of the particular program. These concerns should be made the central theme of the proposal.

The motivation of some of those who champion construction programs is apt to be provincial. If their own institution needs funds to construct new facilities for clinical research, they may be led to exhort the NIH and Congress by pleading the dire necessity of such facilities.

Once the basis of the program is fully understood, the proposal can be drafted in rough form. This draft should be sent to the Program Director in the form of a one- to two-page letter, followed up with a telephone contact to assess the Director's reaction. Most Program Directors realize that the success of their programs, indeed their success as directors, is dependent on the quality of the proposals submitted to them. They are usually generous with their time and their comments to direct you onto the best path and away from distractions in your proposals. Foolish is the

Principal Investigator who fails to take full advantage of all the help available from the concerned bureaucrat.

In this preproposal stage, it is necessary to solidify the support of your own university. This may require surmounting an in-house review and competition, particularly in the case of those programs limited to a single proposal from an institution. All proposals are submitted by the institution, of course, not by an individual, and require the signature of the appropriate university official and commitment of the appropriate matching funds.

Matching funds are required for most Construction grants. These proposals represent a great deal of time and effort, and are expensive to put together since they require the services of an architect. Matching funds should be identified and, if possible, secured before the project gets very far underway. Ogden still remembers with considerable emotion the culmination of his first successful construction project. His proposal received the highest priority among those reviewed, and in due time he was notified that it would be funded, only to learn that his institution had decided not to provide the promised matching funds, and declined a grant of over $500,000!

To avoid such a disaster, you must be sure that your efforts accurately reflect the priorities and goals of your institution. It is not unreasonable to request a memo from a responsible official, such as the Dean, or even the University President, stating support for the project, assuring matching funds will be available, and requesting that you go ahead with the project. It is unlikely that you will obtain this type of support unless your project properly supports institutional goals.

Construction grants also require a commitment from the university that the new space will be used for at least 20 years for the stated purpose (generally, biomedical research). This commitment actually is not as harsh as it seems. It requires only that, if the space should be removed from its stated service, it be replaced with equivalent dedicated space at university expense, and approved by NIH staff.

PLANNING IS ESSENTIAL

Faculty support for the construction project is an important review criterion. As the proposal materializes, it should reflect a wide faculty input. Start the process by circulating a memo to all concerned faculty members seeking their support and input. This should be followed by contact with respondents and, if possible, scheduling of meetings. The initial interaction of interested faculty should provide an acceptable consensus about the general features of the project. Responsibility for different portions of the proposal should be assigned to the most qualified individuals. The initial planning of a construction project will proceed smoothly if the prime motivator is also the PI. In this case, the nature of the project is obvious from the outset. The PI can provide clear definition of the space, its use, and a realistic estimate of its cost to prospective supporters. The main challenge is to get sufficient faculty behind the project to convince officialdom of the likelihood of successful funding and the value of the project to the institution.

Often, however, an investigator is asked by the university to be PI on a project that represents the development of a new area designed to support recruitment of new faculty. For instance, consider the following scenario. A medical school decides to make a major commitment to molecular biology with a new building and 20–30 new faculty positions. Molecular biologists currently work in a variety of departments with their own research space, and will not directly benefit from the new development. An eminent scientist has agreed to head up the program when space becomes available. The project will cost millions and the development office has already raised much of the funds. The Dean would like a federal contribution and an appropriate RFA is current. Although the Dean's office will submit the proposal, a faculty member has the honor of being Project Director and putting it together. The following is the abstract of a typical and recently funded Construction grant, accessed through the CRISP database of the NIH.

Abstract: The proposed construction is a renovation of an existing laboratory building at the Oklahoma Medical Research Foundation (OMRF) to replace scientific offices and research laboratories that support 15 current faculty in the Department of Immunobiology and Cancer and the Department of Arthritis and Immunology. The proposed construction is an integral part of a multiple phase master plan to modernize this portion of the OMRF laboratory facilities over a 10 year period with the intent of providing research space that adheres to current safety standards for biomedical research laboratories. The first phase is under construction and will be completed on April 1, 1999. All funds have been raised from donations to complete this additional 8,000 square feet of new research space. In previous years, OMRF completed renovation of over 48,000 square feet (1,2, 3 west and south wings) of outdated 1950 era research space. OMRF's next construction project represents phase 2 of the current master plan. Phase 2 construction will begin on 4/15/99 and include a new ADA-compliant entrance, handicapped bathrooms, and shared conference and research office space to connect the newly renovated south wing to the east wing of the OMRF building on the 3rd and 4th level. OMRF requests a NIH Facilities Grant for the 3rd phase of our existing master plan. The specific aim of this proposal is to provide modern, safe research facilities for scientists with research programs in molecular immunology and genetics, located on the 3rd and 4th floors of the east wing. Important safety and environmental improvements need to be made in this research building. The cellular and genetic research requires new improved core Lab support and some additional biosafety level 2 laboratories. In addition, this project will support improved scientific interaction by connecting this newly renovated space in the east wing to the research activities in the south wing through the completion of the phase 2 project that is described above. Safety and environmental improvements are currently necessary. Handicap accessibility will be addressed in the phase 2 project that will be completed prior to the construction of the 3rd phase renovation of the proposed 3rd and 4th floor east wing. This proposal for phase 3 construction will provide fire sprinklers, new ventilation systems, additional ADA-compliant bathrooms and core lab support to improve research efficiency.

The strength of such a proposal will depend largely on the enthusiasm of the existing faculty for the project, and the challenge to the PI is to produce a plan with broad-based faculty support. In these circumstances, a committee of faculty, chaired by the PI, should outline the project with the help of its future director. Faculty members are most easily involved if they stand to gain new space from the project. However, construction projects are not persuasive if they do not expand existing research capacity. To the extent that existing productive research space is replaced by the new space, the proposal is weakened. The best arrangement is for the new facility to provide new capabilities for current faculty and for additional faculty whose expertise and productivity are strong and whose activities are very well described. As an example, special animal facilities to support a core colony of transgenic mice might strengthen and expand existing programs. The goal of the initial planning process is to produce a project, or a piece of a larger project, that fits an existing RFA, has the enthusiastic support of NIH-funded faculty, and meets institutional priorities.

A construction committee may lead to a stronger proposal. It will be better prepared and stronger if it reflects the input of numerous faculty members. This input is conveniently obtained by constituting a committee, by having regular meetings, by partitioning work among the members, and by obtaining reviews of the developing document. Unfortunately, the burden of preparation always falls to one individual. In the best circumstances, each member of the committee will take responsibility for and write a different section. The purpose of the meetings is to provide motivation for each member to complete the assigned work and to review progress. These proposals are usually prepared with inadequate time, so continuous progress is essential if a last minute rush is to be avoided. This is best accomplished by setting hard deadlines for each component and holding regular meetings to ensure that the deadlines will be met.

In a well-balanced committee, each member will represent and have the authority to act for a separate constituency, the sum of which includes all possible users. The PI should provide the necessary administrative support for all members if necessary. An important criterion of project strength is the effectiveness of its administration. This is best evaluated from the perspective of the proposal itself and how well the writing was organized.

A serious liability of writing a proposal by a committee is fragmentation of the presentation. The product may look like a committee wrote it. The PI should rewrite all portions of the proposal sufficiently to give it a consistent presentation. It is essential that every page, including the many Biosketches, feature the same font and format. This needs to be organized at the outset, with identification of who will be responsible for the final product (usually the PI).

Time Is of the Essence

Construction proposals must be supported by professional architectural drawings, cost estimates, and city, county, and state approvals, and must be cleared by the state clearing house or "Single Point of Contact" (SPOC). This takes time. The approvals must be completed within 60 days of submission.

THE PROPOSAL PLAN

Preparation of an institutional proposal is greatly simplified if the process begins with a detailed plan. This should follow exactly whatever guidelines are provided. When detailed guidelines are supplied to the applicants, they may also be given to the reviewers, who may take them quite literally. Some guidelines, for instance, recommend that a particular style of table be used to summarize certain information. When the tables are numbered, as they usually are, it is common for the "Instructions to Reviewers" to refer to a particular table by number. The following is an excerpt from such an instruction: "Nature and breadth of the research conducted by participating faculty (see Table 1)." If the suggested format is not followed and Table 1 is something else, reviewers must search for the appropriate table or, worse yet, try to extract the data from a narrative. This extra work has a very negative effect on the attitude of a reviewer toward a proposal and may adversely influence a priority score. If the suggested format is carefully followed, the reviewer can turn directly and gratefully to the required data. It is worthwhile being slavish in adherence to recommended tables and their numbers, even if this means table numbers will not be consecutive because a particular table is inappropriate for the proposal. Start with a table of contents and develop an outline, including headings and paragraph content, for each separate section. Require that the writers of each section adhere to the content and agreed-upon format.

The first draft of the proposal plan should identify every heading in the proposal and list under each heading the points to be discussed. Each item on these lists will eventually be one or more paragraphs of text. This draft should be sent to the NIH Program Director for an initial reaction and suggestions. This will result in a modified draft that can be used as a guide for the first construction committee meeting. It should also be circulated to interested faculty to gain their reactions and support.

Staffing is an important part of putting together a successful proposal. Usually, the individual contributors use their staff, but the final assembly of the proposal should be done by one word processing facility. If this will overload existing resources, consider hiring a professional word processor specifically for this project. Most institutions have a few experts that may be willing to do an extra job for pay. Such a person is far more satisfactory than hiring someone from a temporary service, which can turn out to be a disaster. It is common for university funds to be available for preparation of large proposals.

Identify the word processing software to be used by the contributors at the outset. The program to be used for the final product should also be identified and, if necessary, arrangements made to convert files. A document that was obviously prepared by a committee is a poor testimony for good administration. We have seen proposals prepared on several different printers (some laser, some ink jet), with two or three different fonts, and with printed pages intermingled with obviously photocopied pages— some even bearing the imprint, "Duplicate copy - Use if needed." Such proposals are usually poorly written in several different styles, sloppily proofed, lacking intelligent transition paragraphs between sections, incorrectly paginated with addition of extra pages (pages 16A, 16B, 16C, etc.), and containing sections obviously pasted in from other proposals. All of these practices show a lack of a unified administration and bode poorly for the success of the project.

Administration is very important to the success of a construction project. Proper design, construction, and finishing require close supervision. A responsible administrator will make certain that the appropriate faculty members critically review the design details. Without this supervision, it is unlikely that electrical outlet placement, for instance, will be appropriate for all of the new appliances. Reviewers will not be enthusiastic about a poorly administered project even though (or especially if) the PI is a Nobel laureate.

Alteration and renovation (A and R) of existing space requires much less in the form of approvals, and small projects can be undertaken by any Institute without matching funds by means of Individual Research Grant Application Form NIH 398 (R01). Large alteration and renovation projects, like construction projects, generally require matching funds. However, unlike construction projects, alteration and renovation projects do not require extensive environmental impact statements or state and federal approvals.

Construction RFAs come with specific instructions and forms for proposal preparation. They are directed to the NCRR and use Standard Form SF-424. This is available on the Internet at <www.ncrr.nih.gov/resinfra/rinotice.htm>; click on "applicant information and supplemental instructions." In the *Abstract* and *Specific Aims,* the Program Overview should simply state the project goals. Based on the goals, the dimensions of the project are stated in general terms, including the total cost of the project, the amount requested, and need or justification for the new facilities. Project goals should correspond closely with those stated in the RFA.

The *budget* is only approximate at this stage of development and can be justified as dollars per square foot. A typical figure for animal space (A and R) in Los Angeles is $300 per square foot but costs may range as high as $500 per square foot or more. The estimate should include, as appropriate, grading, foundations, all utility connections and permits, architect fees, demolition costs, and construction costs. Generally, costs are not a point of contention in the review process, providing the need for the new facilities is adequately justified and the materials requested are warranted. A proposal for fume hoods might be well justified and approved, for instance, but the request that they be custom built of stainless steel at great expense would be denied if the Study Section felt that commercially available laminated hoods were sufficient.

A proposal is probably more authentic if the amount requested is not exactly half the cost of the project in the case of a requirement for a 50–50 match—otherwise the suspicion is raised that costs were inflated to meet the limit of the grant. It is better if the cost of the project substantially exceeds the amount the NIH will pay, with an assurance that the institution will make up the deficit. This provides convincing evidence of the institutional commitment to the project.

Official cost estimates must be provided, along with a scaled drawing on 8.5 × 11-inch paper by the architect. This should be in the form of a signed letter on the architect's stationery.

Salaries are generally not supported by Construction grants. However, for a large project, a Project Coordinator may be funded, but the Program Director should first be consulted. Consultants may also be supported, but this may be at the expense of some construction dollars. These are best considered part of the matching funds to be provided by the institution.

Equipment must be fully justified and identified as to model, manufacturer, and price. The directions must be carefully followed, especially with respect to fixed vs. movable equipment. If there is a budget limit, as there usually is, the entire budget should be attributed to construction costs since it is less likely that these will be cut. Many programs, however, like the NCRR program to enhance animal facilities, specify limits to construction and/or equipment costs. Items of equipment should be requested if appropriate to derive the maximum benefit from the program. Equipment must be fixed or built in to be included in a Construction grant. Typical examples of fixed equipment are attached fume hoods, autoclaves, dishwashers, coldrooms, production stills, water filter systems, benches and cupboards, and surgical lights.

PROGRAM NARRATIVE

Construction projects are usually justified on the basis of an increase in the quantity and quality of research at the institution as a direct result of the project. These projects are intended to support funded investigators. If the construction focuses on cancer research, for instance, the strongest support for the project is a statement of the number of NCI-funded R01 grants that will benefit. There is usually a minimum of 3 to 5 such projects required, but a strong proposal will list 10 or more projects funded by the NCI, and most with renewal dates at least 24 months after the submission deadline for the proposal. The funding strength of the faculty is best indicated in a table. This kind of faculty is obviously among the top 10–20% in their field since they are all funded. Their credentials will not be questioned. Different sources of funds may carry less clout. Other NIH funds offer good support; NSF support is almost as good as NIH support, but research support from private sources does little to strengthen a construction proposal to the NIH.

The extent of use of the facility by each of the funded faculty will be scrutinized very carefully since it is a common practice to pad the faculty with funded nonusers. The best evidence of use is publications indicating the use of similar facilities. If statements of use are provided without such support, they should be detailed enough to show the identity of the users, the expected use or procedures to be done, and the time involved. This is best presented in terms of current usage of a (unsatisfactory) facility or expanded use beyond the capability of current facilities.

Replacement of existing facilities with new structures with the same capacity or capability will not be approved. *There must be expansion.* Also, remodeling of existing research space to suit a different type of research does not expand facilities and is not a good approach. It should be stated that facilities to be remodeled are not currently in use for research, so that the renovation represents an increase in research capacity. New construction must never result in the removal of space from a research purpose. If faculty members are to be moved into new space, detailed plans must be provided for the use of the vacated space, proving that it will still be used for research.

New facilities may be required to support recruitment of new faculty. This is a strong project only if the existing faculty can also benefit and the new faculty members can be convincingly identified as to type of research and university support. A successful project of this sort concerned the construction of a clinical research center for eye research. A strong clinical faculty successfully argued that their increasing daily patient loads had saturated existing facilities to the extent that research patients could not be seen. The project consisted of remodeling office space into four ophthalmic examination rooms, a computer/data analysis room, and a record office. Care was taken to produce convincing data and assurances that the new space would be used only for research patients, and that existing NIH-supported clinical trials would benefit, that new clinical studies would result from the availability of the unit, and that new clinical research faculty could be recruited as a result of the expansion.

Project design must be based on a clear statement of project goals. It should be obvious that the design will meet the goal, for example, of bringing a vivarium up to new federal standards. It is very important that facility design conserves space and is efficient. Designs based on new developments in other institutions are most easily defended. What is needed is to establish the perception in the minds of the reviewers that the new facility will be state-of-the-art and efficient, and will accomplish the stated goals.

Shell space is a no-no, but proposals to complete existing shell space are acceptable. An architect must do the actual design to establish the credibility of the proposed construction in terms of facilities and permits. A design for a laboratory on the 3rd floor of a 10-story building that includes vented chemical hoods but does not include the engineering required for venting will do badly. This kind of oversight is avoided by involving a qualified architect who should prepare the $8\frac{1}{2} \times 11$-inch drawings submitted in support of the project. Not all architects are created equal. Those used should be experienced with laboratory design and frequently employed by the university. Only such experienced personnel will, for instance, know what type of ceiling material should be used in a sterile surgery. The priority score will suffer if the Study Section picks up a mistake in design.

The general process is to achieve funding and then obtain the finished drawings, which are submitted for an initial, and then a revised, final review, at which time the project may be put out for bid. Normally, contracts for construction should be completed within a year, but extensions may be requested. All funds must be obligated within 5 years.

Substantial departures from the design reviewed originally may be taken, but approval from the NCRR program and engineering staffs is required. Design changes should not reflect goal changes. Thus, if animal housing for 400 rabbits was requested, reviewed, and approved, this should not be reduced to 200 rabbits so that a primate facility could be added. Such a change would probably require rereview. It is far better to change the design but keep the goal unchanged. Once the project is finished, how it is used has, in the past, not been closely monitored. With the instigation of the 20-year rule, however, the NIH may actually be forced to monitor the use of construction projects well into the future.

24

T32 Institutional Research Training Program Grants

The T32 Training grant is made to an institution. The PI is usually a department chair, a senior investigator, or even the Dean. Most NIH Institutes fund these fellowships. The award provides funds to the institution, which selects the fellows. Both predoctoral and postdoctoral positions are allowed. The stipends are the same as those of the F32 fellowships, determined by the number of postdoctoral years and experience of the candidate (see Table 18.1). Thus, there is not a proper NIH peer review for selection of awardees, which are selected usually by a committee of the institution or department.

The goal of a particular NIH Institute in supporting a National Research Service Award (NRSA) Training grant is to ensure a continued supply of researchers interested in the programs of the Institute. The NIH found that investigators tend to stay in the research field of their thesis. To provide predoctoral support for students working in a field of interest increases the probability that research workers in that area will be available in the future. Similarly, to provide postdoctoral fellowships in a particular field ensures continued work in that area. What it does not ensure is the recruitment of the best minds into the field. Only the F32 program, in which a Study Section individually reviews candidates, can guarantee selection of the best. The potential weakness of T32 Training grants is found in the institution applicant pool size and nature. If the pool is large and of high quality, the trainees will be of high quality. If the applicant pool is limited, substandard trainees may be selected in order to fill the vacancies. Unfortunately, the current stipends (predoctoral, $16,500; first-year postdoctoral, $28,260) cause budding scientists to question why they did not go into a more lucrative career. Fortunately many institutions find ways to supplement these stipends.

277

The NIH Institutes award many different individual and institutional Training grants. The NIH web page (<www.grants.nih.gov/grants/oer.htm>) lists 81 different Training grant mechanisms; 44 of these are specific for either minority or disabled candidates. Each Institute supports different combinations of the mechanisms, so mentors and potential trainees should search for the best choice by going to the appropriate Institute home page and talk to Institute Program Directors.

THE APPLICATION

Section V of the PHS 398 form, "Institutional National Research Service Award," is used for T32 Training grant applications. F32 application packets (PHS 416-1) are different and should be obtained from the Office of Contracts and Grants of your university or the NIH web site (<http://grants.nih.gov/grants/funding/416/phs416.htm>).

Criteria for review of T32 Training grants are very different from those of other applications. Foremost in consideration are the qualifications of the faculty: their research experience, productivity, funding, and previous training experience. The nature of the applicant pool, its qualifications, and recruitment are also very important. A well-defined training program and strong administrative support are necessary; sections of the proposal must present an affirmative action plan for recruiting underrepresented minorities and must include instruction in ethical principles of research.

The *Program Director* should be a senior scientist with a solid list of publications and previous experience as a preceptor. Former trainees should include many individuals who have become independent, funded PIs. The Program Director need not be the Principal Investigator if there are internal reasons for a difference. In some situations it may be better for the PI to be the Dean or an Associate Dean of a school, or a department chairperson. Such individuals lend credibility to a claim of university involvement, but are liabilities as Program Directors due to their other time commitments. The Program Director should be presented as someone with a long-term interest in teaching, a good teaching record, experience in administration, and time to be a conscientious Program Director.

Training grants are notoriously inadequate in providing staff for the program, so the Program Director should be perceived as having the university support to provide staffing. Program administration includes publicizing its availability, generating and distributing descriptive brochures, contacting graduate advisers in local institutions, handling correspondence, and assisting with course selection and registration, housing, and finances. The administration may also assist the student in identifying a suitable preceptor, and should provide counseling services as needed. Students in the program should be followed to ensure their success and contacted regularly in a social context to maintain open channels of communication. These services are essential to program success but are rarely supported. Nevertheless, the services should be described and attributed to some other administrative unit if necessary.

Continued funding for a Training grant is dependent on its success. The only measure of success that counts is what happens to its graduates. It is essential that they be tracked. Those that achieve academic appointments with NIH funding provide great support for the program. It is particularly impressive when one of your chickens comes to roost in a departmental chair. However, these bragging rights require a long-term commitment to tracking fellows.

The Training grant proposal itself provides the best evidence of the strength of the administration. The proposal should follow the guidelines exactly, be clearly and succinctly written, contain no typos or spelling errors, and contain up-to-date Biosketches for each of the faculty, and every page should be printed on the same printer using the same font. These proposals require input from many individuals. The administration must obtain faculty input in a timely manner and develop an integrated consistent document. Most groups that are not this well organized lack the staff support to unify the proposal and submit a conglomeration of pages pasted in and photocopied from a variety of printers using many fonts. There is usually repetition in such proposals and important sections may be omitted. A well-written proposal is the exception rather than the rule, and will be much appreciated by the Study Section.

The *preceptor faculty* will be evaluated carefully. Each member should be obviously successful in the area of training, and ideally will have past fellows who have become successful as independent investigators. Since the training is in research, every preceptor should have a funded NIH R01 or equivalent grant, hopefully with a termination date at least 2 years after the date of Training grant submission. If the faculty are successful in peer review, it is unlikely that the Study Section reviewing the Training grant will be concerned about faculty expertise. Nonfunded investigators should not be included as preceptors, even though they may be excellent teachers or clinicians. There will certainly be concern about faculty commitment to teaching. This is best handled with a table showing each preceptor and listing the names of every past and present student, position (pre- or postdoctoral), inclusive dates if appropriate, and current position. The distribution of MCAT and GRE scores and undergraduate GPAs of past fellows should be provided without identifying individuals (this is probably privileged information). The strongest and most successful past student is one that holds a faculty appointment and a current R01 grant, and these should be especially noted.

A major concern of the Study Section is the number of fellowship positions appropriate to a given faculty. This judgment is based on the size and strength of the faculty, and existing commitments to other students. Before preparing a proposal for a T32, discuss this issue with the Training Officer of the NIH Institute. Be sure to discuss Institute biases (recommendations) with respect to balance between numbers of predoctoral and postdoctoral stipends, and any special considerations or preferences for research fellows who hold clinical degrees.

Training grants are designed to provide a source of young research talent for specific NIH programs. The most modern and powerful studies in most areas today are conducted at the molecular, the genetic, or the cellular level. A strong training program should be multidisciplinary and should include several faculty members working at each of these basic levels. When the program is organized, the available faculty should be organized in conceptual groups. As an example, one such NIGMS-funded program had multidisciplinary groups centered on diabetes and hypertension, wound healing, cancer biology, and autoimmune disease. Each area had 8–10 faculty whose research involved biochemistry, molecular biology, cell biology, immunology, pharmacology, and, in some cases, clinical applications. Data were available for past pre- and postdoctoral fellows, and the programs were closely integrated with common seminars and discussion sessions. In another outstanding and successful program funded by the NEI, the proposal focused on 8 PIs who studied the molecular biology of the visual system and requested 4 postdoctoral and 2 predoctoral positions. The details may vary among programs in various universities, but a strong, closely integrated faculty characterizes the successful ones.

Recruitment is an important part of a training program to ensure a superior applicant pool. An organized program is needed. If an existing program is available, it should be used. Elements of a program designed to attract medical students, for instance, can be modified to recruit predoctoral Ph.D. students for a medical school. Such programs are usually well staffed and much more effective than a small program based on a single department. Key elements of recruitment programs include distribution of brochures and announcements, contacts with student advisers and placement centers at national meetings, advertisements in national journals such as *Science,* and recruiting visits to local campuses. An excellent recruitment stratagem is to provide summer fellowships for outstanding undergraduate students.

Minority recruitment is required of all programs. This is a complex well-organized effort at all universities, and involves contacts with high schools, summer outreach programs, and special tutoring programs. It is not realistic for each training program to launch a detailed minority recruitment effort, but the institution's efforts can be used. Details of the institution's program can be obtained from the individual responsible for administering the program and adapted to the training proposal.

Applicant pool quality and size is a limiting factor in the success of a training program. A new program has no applicant pool, but each proposed preceptor should have had previous predoctoral students and postdoctoral fellows who will be listed in the table described above. Reference to this table and the average GPA or GRE scores can be used to support a claim that a quality applicant pool will be available. Competing renewals of Training grants are required to list all trainees and their accomplishments during and after training. It is required also to provide data on the number of applicants, the number who were offered positions, and the number who accepted the offer, including the range of their GPA and GRE scores. The best programs offer positions only to the best students and have a high (better than 75%) acceptance rate.

PROGRAM CONTENT AND GOALS

In 1989, a task force chaired by Claude Lenfant reviewed all NIH Biomedical Research Training Programs, particularly M.D./Ph.D. programs. The task force made a number of recommendations, many of which should be incorporated into new proposals.

1. Professional pre-doctoral students (e.g., medical students) should be eligible for training on institutional training grants during the summer or elective time for periods of between three and 12 months with a maximum of 12 months. A minimum of six months should be encouraged.

The revised research training structure can be effectively integrated with the requirements for clinical training. The existing investigator track for board certification permits research training and satisfies the requirements for both board certification in internal medicine and subspecialty certification within the normal clinical training period. Differing approaches to integrating research training with clinical training are likely to exist, and they can be permitted as long as NRSA training grant appointments are not used to support clinical training.

2. Multiple pathways should be permitted to accommodate the needs for clinical certification within the context of the research training experience of two or more years.

3. A minimum of two years of training should be required for all professional doctorate appointees to institutional NRSA grants. Trainees should be encouraged to apply for further research training and career development through national competition. Training grant appointments may be extended beyond two years upon the recommendation of the training director and with the concurrence of the NIH.

4. Review of competing renewals for NRSA training grants should focus upon performance, in terms of the preparation of trainees for productive research careers.

5. Numbers of trainees in training programs should be consistent with individual Institute policies and the institution's resources.

6. The presence of both MD and PhD trainees in the same program should be considered favorably in the review of NRSA training grant applications.

7. Special training experiences away from the training institution may be proposed as part of the training grant application or subsequently to NIH staff.

The task force proposed a number of changes in NIH Training grant policy. Some programs now place much greater emphasis on predoctoral training. This is a response to a widespread perception that there has been a decline in both quality and quantity of biomedical trainees, and to the realization that fellows trained on individual F32 awards are more successful than their colleagues trained on institutional T32 awards. Although there is still a prohibition against clinical training in most programs, NIH-supported physician/scholar (M.D./Ph.D.) programs exist in many medical colleges, and there is interest in promoting residencies that permit extended research activity. In addition, the various NIH Institutes also support short-term training in research for professional-degree candidates (doctors, dentists, optometrists, etc.) both under the scope of institutional T32 awards and under separate institutional T35 program awards that are specific for this purpose.

The specific goals and structure of a program should be adapted to the needs of the funding Institute. The Institute Program Director responsible for Training grants should be closely questioned about the perceived need for another training program, the availability of funds, and the nature of the competition. Some directors will respond to a letter of intent with detailed and helpful advice. Although all training programs share a common interest in the quality of the faculty and applicant pool, there are substantial differences among NIH Institutes and among programs within a single Institute in the nature of the programs sought. The training goals of a specific program must be understood and a program assembled that will satisfy these goals. If a program's goal is to produce epidemiologists who will study risk factors in age-related diseases, for instance, a highly structured program with course work in epidemiology and biometry associated with appropriate clinical experience, and access to a large controlled population of elderly subjects, would be appropriate. It must be argued convincingly that the proposed training program will produce the desired product. This is best accomplished if the program has already been successful, even if that success was achieved at a different university.

Instruction in research ethics is required in all T32 programs and must be described in detail. This is easily handled as a seminar series involving the ethical use of human subjects and animals, responsibilities of data management and recording, joint authorship, traditions of authorship, scientific misconduct, and conflict of interest. Successful grantsmanship is a requirement for success in biomedical research and it is appropriate to include course work in scientific writing and grantsmanship in the program plan. Flexibility of programs is also important since candidates present themselves with widely varying backgrounds. This should be specifically acknowledged and alternative paths described, for instance, for a trainee with a M.D. and a trainee with a liberal arts college background.

The criteria for review expressed in most Training grant announcements provide excellent insight into what is considered important program content:

A. *Program Director.* Research experience and leadership capabilities of the program director. Adequacy of the program advisory structure and administration. Origin and development of the program.

B. *Training Faculty.*

1. Nature and breadth of research, numbers of assistant, associate, and full professors, and department affiliation of the faculty can be presented as a table.

2. Funding of the faculty with a list of NIH grant numbers, start and end dates, grant titles, and annual and total awards should be presented as a table.

3. The publication record for the faculty is best shown as a table listing the total number of publications of each member, the number of publications in the past 5 years, and the papers in press. The actual publications will be listed in the standard NIH Biosketch.

4. Evidence of collaboration among the faculty is easily demonstrated with a scatter chart in which the faculty members are listed across the top and down the side of a graph. An "X" is placed wherever two members are coauthors of a paper. A large and scattered distribution of X's indicates widespread collaboration.

5. Teaching experience of each member can be shown with a table listing every student of every member. The table should indicate whether the student was a predoctoral or a postdoctoral fellow, where the undergraduate work was done, and what the current position is. Current NIH support, other grant support, and number of recent research publications should be especially noted.

C. *Training Candidates or Current Applicants (Predoctoral).* Undergraduate institution, GPA, MCAT, and GRE scores, source of support, and potential preceptor should be listed in a table. This information establishes the qualifications of current candidates. New programs should submit data from existing programs in the school as examples of the expected student quality.

D. *Applicant Pool.*

1. List in a separate table the names and GPA, MCAT, and/or GRE scores of all past students or, for new programs, all past students in other training programs of the school. Publications of past students should be listed in a separate table to indicate their scholastic success.

2. Recruitment success should be indicated in the same table by listing the names and credentials of applicants, indicating if each was offered a position and whether matriculation occurred.

3. The training program will be evaluated as to goals, rationale, degree requirements, research opportunities, cohesiveness, balance, integration of different units, self-assessment, trainee counseling, opportunities for collaboration, and unique features.

F. *Training Record.* The training record will be evaluated in terms of number, quality, current position, publications, and funding of each trainee.

G. *Resources and Environment.* Resources and environment are evaluated as to ability to absorb new students, freedom from isolation, collegiality, collaboration, institutional support, and quality of the facilities and equipment in preceptors' laboratories.

Each NIH Institute issues guidelines for Training grant review that are given to applicants and reviewers. The reviewers will have to comment on each criterion of review, and greatly appreciate proposals that devote a titled section to each criterion in the order presented in the guidelines. Such a proposal is easy to review, and this has a positive impact on priority scores. It is a common observation that T32 Training grants rarely are funded on the first submission. The resubmission has the benefit of corrections of deficiencies and omissions noted by the initial review, and is a vastly better proposal, even though the programs are probably unchanged. This suggests the benefit of preparing a careful, thoughtful, well-written, and well-reviewed proposal the first time!

25

Instrumentation Grants

Instrumentation is essential for most research projects. Many instruments cost in excess of $25,000, the threshold of imbalance for an R01 research proposal. Requests for expensive instruments are bad for these proposals because they imply that the investigator does not have the capability of currently doing the research. The claim that a borrowed instrument is no longer available is so common that it lacks credibility. Requests for large equipment items invariably weaken research proposals. Certainly, some proposals are so strong that they can survive such requests, and we know of instances (admittedly some years ago) where an electron microscope (EM) costing well in excess of $100,000 was awarded on a research grant. Such awards are now very rare and virtually impossible for new investigators to obtain. The need for instrumentation remains, and can be satisfied with an Instrumentation grant from the NSF, the NIH, or a private foundation. It is worth restating what was said to young investigators in Chapter 19. When you take a new job and set up a new laboratory you require equipment to be productive. You need to get this from your institution as part of your hiring package. You certainly will not get it from the NIH. This is particularly true of large equipment.

The NIH has several mechanisms for instrumentation awards. Any Institute may periodically offer Instrumentation grants. For example, in FY 2000, the NIGMS had a special initiative related to acquisition and research with advanced instrumentation for high-resolution EM. In FY 2001, a number of Institutes accepted proposals for competing supplements to expand microarray facilities in their areas of interest.

The NIH regularly offers Shared Instrumentation Grants (SIGs) for instruments costing $100,000 and up, through annual competition. These SIGs are funded as S10 awards by the NCRR. These grants do not require matching funds but the maximum award is $500,000, and if the cost is greater, then the availability of the remainder of the funding must be documented. More than one proposal may be submitted at the same time by an institution. (However, from a grantsmanship standpoint, this is a bad idea.) The NIH budget for these grants was about $45 million in 2001. Funds for instrumentation vary from year to year, but are always in short supply. Competition for the few available dollars is keen.

The NSF also has a Multi-User Biological Instrumentation Program and some programs at the NSF also make individual equipment awards. The Multi-User awards range from $40,00 to $400,000 and can even be used to supplement an NCRR–SIG award. However, the NSF has fewer dollars than the NIH; the research and education objectives of the NSF are not often the same as the biomedical research objectives of the NIH. Investigators should consult with NSF staff at <www.nsf.gov/bio/dbi> before considering a proposal.

Typical instruments suitable for the NCRR–SIG program are computer systems, NMR systems, mass spectrometers, protein sequencer/amino acid analyzers, flow cytometers, confocal microscopes, DNA synthesizers, micro-assay arrays, etc.

SIG awards are made on the basis of the strength of the faculty, their current research support, the coherence of the program, and a compelling presentation that the group will be strengthened and become more productive of better research as a result of the award. Administration of the project is important, as is periodic external review. A special section should convince the reviewers that the instrument would actually foster new interdisciplinary research. There may be a tendency for these programs to give awards to smaller, rather than larger, universities, all other criteria being equal. The FY 2001 instructions state,

> Applications are evaluated for scientific and technical merit by specially convened instrument specific initial review groups of the Center for Scientific Review (CSR) . . . and receive a second level review by the National Advisory Research Resources Council. Funding decisions . . . will not be made until the program receives an appropriation for FY-2002.

CRITERIA FOR REVIEW

Criteria for review of SIG applications include the following:

1. The extent to which an award for the specific instrument would meet the scientific needs and enhance the planned research endeavors of the major users by providing an instrument that is unavailable or to which availability is highly limited.

2. The availability and commitment of the appropriate technical expertise within the major user group or the institution.

3. The adequacy of the organizational plan and the internal advisory committee for oversight of the instrument, including sharing arrangements.

4. The institution's commitment for the continued support of the utilization and maintenance of the instrument.

5. The benefit of the proposed instrument to the overall research community it will serve.

Unfortunately, these grants support the maxim, "the rich get richer." Well-established, well-funded researchers in strong departments are more likely to be successful in an intense competition. It is not unusual for as many as 200 proposals to be reviewed by the sections on microscopy or computers, for instance. All major users should be funded by NIH grants for strongest presentation. At the least, there must be 3 such users, and the equipment must be used at least 75% of the time for NIH-supported research. A strong proposal will have 7–10 funded users. Unfunded major users add little strength and may well detract from the proposal. Use should be forecast to be about 70–80% of a reasonable capacity (32 hours per week). This will allow expanded use by new faculty, or for new collaborative projects. These grants do not provide for maintenance or continued support funds, without which the instrument would soon be useless. Thus it is essential to provide detailed evidence that such support will be provided by the institution (not by other grants). It must be clear that the institution holds the research team in high regard as evidenced by active support.

Administrative details will be scrutinized carefully for evidence that the PI is familiar with managing a shared facility. These details should include scheduling, supervision, user training, quality control, and maintenance. A committee should arbitrate disputes and advise the PI concerning operations. The facility should be reviewed annually by a disinterested expert from another department or institution.

Instrumentation proposals are most likely to succeed if the requested instrument is being added to an existing facility and a group of users already exists. Perhaps the capacity or scientific utility of the existing equipment has been exceeded, because the group is increasingly productive, successful, and growing. Such a group certainly will have established procedures for *scheduling* already, and these should be described. A typical sign-up sheet should be shown and tabular data provided to show usage hours by each funded user. Heavy usage implies use during the evening hours and on weekends. However, the best proposals will feature a new instrument that will extend the research capability of the group into new areas of research.

Supervision should be provided by a highly trained senior technician. Some proposals assign supervision to a faculty member who is a user. This does not have credibility with the reviewers. The supervisor must oversee use, train users, monitor output, and maintain the instrument. A faculty member who does these things is functioning like an overpaid technician. This probably happens sometimes, but the reviewers will suspect that the instrument simply will not be properly supervised. A Biosketch for the supervisor should be included.

Training of users should be taken seriously. The minimum skills required to properly operate the instrument should be listed, and a program to establish that all users will have these skills should be described. The program should be described in sufficient detail to show actual contact hours involved with each facet of training, and the level of supervision required.

Quality control is also an important criterion of review. The supervisor should monitor the quality of the data or material produced by each user. In the case of electron microscopy, for instance, the electron micrographs produced should meet minimum standards, and a plan to rectify a defective product should be described; this is usually done in a retraining session. It should be stated emphatically that the instrument will be operated only to the highest standards, and that this will be ensured by frequent quality checks.

External review procedures should be described. A prominent scientist in the community should be named and an annual program of review presented. The purpose of the review is to ensure that quality has been maintained and that all potential users have full access to the instrument. A letter from the external reviewer expressing willingness to serve should be appended to the proposal.

Maintenance procedures vary from instrument cleaning and calibration to complete disassembly. It is not enough to state simply that a maintenance contract will be purchased. Daily maintenance is required of all instruments. This should be described in detail, and methods of calibration, alignment, fluid replacement, etc., included. Funding of instrument maintenance, supervision, and operation must also be described in detail. This may be done in terms of user fees, charged at the rate of so much per hour or use. However, many successful proposals list this type of support as part of the institution's contribution to the group of investigators and the instrumentation project.

As noted before, the best indication of administrative expertise available to the reviewers is the research proposal itself. It must be well prepared, well written, thoughtful, and thorough. It must look nice, and all pages must be printed on the same printer with one font style. The Biosketches must be identically prepared. Photocopying Biosketches is a real time saver but is bad grantsmanship because they always look ragged and use a variety of print fonts and formats. Proposals that look like a committee prepared them witness to the world that this group lacks a good central administration.

Private foundations are an excellent source of equipment support. Many foundations that will not fund research projects will provide $50,000–100,000 for purchase of major equipment. Access to foundations varies with institutions, but if you have such access, it should be used. Prospects for funding are better than through NSF or NIH grants. Instrumentation funds are made available by the individual NIH Institutes on an irregular basis, but announced by a request for proposals. Some Institutes will provide instrumentation funds through their Core Center grants. The RFP is released by the Institute following a decision by its council (or by the U.S. Congress) that a need exists. As noted above, the time from official announcement of the RFP to the application deadline is usually too short to permit generation of a strong proposal *de novo*. If your institution is to benefit from these ad hoc programs, it must maintain close contact with the various councils. The individuals most able to keep up with council decisions are the senior staff of the NIH Institutes and scientists who either are on the council or know people who are. Through this close liaison it is often possible to learn of an impending RFP several months before it is released—enough lead time to foster a really good proposal.

Instrumentation grants from a particular NIH Institute are designed primarily to benefit the grantees of that Institute. Thus justification of your need for the instrument must be based on the collective needs of grantees supported by the same Institute. Grants from other Institutes and from private sources may provide evidence of a strong research group but should not be given prominence in the proposal.

Table 25.1 shows the Specific Aims and Introduction from a successful proposal for a scanning electron microscope that Ogden submitted

Table 25.1 *Example Construction Grant*

A. SPECIFIC AIMS

The specific aims of this proposal are to strengthen our programs of research-in ultrastructure by acquiring a new scanning electron microscope (SEM).

The long range goal of the Estelle Doheny Eye Foundation (EDEF) is to build a broadly based program of vision research of excellence second to none. Achievement of this goal requires provision of modern laboratories, state-of-the-art equipment, and a superior faculty of scientists. This proposal, in requesting funds for a new SEM, supports these goals. Acquisition of a modern SEM (Hitachi S-570) will facilitate recruitment of new faculty and will provide our researchers with badly needed equipment.

B. INTRODUCTION

Funds are requested by EDEF and the Department of Ophthalmology of the University of Southern California (USC) for the purchase of an Hitachi S-570 scanning electron microscope (SEM). The new microscope will replace an outdated 1974 JEOL JSM-35 SEM. Its approaching obsolescence is clearly revealed by the difficulty we have experienced in obtaining proper maintenance and parts. The limitations of our JEOL include excessive downtime and inadequate servicing, the need for such extensive user training that use is inhibited, limited resolution, non-programmable stage, and absence of automatic focus and exposure. These limitations result in long and unpredictable delays in access to the JEOL. Our need is for ready access to a user friendly, reliable modern instrument. A large backlog of work, our inability to start new studies involving SEM and the imminence of the addition of new faculty add urgency to our need for a new instrument.

EDEF is the research arm of the Department of Ophthalmology. It is a private non-profit foundation affiliated with USC. The EDEF building, located on the health sciences campus of USC, has 4 floors totaling about 40,000 net square feet of space. It provides outpatient facilities and office space for the Department of Ophthalmology on the first floor, 11 research laboratories on the second and third floors, and a research vivarium in the basement. The fourth floor is occupied temporarily by USC personnel of other departments. Over the past 10 years, EDEF has grown into a major center of vision research with 28 current NEI funded research projects involving 11 clinicians and 9 basic scientists on the regular faculty.

EDEF is experiencing rapid growth. The 35-bed Estelle Doheny Eye Hospital, located adjacent to the EDEF building, opened for patients on April 15, 1985. Four new basic science faculty will be added during the coming year. Funds to provide 4 new laboratories devoted to ocular pharmacology and immunology are currently being sought. These funds will be used to remodel existing administrative space and renovate and expand our EM facility. The faculty recruited for the hospital and these laboratories will also use the SEM to further aggravate the inadequacy of the JEOL.

From the following review of the use of SEM by our faculty, it is apparent that our staff is heavily oriented toward quantitative morphology, that SEM is a vital part of our projects, and that we are well qualified in its use. The inadequacies of our JEOL are documented. A review of funded research at EDEF is included and an indication is given of the expanded use of SEM that will be supported by a new instrument.

---

about 12 years ago. The proposal was brief, but included copious documentation of the expertise of the users in the appendix. Also provided is a diagram (Figures 25.1 and 25.2) used to show the laboratory in which the microscope would be housed.

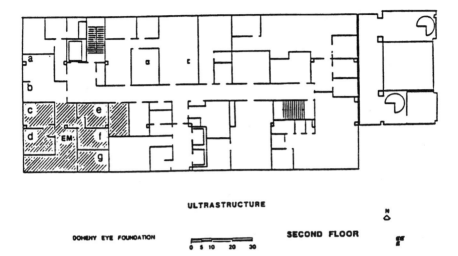

ULTRASTRUCTURE

DOHENY EYE FOUNDATION

SECOND FLOOR

Figure 25.1. Example floor plan.

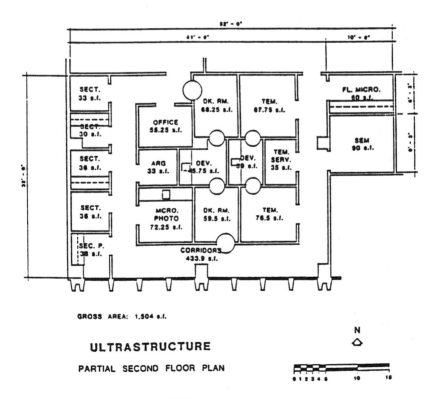

GROSS AREA: 1,504 s.f.

ULTRASTRUCTURE

PARTIAL SECOND FLOOR PLAN

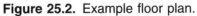

Figure 25.2. Example floor plan.

APPLICATION PROCEDURES

The following paragraphs are excerpted from the NIH instructions:

Awards under this Program Announcement (PA) will use the SIG mechanism (S10). SIG provides support for expensive state-of-the-art instrumentation utilized in both basic and clinical research. Applications are limited to instruments that cost at least $100,000 per instrument or integrated instrument system. The maximum award is $500,000. Since the nature and scope of the instruments that may be requested will vary, it is anticipated that the size of an award will vary also. Awards will be made for the direct costs only. The institution must meet those costs (not covered in the normal purchase price) required to place the instrumentation in operational order as well as the maintenance, support personnel, and service costs associated with maximum utilization of the instrument. There is no upper limit on the cost of the instrument, but the maximum award is $500,000. Grants will be awarded for a period of one year and are not renewable. Supplemental applications will not be accepted. The program does not provide facilities and administrative (F&A) costs or support for construction or alterations and renovations. Cost sharing is not required. If the amount of funds requested does not cover the total cost of the instrument, the application should describe the proposed sources(s) of funding for the balance of the cost of the instrument. Documentation of the availability of the remainder of the funding, signed by an appropriate institutional official, must be presented to NCRR prior to the issuance of an award.

A major user group of three or more investigators should be identified. A minimum of three major users must be PIs on NIH peer-reviewed research grants at the time of the application and award. . . . The application must show a clear need for the instrumentation by projects supported by multiple NIH research awards and demonstrate that these projects will require at least 75% of the total usage of the instrument. Major users can be individual researchers, or a group of investigators within the same department or from several departments at the applicant institution. NIH extramural awardees from other institutions may also be included.

If the major user group does not require total usage of the instrument, access to the instrument can be made available to other users upon the advice of the internal advisory committee. These users need not be NIH awardees, but priority should be given to NIH-supported scientists engaged in biomedical or behavioral research. . . . The application must include a plan for the day-to-day management of the instrument including designation of a qualified individual to supervise the operation of the instrument and to provide technical expertise to the users. Specific plans for sharing arrangements and for monitoring the use of the instrument should be described.

The application also requires the following:

1. Inventory similar instruments existing at the institution or otherwise accessible; describe why they are unavailable or inappropriate for the pro-

posed research and provide a clear justification why new or updated equipment, including accessories, is needed.

2. Have the major users describe their research projects and indicate how the requested instrumentation and/or accessories would enhance the progress of their research projects. While most projects are included in currently funded applications, some represent new directions. *In the case of funded projects, the description should not exceed four pages per user,* but should point out the benefit of the proposed instrument to the research objectives of each major user. New directions and their requirements for the proposed instrumentation should be described in sufficient detail to allow adequate review (including preliminary data or supplemental materials). Use a table to list the names of the users, brief titles of the projects, the PHS grant numbers, and the estimated percentage of use. Make a separate table to indicate the major users' needs for requested accessories. If possible, each user should highlight those publications that demonstrate the user's expertise in using the requested instrumentation.

If appendix material is submitted, four collated sets must be included with the application package for the CSR. Applications (Form PHS 398) must typically be received by a date in March, which changes from year to year. Applications received after this date will not be accepted for review in the current competition. The original and four copies should be sent to

Application Receipt Office
Center for Scientific Review
National Institutes of Health
6701 Rockledge Drive
Room 1040-MSC 7710
Bethesda, MD 20892-7710 (or 20817 for express/courier service)

One copy of the application and one copy of any appendix material also should be addressed to

Shared Instrumentation Grant Program
Biomedical Technology Area
National Center for Research Resources
6705 Rockledge Drive, Room 6148-MSC7965
Bethesda, MD 20892-7965

For information call Marjorie Tingle, Ph.D., at 301-435-0772, or e-mail at SIG@ncrr.nih.gov. The web page for the fiscal 2002 Program Announcement is <http://grants.nih.gov/grants/guide/pa-files/PAR-02-036.html>.

Appendix A
Information Sources: Private Foundation and Government Web Sites, and Study Section Contacts

Without question, the world is different than 5 years ago. In prior editions, this first appendix was a list of names, addresses, and telephone numbers of contacts and offices at the NIH. The second appendix included 118 pages with descriptions of the categorical programs of the NIH Institutes. All of this information is now available on the Internet. So, in the various chapters we "modernized" the text by providing URLs wherever we could. Below is a summary of those information sources.

The list is far from complete. We are certain that our readers—especially those who grew up with computers and the Internet—are savvy enough to pursue and find further information about grants and research funding.

Agency	URL
National Institutes of Health	
NIH home page	www.nih.gov
Institute directory and links to programs and staff	www.nih.gov/icd
NIH Guide—links to RFAs, Notices, and Program Announcements	http://grants.nih.gov/grants/guide/index.html
NIH links to instructions and forms for all grant programs	http://grants.nih.gov/grants/forms.htm
Application forms for various federal agencies in Mac and PC format	http://tram.east.asu.edu
DHHS Office for Human Research Protections	http://ohrp.osophs.dhhs.gov

Agency	URL
NIH Office of Laboratory Animal Welfare	http://grants.nih.gov/grants/olaw
NIH CRISP database of information and abstracts of funded grants	www-commons.cit.nih.gov/crisp
NIH modular grant web page	http://grants.nih.gov/grants/funding/modular/modular.htm
NIH—CSR Study Section descriptions	www.csr.nih.gov/review/irgdesc.htm
NIH—CSR Study Section membership rosters	www.csr.nih.gov/ASPDocs/Committees/rosterindex.asp
NCRR—NIH Construction Program	www.ncrr.nih.gov/resinfra/rinotice.htm
NCRR—NIH Shared Instrumentation Grant Program (FY 2002 guidelines)	http://grants.nih.gov/grants/guide/pa-files/PAR-02-036.html
NIH Grants Policy Statements	http://grants.nih.gov/grants/policy
NIH Small Business Research Grant Programs (SBIR and STTR)	www.grants.nih.gov/grants/funding/sbir.htm
National Science Foundation	
NSF home page	www.nsf.gov
NSF Directorate for Biological Sciences	www.nsf.gov/bio
Electronic submission of NSF grant proposals	www.fastlane.nsf.gov
U.S. Department of Defense	
U.S. Army Research Office	www.aro.army.mil
U.S. Army Congressionally Directed Medical Research Programs	http://cdmrp.army.mil
U.S. Air Force Office of Scientific Research	www.afosr.af.mil
U.S. Office of Naval Research	www.onr.navy.mil
Various private foundations	
American Heart Association	www.americanheart.org/research
American Cancer Society	www.cancer.org
Alzheimer's Association	www.alz.org/research
National Parkinson Foundation	www.parkinson.org/grants.htm
American Diabetes Association	www.diabetes.org/research
Juvenile Diabetes Research Foundation International	www.jdf.org

The rest of this appendix is a listing (current as of 8/04/01) of contacts for the various Study Sections of the Center for Scientific Review (CSR).

Center for Scientific Review (CSR)
National Institutes of Health
6701 Rockledge Drive
Bethesda, MD 20892
Dr. Ellie Ehrenfeld, Director
Dr. Brent Stanfield, Deputy Director

The Center for Scientific Review at the National Institutes of Health is the focal point for the conduct of initial review, which is the foundation of the NIH grant and award process. The CSR carries out peer review of the majority of research and research training applications submitted to the NIH. In addition, the Center serves as the central receipt point for all Public Health Service (PHS) applications and refers those applications to Integrated Review Groups (IRGs) for scientific and technical merit reviews, and to funding components for potential award. To this end, the Center develops and implements innovative and flexible ways to conduct referral and review for all aspects of science. Below is a listing of professional staff, with telephone numbers (or e-mail addresses in some cases), in the Division of Receipt and Referral and in the three review divisions (Division of Molecular and Cellular Mechanisms, Division of Physiological Systems, and Division of Clinical and Population-Based Studies). Each review division consists of several IRGs and their constituent Study Sections where review for scientific and technical merit takes place.

DIVISION OF RECEIPT AND REFERRAL

Dr. Suzanne Fisher, Director 301-435-0715
Dr. M. Janet Newburgh, Deputy Director 301-435-0715
Ms. Carol Campbell, Health Scientist Administrator 301-435-1080
Dr. Narayani Ramakrishnan, Assistant Chief 301-435-0715
Dr. Kalman Salata, Assistant Chief 301-435-0715

DIVISION OF MOLECULAR AND CELLULAR MECHANISMS

Dr. Donald Schneider, Director 301-435-1727

Biochemical Sciences IRG (BCS)

Dr. Zakir Bengali, Chief 301-435-1742

Biochemistry (BIO)
Dr. Chhanda Ganguly 301-435-1739

Medical Biochemistry (MEDB)
Dr. Alec S. Liacouras 301-435-1740

Pathobiochemistry (PBC)
Dr. Zakir Bengali 301-435-1742

Physiological Chemistry (PC)
Dr. Richard Panniers 301-435-1741

Special Reviews 2 (SSS-2)
Dr. Prabha Atreya 301-435-8367

Biophysical and Chemical Sciences IRG (BPC)

Dr. John Bowers, Chief 301-435-1725

Bioanalytical Engineering & Chemistry (BECM)
Dr. Noni Byrnes 301-435-1217

Bio-organic & Natural Products Chemistry (BNP)
Dr. Mike Radtke 301-435-1728

Biophysical Chemistry (BBCB)
Dr. Arnold Revzin 301-435-1153

Medicinal Chemistry (MCHA)
Dr. Ronald Dubois 301-435-1722

Metallobiochemistry (BMT)
Dr. John Bowers 301-435-1725

Molecular & Cellular Biophysics (BBCA)
Dr. Nancy Lamontagne 301-435-1726

Physical Biochemistry (PB)
Dr. Gopa Rakhit 301-435-1721

Special Reviews 6 (SSS-6) BEHARM@csr.nih.gov

Special Reviews A (SSS-A)
Dr. Arnold Revzin 301-435-1153

Special Reviews L (SSS-L)
Dr. Janet Nelson 301-435-1723

Cell Development and Function IRG (CDF)

Dr. Marcia Steinberg, Chief 301-435-1023

Cell Development and Function 1 (CDF-1)
Dr. Michael Sayre 301-435-1219

Cell Development and Function 2 (CDF-2)
Dr. Ramesh Nayak 301-435-1026

Cell Development and Function 3 (CDF-3)
Dr. Gerhard Ehrenspeck 301-435-1022

Cell Development and Function 4 (CDF-4)
Dr. Marcia Steinberg 301-435-1023

Cell Development and Function 5 (CDF-5)
Dr. Sherry Dupere 301-435-1021

Cell Development and Function 6 (CDF-6)
Dr. Richard Rodewald 301-435-1024

International Cooperative Projects (ICP)
Dr. Sandy Warren 301-435-1019

Special Reviews U (SSS-U)
Dr. Eugene Vigil 301-435-1025

Genetic Sciences IRG (GNS)

Dr. Camilla Day, Chief 301-435-1037

Biological Sciences 1 (BIOL-1) VACANT@csr.nih.gov

Ethical, Legal, & Social Issues of Human Genetics (ELSI)
Dr. Cheryl Corsaro 301-435-1045

Genetics (GEN)
Dr. David Remondini 301-435-1038

Genome (GNM)
Dr. Cheryl Corsaro 301-435-1045

Mammalian Genetics (MGN)
Dr. Camilla Day 301-435-1037

Special Reviews Y (SSS-Y)
Dr. Sally Ann Amero 301-435-1159

Infectious Diseases and Microbiology IRG (IDM)

Dr. Rona Hirschberg, Chief 301-435-1150

Bacteriology and Mycology 1 (BM-1)
Dr. Tim Henry 301-435-1147

Bacteriology and Mycology 2 (BM-2)
Dr. Lawrence Yager 301-435-0903

Experimental Virology (EVR)
Dr. Robert Freund 301-435-1050

Microbial Physiology & Genetics 1 (MBC-1)
Dr. Martin Slater 301-435-1149

Microbial Physiology & Genetics 2 (MBC-2)
Dr. Rona Hirschberg 301-435-1150

Special Reviews K/SBIR (SSS-K)
Dr. Clare Schmitt 301-435-1148

Tropical Medicine & Parasitology (TMP)
Dr. Jean Hickman 301-435-1146

Virology (VR)
Dr. Rita Anand 301-435-1151

Immunological Sciences IRG (IMM)

Dr. Calbert Laing, Chief 301-435-1221

Allergy and Immunology (ALY)
Dr. Samuel Edwards 301-435-1152

Experimental Immunology (EI)
Dr. Calbert Laing 301-435-1221

Immunobiology (IMB)
Dr. Betty Hayden 301-435-1223

Immunological Sciences (IMS)
Dr. Alexander Politis 301-435-1225

Special Reviews 4 (SSS-4)
Dr. Stephen Nigida 301-435-1222

Molecular, Cellular, and Developmental Neuroscience IRG (MDCN)

Dr. Carole Jelsema, Chief 301-435-1248

Molecular, Cellular, & Developmental Neuroscience 1 (MDCN-1)
Dr. Carl Banner 301-435-1251

Molecular, Cellular, & Developmental Neuroscience 2 (MDCN-2)
Dr. Gillian Einstein 301-435-4433

Molecular, Cellular, & Developmental Neuroscience 3 (MDCN-3)
Dr. Michael Lang 301-435-1265

Molecular, Cellular, & Developmental Neuroscience 4 (MDCN-4)
Dr. Mary Custer 301-435-1164

Molecular, Cellular, & Developmental Neuroscience 5 (MDCN-5)
Dr. Syed Husain 301-435-1224

Molecular, Cellular, & Developmental Neuroscience 6 (MDCN-6)
Dr. Michael Nunn 301-435-1257

Molecular, Cellular, & Developmental Neuroscience 7 (MDCN-7)
Dr. Joanne Fujii 301-435-1178

Special Reviews P (SSS-P)
Dr. Carole Jelsema 301-435-1248

Special Reviews Q (SSS-Q)
Dr. Anne Schaffner 301-435-1239

Special Reviews R (SSS-R)
Dr. Luigi Giacometti 301-435-1246

Visual Sciences A (VISA)
Dr. Michael Chaitin 301-435-0910

Visual Sciences C (VISC)
Dr. Carole Jelsema 301-435-1248

DIVISION OF PHYSIOLOGICAL SYSTEMS

Dr. Michael Martin, Director 301-594-7945

Cardiovascular Sciences IRG (CVS)

Dr. Jeanne Ketley, Chief 301-435-1789

Cardiovascular (CVA)
Dr. Gordon Johnson 301-435-1212

Cardiovascular and Renal (CVB)
Dr. Russell Dowell 301-435-1850

Clinical Cardiovascular Sciences (CCVS)
Dr. Russell Dowell 301-435-1850

Experimental Cardiovascular Sciences (ECS)
Dr. Anshumali Chaudhari 301-435-1210

Hematology 1 (HEM-1)
Dr. Robert Su 301-435-1195

Hematology 2 (HEM-2)
Dr. Jerrold Fried 301-435-1777

Pathology A (PTHA)
Dr. Larry Pinkus 301-435-1214

Pharmacology (PHRA)
Dr. Jeanne Ketley 301-435-1789

Endocrinology and Reproductive Sciences IRG (ENR)

Dr. Sooja Kim, Chief 301-435-1780

Biochemical Endocrinology (BCE)
Dr. Debora Hamernik 301-435-4511

Endocrinology (END)
Dr. Syed Amir 301-435-1043

Human Embryology & Development 1 (HED-1)
Dr. Michael Knecht 301-435-1046

Reproductive Biology (REB)
Dr. Dennis Leszczynski 301-435-1044

Reproductive Endocrinology (REN)
Dr. Abubakar Shaikh 301-435-1042

Integrative, Functional, and Cognitive Neuroscience IRG (IFCN)

Dr. Christine Melchior, Chief 301-435-1713

Alcohol and Toxicology 3 (ALTX-3)
Dr. Christine Melchior 301-435-1713

Integrative, Functional, & Cognitive Neuroscience 1 (IFCN-1)
Dr. Gamil Debbas 301-435-1018

Integrative, Functional, & Cognitive Neuroscience 2 (IFCN-2)
Dr. Richard Marcus 301-435-1245

Integrative, Functional, & Cognitive Neuroscience 3 (IFCN-3)
Dr. Richard Marcus 301-435-1245

Integrative, Functional, & Cognitive Neuroscience 4 (IFCN-4)
Dr. Daniel R. Kenshalo 301-435-1255

Integrative, Functional, & Cognitive Neuroscience 5 (IFCN-5)
Dr. John Bishop 301-435-1250

Integrative, Functional, & Cognitive Neuroscience 6 (IFCN-6)
Dr. Joseph Kimm 301-435-1249

Integrative, Functional, & Cognitive Neuroscience 7 (IFCN-7)
Dr. Bernard Driscoll 301-435-1242

Integrative, Functional, & Cognitive Neuroscience 8 (IFCN-8)
RAWLINGS@csr.nih.gov

Visual Sciences B (VISB) JAKUBCZL@csr.nih.gov

Musculoskeletal and Dental Sciences IRG (MSD)

Dr. Daniel McDonald, Chief 301-435-1215

Chronic Fatigue Syndrome (CFS)
Dr. J. Terrell Hoffeld 301-435-1781

General Medicine A 1 (GMA-1)
Dr. Harold Davidson 301-435-1776

General Medicine B (GMB)
Dr. Shirley Hilden 301-435-1198

Geriatrics & Rehabilitation Medicine (GRM)
Jo Pelham 301-435-1786

Oral Biology and Medicine 1 (OBM-1)
Dr. J. Terrell Hoffeld 301-435-1781

Oral Biology and Medicine 2 (OBM-2)
Dr. Priscilla Chen 301-435-1787

Orthopedics and Musculoskeletal (ORTH)
Dr. Daniel McDonald 301-435-1215

Skeletal Muscle Biology (SMB)
Dr. Paul Wagner 301-435-6809

Special Reviews 5 (SSS-5)
Dr. Nancy Shinowara 301-435-1173

Special Reviews M (SSS-M)
Dr. Jean D. Sipe 301-435-1743

Urology (UROL)
Dr. Shirley Hilden 301-435-1198

Nutritional and Metabolic Sciences IRG (NMS)

Dr. Sooja Kim, Chief 301-435-1780

Metabolism (MET)
Dr. Krish Krishnan 301-435-1041

Nutrition (NTN)
Dr. Sooja Kim 301-435-1780

Special Reviews (SSS-T)
Dr. Ann Jerkins 301-435-4514

Pathophysiological Sciences IRG (PPS)

Dr. Mushtaq Khan, Chief 301-435-1778

Alcohol and Toxicology 1 (ALTX-1) @csr.nih.gov

Alcohol and Toxicology 4 (ALTX-4)
Dr. Rass Shayiq 301-435-2359

General Medicine A 2 (GMA-2)
Dr. Mushtaq Khan 301-435-1778

Lung Biology and Pathology (LBPA)
Dr. George Barnas 301-435-0696

Respiratory & Applied Physiology (RAP)
Dr. Everett Sinnett 301-435-1016

Special Reviews 3 (SSS-3)
Dr. Gopal Sharma 301-435-1783

DIVISION OF CLINICAL AND POPULATION-BASED STUDIES

Dr. Elliot Postow, Director 301-435-0911

AIDS and Related Research IRG (AARR)

Dr. Ranga V. Srinivas, Chief 301-435-1167

AIDS and Related Research 1 (AARR-1)
Dr. Ranga V. Srinivas 301-435-1167

AIDS and Related Research 2 (AARR-2)
Dr. Sami Mayyasi 301-435-1166

AIDS and Related Research 3 (AARR-3)
Dr. Eduardo Montalvo 301-435-1168

AIDS and Related Research 4 (AARR-4)
Dr. Eduardo Montalvo 301-435-1168

AIDS and Related Research 5 (AARR-5)
Dr. Ranga V. Srinivas 301-435-1167

AIDS and Related Research 6 (AARR-6)
Dr. Sami Mayyasi 301-435-1166

AIDS and Related Research 7 (AARR-7)
Dr. Angela Pattatucci-Aragon 301-435-1775

AIDS and Related Research 8 (AARR-8)
Dr. Angela Pattatucci-Aragon 301-435-1775

Vaccines and Infectious Diseases (VACC)
Dr. Mary Clare Walker 301-435-1165

Behavioral and Biobehavioral Processes IRG (BBBP)

Dr. Anita Miller Sostek, Chief 301-435-1260

Behavioral and Biobehavioral Processes 1 (BBBP-1)
Dr. Julian Azorlosa 301-435-1507

Behavioral and Biobehavioral Processes 2 (BBBP-2)
Dr. Thomas Tatham 301-435-0692

Behavioral and Biobehavioral Processes 3 (BBBP-3)
DIMITROM@csr.nih.gov

Behavioral and Biobehavioral Processes 4 (BBBP-4)
Dr. Cheri Wiggs 301-435-1261

Behavioral and Biobehavioral Processes 5 (BBBP-5) KOZAKM@csr.nih.gov

Behavioral and Biobehavioral Processes 6 (BBBP-6)
Dr. Anita Miller Sostek 301-435-1260

Behavioral and Biobehavioral Processes 7 (BBBP-7)
Dr. Anita Miller Sostek 301-435-1260

Special Reviews (SSS-C)
Dr. Anita Miller Sostek 301-435-1260

Brain Disorders and Clinical Neuroscience IRG (BDCN)

Dr. Elliot Postow, Acting Chief 301-435-0911

Brain Disorders & Clinical Neuroscience 1 (BDCN-1) MARWAHJ@csr.nih.gov

Brain Disorders & Clinical Neuroscience 2 (BDCN-2) TEITELBH@csr.nih.gov

Brain Disorders & Clinical Neuroscience 3 (BDCN-3)
Dr. David Simpson 301-435-1278

Brain Disorders & Clinical Neuroscience 4 (BDCN-4)
Dr. Jay Joshi 301-435-1184

Brain Disorders & Clinical Neuroscience 5 (BDCN-5)
Dr. Jay Joshi 301-435-1184

Brain Disorders & Clinical Neuroscience 6 (BDCN-6)
Dr. Jay Cinque 301-435-1252

Oncological Sciences IRG (ONC)

Dr. Syed Quadri, Chief 301-435-1211

Chemical Pathology (CPA)
Dr. Victor Fung 301-435-3504

Clinical Oncology (CONC)
Dr. Jerry L. Klein 301-435-1213

Experimental Therapeutics 1 (ET-1)
Dr. Philip Perkins 301-435-1718

Experimental Therapeutics 2 (ET-2)
Dr. Marcia Litwack 301-435-1719

Metabolic Pathology (MEP)
Dr. Angela Ng 301-435-1715

Pathology B (PTHB)
Dr. Martin Padarathsingh 301-435-1717

Pathology C (PTHC)
Dr. Elaine Sierra-Rivera 301-435-1779

Radiation (RAD)
Dr. Paul Strudler 301-435-1716

Special Reviews (SSS-1)
Dr. Sharon Pulfer 301-435-1767

Special Reviews 1 (SSS-N)
Dr. Syed Quadri 301-435-1211

Risk, Prevention, and Health Behavior IRG (RPHB)

Dr. Michael Micklin, Chief 301-435-1258

Risk, Prevention, and Health Behavior 1 (RPHB-1)
Victoria Levin 301-435-0912

Risk, Prevention and Health Behavior 2 (RPHB-2)
Dr. Michele Hindi-Alexander 301-435-3554

Risk, Prevention, and Health Behavior 3 (RPHB-3)
Dr. Lee Mann 301-435-0677

Risk, Prevention, and Health Behavior 4 (RPHB-4)
Dr. Michael Micklin 301-435-1258

Special Reviews 1 (SSS-D)
Dr. Karen Sirocco 301-435-0676

Social Sciences, Nursing, Epidemiology, and Methods IRG (SNEM)

Dr. Robert Weller, Chief 301-435-0694

Epidemiology and Disease Control 1 (EDC-1)
Dr. Scott Osborne 301-435-1782

Epidemiology and Disease Control 2 (EDC-2)
Dr. David Monsees 301-435-0684

Epidemiology and Disease Control 3 (EDC-3)
Dr. Robert Weller 301-435-0694

Nursing Research (NURS)
Dr. Gertrude McFarland 301-435-1784

Safety and Occupational Health (SOH)
Dr. Charles Rafferty 301-435-3562

Social Sciences, Nursing, Epidemiology, and Methods 1 (SNEM-1)
Dr. Ellen Schwartz 301-435-0681

Social Sciences, Nursing, Epidemiology, and Methods 2 (SNEM-2)
Dr. Yvette Davis 301-435-0906

Social Sciences, Nursing, Epidemiology, and Methods 3 (SNEM-3)
Dr. Robert Weller 301-435-0694

Social Sciences, Nursing, Epidemiology, and Methods 4 (SNEM-4)
Dr. Gloria Levin 301-435-1017

Social Sciences, Nursing, Epidemiology, and Methods 5 (SNEM-5)
Dr. Robert Weller 301-435-0694

SURGERY, RADIOLOGY, AND BIOENGINEERING IRG (SRB)

Dr. Eileen Bradley, Chief 301-435-1179

Diagnostic Imaging (DMG)
Dr. Lee Rosen 301-435-1171

Diagnostic Radiology (RNM)
Dr. Eileen Bradley 301-435-1179

Special Reviews (SSS) @csr.nih.gov

Special Reviews 7 (SSS-7)
Dr. Tracy Orr 301-435-1259

Special Reviews 8 (SSS-8)
Dr. Nada Vydelingum 301-435-1176

Special Reviews 9 (SSS-9)
Dr. Bill Bunnag 301-435-1177

Special Reviews W (SSS-W)
Dr. Dharam Dhindsa 301-435-1174

Special Reviews X (SSS-X)
Dr. Lee Rosen 301-435-1171

Surgery and Bioengineering (SB)
Dr. Teresa Nesbitt 301-435-1172

Surgery, Anesthesiology, & Trauma (SAT)
Dr. Gerald Becker 301-435-1170

Appendix B
Summary Statements, Reviewer Comments, Assignment, Award, and Triage Letters

═══ Appendix B-1 ═══
Sample NIH Notice
of Grant Award

NOTICE OF GRANT AWARD
RESEARCH Issue Date: 12/26/1998
Department of Health and Human Services
National Institutes Of Health
NATIONAL HEART, LUNG, AND BLOOD INSTITUTE

Grant Number: 1 R01 HL13456-01
Principal Investigator: SMITH, JOHN S, M.D.
Project Title: XXXXXXXXXXXXXX

DIRECTOR, SPONSORED RESEARCH
UNIVERSITY OF XXXXXXXX
1000 MAIN STREET, ROOM 10
ANYTOWN, USA 11111-1111
Budget Period: 01/01/1999 - 12/31/1999
Project Period: 01/01/1999 - 12/31/2003

Dear Business Official:

The National Institutes of Health hereby awards a grant in the amount of $268,200 (see "Award Calculation" in Section I) to UNIVERSITY OF XXXXXXXXXX in support of the above referenced project. This award is pursuant to the authority of 42 USC 241 42 CFR 52 and is subject to attached terms and conditions.

Acceptance of this award including attached Terms and Conditions is acknowledged by the grantee when funds are drawn down or otherwise obtained from the grant payment system.

Award recipients are responsible for appropriate acknowledgment of NIH support when preparing publications, or issuing statements, press releases, request for proposals, bid solicitations, and other documents describing projects or programs funded in whole or in part with NIH support.

If you have any questions about this award, please contact the individual(s) referenced in the attachments.
Sincerely yours,
Grants Management Officer
NATIONAL HEART, LUNG, AND BLOOD INSTITUTE

SECTION I - AWARD DATA - 1 R01 HL13456-01 AWARD CALCULATION
(U.S. Dollars):

Direct Costs	$200,000
F&A Costs	$68,200
APPROVED BUDGET	$268,200
FINANCIAL ASSISTANCE	$268,200

Recommended future year total cost support, subject to the availability of funds and satisfactory progress of the project, is as follows.

02	$241,203
03	$241,203
04	$241,203
05	$241,203

FISCAL INFORMATION:
EIN: 1998877665A1
Document Number: R1HL13456A
IC/CAN FY1999 FY2000 FY2001 FY2002 FY2003
HL/842,4000/
268,200 241,203 241,203 241,203 241,203
NIH ADMINISTRATIVE DATA:
PCC: LLLD ACO/OC: 41.4A/Processed: NHLBIGMS15 981225 1198
Award e-mailed to: nih-nga@XXXXu.edu

SECTION II - PAYMENT/HOTLINE INFORMATION - 1 R01 HL13456-01
For Payment and HHS Office of Inspector General Hotline Information, see the NIH Home Page at http://www.nih.gov/grants/policy/awardconditions.htm

SECTION III - TERMS AND CONDITIONS - 1 R01 HL13456-01
This award is based on the application submitted to, and as approved by, the NIH on the above-titled project and is subject to the terms and conditions incorporated either directly or by reference in the following:
a. The grant program legislation and program regulation cited in this Notice of Grant Award.
b. The restrictions on the expenditure of federal funds in appropriations acts, to the extent those restrictions are pertinent to the award.
c. 45 CFR Part 74 or 45 CFR Part 92 as applicable.
d. The NIH Grants Policy Statement, including addenda in effect as of the beginning date of the budget period.
e. This award notice, INCLUDING THE TERMS AND CONDITIONS CITED BELOW. (See NIH Home Page at http://www.nih.gov/grants/policy/awardconditions.htm for certain references cited above.)
This grant is awarded under the terms and conditions of the Federal Demonstration Partnership Phase III.
This grant is subject to Streamlined Noncompeting Award Procedures (SNAP).
Treatment of Program Income:
Additional Costs

SECTION IV - ADDITIONAL TERMS AND CONDITIONS
STAFF CONTACTS
The Program Official is responsible for the scientific, programmatic and technical aspects of this project. The Grants Management Specialist is responsible for the negotiation, award and administration of this project and for interpretation of Grants Administration policies and provisions. These individuals work together in overall project administration. For up-to-date information, you may access the NIH Home Page at http://www.nih.gov/.
Program: Dr. XXXXXXXX XXXXX (301) 496-5000
Fax Number (301) 480-9999
Grants Management: XXXXX XXXXX (301) 496-8888
Fax Number (301) 480-7777
GRANT NUMBER: 1 R01 HL13456-01
P.I.: SMITH, JOHN S
INSTITUTION: UNIVERSITY OF XXXXXXXX

	YEAR 01	YEAR 02	YEAR 03	YEAR 04	YEAR 05
TOTAL DC	200,000	175,000	175,000	175,000	175,000
TOTAL F&A	68,200	66,203	66,203	66,203	66,203
TOTAL COST	268,200	241,203	241,203	241,203	241,203

	YEAR 01	YEAR 02	YEAR 03	YEAR 04	YEAR 05
F&A Cost Rate 1	40%	45.5%	45.5%	45.5%	45.50%
1. F&A Cost	170.500	145,500	145,50	145,500	145,500
F&A Costs	68,200	66,203	66,203	66,203	66,203

Appendix B-2
Sample NIH
Application Number

The application number "1 R01 HL 12345-01A1" is made up of the following components:

Application Type	Activity Code	Awarding Unit	Serial Number	Year of Support	Suffixes
1	**R01**	**HL**	**12345**	**01**	**A1**
New grant application	Regular research	NHLBI	12,345th NHLBI proposal	First year	First amended proposal

═══ Appendix B-3 ═══
Sample NIH Application Receipt Letter

October 1, 2000
Dear Dr. Writer:

Your grant application entitled "LIPID-MEDIATED GENE TRANSFER TO VASCU-LAR ENDOTHELIUM" has been received by the National Institutes of Health and assigned to a Scientific Review Group (SRG) for scientific merit evaluation and to an Institute/Center for funding consideration. Specific information about your assignment is given below. The initial peer review should be completed by November 1999, and a funding decision made shortly after the appropriate National Advisory Group meets in January 2000. Questions about the assignment should be directed to the Scientific Review Administrator (SRA) or the Division of Receipt and Referral, Center for Scientific Review (formerly Division of Research Grants), at (301) 435-0715. Other questions prior to review should be directed to the Scientific Review Administrator, and questions after the review to the program staff in the Institute/Center.

Principal Investigator: WRITER, GRANT

Assignment Number: 1 R01 HL12345-01A1
Dual Assignments: DK

Scientific Review Group:
CENTER FOR SCIENTIFIC REVIEW ECS-7
Information about SRGs may be found on the CSR Home Page
(http://www.csr.nih.gov)

Scientific Review Administrator:
DR. WILLIAM SMART, SRA
CENTER FOR SCIENTIFIC REVIEW
6701 ROCKLEDGE DR, RM 4321-MSC7818
BETHESDA, MD 20892
(301) 435-0715

<u>Institute/Center</u>
NATL HEART, LUNG, & BLOOD INST
DIV/EXTRAMURAL AFFAIRS RKL2 7100
NATIONAL INSTITUTES OF HEALTH
BETHESDA, MD 20892
(301) 480-5295

NIH announced implementation of Modular Research Grants in the December 18, 1998, issue of the NIH Guide to Grants and Contracts. The main feature of this concept is that grant applications will request direct costs in $25,000 modules, without budget detail for individual categories.

Further information can be obtained from the Modular Grants Web Site at http://www.nih.gov/grants/funding/modular/modular.htm

Appendix B-4

Sample NIH Notice of Study Section Review

03/19/01

Dear Dr. Writer:

The first phase of the dual review of your application (1 R01 HL12345-01A1) is complete. The Scientific Review Group (SRG) accorded your application a PRIORITY SCORE of 175 and a PERCENTILE of 18.6. A Summary Statement containing important evaluative comments and budget recommendations will automatically be sent to you in approximately eight weeks. Until then, no specific information regarding the review will be available.

After receiving your Summary Statement you may wish to call the program staff at the contact number listed below to discuss the contents and for advice regarding the likelihood of funding or a possible resubmission. Should a revised application be indicated, you must follow the instructions in the application kit and respond specifically to the comments in the Summary Statement. Please note that current NIH policy limits the number of amended versions of an application to two and these must be submitted within two years of the unamended version of the application.

Contact:
MARY T. NICELY, PH.D.
NATL HEART, LUNG, & BLOOD INST
DIV/EXTRAMURAL AFFAIRS RKL2 7100
NATIONAL INSTITUTES OF HEALTH
BETHESDA, MD 20892
(301) 480-5295

Appendix B-5

Sample NIH Notification of Scientific Review Action

December 22, 1999

HAPLESS, HARRY L, Ph.D.
AGGRESSIVE BIOLOGICAL, INC.
12345 LIND BURGH DRIVE
ST. LOUIS, MO 63129

Our Reference: 1 R43 DK56789-01 ZRG1 HEM-7

The scientific merit review of your application, referenced above, is complete. As part of this initial review, reviewers were asked to provide written evaluations of each application and to identify those with the highest scientific merit, generally the top half of applications they customarily review, for discussion at the meeting and assignment of a priority score. Your application did not receive a score. Unscored applications are neither routinely reviewed at a second level by a national advisory council nor considered for funding.

Enclosed is your Summary Statement containing the reviewers' comments. You should call the program official listed below to discuss your options and obtain advice.

Dr. Ira T Helpful
Diabetes, Digestive, Kidney Diseases
(301) 594-7726
HELPFUL@EXTRA.NIDDK.NIH.GOV

If you choose to resubmit, it is important to respond specifically to comments in the Summary Statement, as outlined in the instructions for submission of applications under the Small Business Innovation Research Grants (SBIR) program.

Enclosure

cc: Business or institutional official of applicant organization

═══ Appendix B-6 ═══
NIH Description of the Process
of Proposal Assignment

The following is the view of the NIH about the process of proposal assignment (from <www.csr.nih.gov/review/peerrev.htm>).

A Straightforward Description of What Happens to Your Research Project Grant Application (R01/R21) after It Is Received for Peer Review

On a major grant application receipt day, delivery trucks unload thousands of packages containing grant applications at the loading docks of the Rockledge 2 Building, the home of the NIH Center for Scientific Review (CSR). Each package is opened; the application is date-stamped and logged into the NIH database for tracking.

Over a dozen Referral Officers review the contents of some 10,000 applications each grant cycle and, using written guidelines, decide first which Integrated Review Group (IRG) would be most appropriate for assessment of scientific merit. IRGs are clusters of study sections that review similar science. Once the IRG is identified, the application is then assigned to one of the constituent study sections within the IRG. In addition to the IRG assignment, Referral Officers also identify which Institute(s)/Center(s) (I/C) of the NIH would be most suitable to fund the application, should it be considered sufficiently meritorious. Once the I/C is identified, a unique application number is assigned to each application. The Referral Office seriously considers written requests from applicants for both study section and Institute assignments (just include a cover letter with the application). The assignment process is a collegial one, with interaction, when necessary, on a case-by-case basis among Referral Officers, study section Scientific Review Administrators (SRAs), Institute program representatives, and applicants.

Within 10 days of the completion of application assignment, a computer-generated letter is mailed to each applicant and sponsored research office, listing the study section and potential funding Institute. Upon receipt of this notice, applicants can question the study section or I/C assignments by contacting either the study section SRA or the Referral Office (301-435-0715). There are official guidelines defining the content and boundaries of the science reviewed in each study section, but because of the broad scope of today's research projects, often a particular application may be reviewed by a number of different study sections. The assignment of all 10,000 applications for a given review round may take up to six weeks. If applicants have not received notification at that time, they should contact the Referral Office.

As applications are assigned to a study section, the SRA begins to read through them, analyzing content, checking for completion, and deciding which study section members would be best suited to review each application, or act as discussants. Approximately six weeks before the study section meeting, packages are mailed to members who include all of the applications to be reviewed at the meeting (with the exception of those applications for which a particular member is in conflict.) Typically, two or three members are assigned to provide written reviews of each application, and one or two additional members to serve as discussants.

NOTE: A chartered CSR study section is composed generally of 18 to 20 individuals, nominated by the SRA from among the active and productive researchers in the biomedical community, to serve for multi-year terms. The goal is to have the group's combined knowledge span the diversity of subject matter assigned to the study section for review. However, this is difficult to accomplish, and the study section's membership is frequently supplemented by temporary members and written outside opinions. In some instances, Special Emphasis Panels (SEPs) are formed on an ad-hoc basis to review applications requiring special expertise, or due to special circumstances (such as when a conflict of interest occurs).

Because of the multi-month period between submission and review of an application, applicants often wish to submit supplementary materials. However, each study section has policies for acceptance of such additional material (e.g. length; time of submission). SRAs should be contacted prior to submission, both as an alert for the SRA, and to ascertain acceptable content, format, and deadline.

One week before the convening of a study section, the SRA solicits, from all members, a list of R01 applications believed not to rank in the top half for scientific merit. The individual lists are coalesced, and a final list is established at the outset of the study section meeting. Those R01 applications in the lower half are "streamlined". They are not scored or discussed at the meeting, but reviewers' written critiques are provided, and the applicant may subsequently revise and resubmit the application. "Streamlining" is not equivalent to disapproval, but rather represents a decision by the study section that the application would not rank in the top half of applications generally reviewed by that study section.

With some minor variations, all regular CSR study section meetings follow the same format. The meetings usually last two days. Members convene around a conference table to maximize interaction. The chairperson (a member of the study section) and the SRA sit together and are responsible for jointly conducting the meeting. Representatives from the various NIH Institutes are encouraged [to] attend, but must sit in chairs set back from the conference table and may not participate in the discussions. After the assigned reviewers and discussants provide their evaluations, any outside opinions are read. After general discussion, members mark their priority scores privately for each application on scoring sheets provided by the SRA. These sheets are collected by the SRA or an administrative assistant at the conclusion of the meeting.

Within a few days after the meeting, all priority score information is entered into the application database. Computer generated priority scores and percentiles are then automatically mailed to applicants. Feedback to applicants is important. However, it requires approximately six weeks to generate an average of 80 summary statements. Once summary statements are produced and transmitted to the appropriate NIH Institute for funding consideration, the SRA's control over the review of those applications ends, and his/her attention turns to the next grant application cycle. At this junction, it is the Institute program officials who become the applicant's link to the NIH with regard to interpretation of the reviews and the disposition of the application.

There is a flow to the review process, repeated cycle after cycle. For example, applications submitted for the October/November receipt dates will be assigned to CSR study sections by early December, and sent out to members of the study section for scientific review in late December/January.

Study sections meet between mid-February and mid-March, and summary statements are prepared by late April/May. Institute Advisory Councils, the second step in NIH peer review, meet in May/June to consider the study sections' recommendations, and successful applicants can begin to receive funding several months later.

While this introduction describes R01/R21 applications, other types of grant applications reviewed in CSR are handled in a similar manner, but there are some differences. Several types of applications (e.g. Small Business Innovation Research (SBIR) and fellowships) receive expedited review and have receipt deadlines one to two months later than R01s. Also, SBIRs are always reviewed by Special Emphasis Panels and fellowships are not "streamlined."

Appendix B-7
Summary Statement
Comments

The following comments are excerpted from Summary Statements.

- "... most of the experiments duplicate work already done in other systems."
- "... the application remains rooted in descriptive analysis, with only vague statements regarding hypotheses."
- "There is very little explanation of the importance of these experiments."
- "... of limited importance because it focuses on a drug found to be unsuccessful in humans."
- " One of the weaknesses of this proposal is that the PI's hypotheses are supported only by circumstantial evidence."
- "... the figures are poor in quality."
- "... what constituted normal controls is not mentioned."
- "... the conclusion drawn from the preliminary data does not support the hypothesis."
- "... the quality of staining for TNF receptor is poor."
- "... the experiments are directed largely by techniques, without critical analysis of advantages and pitfalls of each technique."
- "... the Experimental Design does not provide information about design."
- "... as a stylistic issue, this application contains many unclear sentences, and this makes it difficult to read through."
- "... despite the attempt to address many of the pitfalls of the previous application, the current proposal still has the same defects."

Appendix C
Examples of Figures from Preliminary Data

The following are examples of typical figures from the Preliminary Data section of several successful R01 proposals.

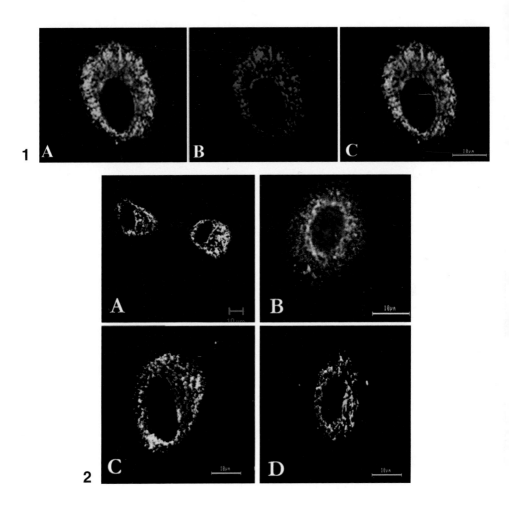

FIG. 1. Subcellular localization of protein disulfide-isomerase (PDI) and prolyl 4-hydroxylase (P4-H). Cells were fixed, permeabilized, and stained with sheep anti-P4-H antibody and mouse anti-PDI antibody as described in the text. (A) CEC stained for P4-H; (B) CEC stained for PDI; (C) superimposed signals of A and B. Bar, 10 μm. The data are representative of the four experiments.

FIG. 2. Colocalization of procollagen I and type IV collagen with PDI and P4-H. Cells were fixed, permeabilized, and stained as described in the text. Control experiments, as described in the text, were performed in parallel. (A) Procollagen I (red) with PDI (green); (B) procollagen I (red) with P4-H (green); (C) type IV collagen (green) with PDI (red); (D) type IV collagen (red) with P4-H (green). Bar, 10μm. The data are representative of the six experiments.

pletely colocalized (Fig. 3A), with a profile very similar to that observed in the untreated cells (Fig. 2A). Double-staining of the underhydroxylated procollagen I and P4-H demonstrated colocalization of the two proteins at the perinuclear site (Fig. 3B, the cell in the center), as observed in the untreated cells (Fig. 2B) Another cell in Fig. 3B showed a strong colocalization of the two proteins throughout the ER; however, our unpublished data show that this pattern of colocalization is a lesser event compared to the coincidental perinuclear sites. The underhydroxylated type IV collagen showed a large degree of colocalization with PDI (Fig. 3C), unlike the profiles observed in the untreated cells (Fig. 2C), and demonstrated colocalization at the perinuclear site with P4-H in addition to the other compartment of the ER (Fig. 3D). The perinuclear localization of the underhydroxylated collagens (both procollagen I and type IV collagen) with P4-H suggests that procollagen I synthesized in normal CEC may be underhydroxylated.

e). Phosphorylated (activated) MAPK is present in RPE of human PVR membrane.

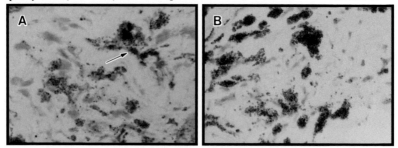

Immunohistochemistry for phosphorylated (activated) MAPK using monoclonal antibody to ERK-1 and ABC detection. (A) Epiretinal membrane from a 10 year old with traumatic PVR. Red stained cells (arrow) are positive for phosphorylated MAPK (in serial sections these cells are positive for cytokeratin showing that they are RPE). (B) Adjacent no primary control section showing pigmented RPE but no reaction product. (X380)

f). Human cultured RPE activate MAPK when stimulated by PDGF.

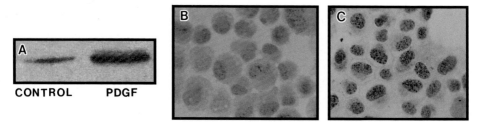

A). Serum starved RPE were stimulated with PDGF for 10 minutes. Immunoprecipitates of protein lysates were prepared with monoclonal ERK-1 antibody (p44 MAPK). In vitro phosphorylation reaction performed with cold ATP and glutathione Elk-1 fusion protein as substrate. After phosphorylation reaction, the mixture was run on a polyacrylamide gel, transfered to nitrocellulose and probed with an antibody recognizing phospho-Elk-1 (Ser383). Note the prominent increase in MAPK activity after PDGF stimulation. B,C). Immunohistochemistry of similarly treated RPE cells stained with an antibody against phosph-MAPK. In unstimulated RPE (B) only punctate nuclear staining is present. After PDGF (C), note the prominent increase in nuclear phosph-MAPK. (X650)

g). PDGF stimulated RPE migration is markedly inhibited by the MAPK inhibitior.

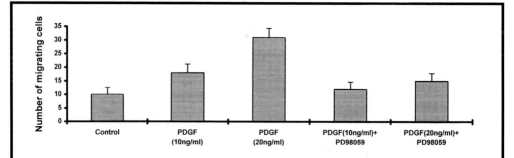

Chemotactic migration measured in a Boyden chamber (500,000 cells in upper compartment). PDGF in the lower chamber strongly stimulated chemotactic migration in a dose responsive manner. The MAPK inhibitor PD 98059 almost completely inhibited the PDGF stimulated increase. Checkerboard analysis revealed that PDGF also stimulated chemokinesis however this was not inhibited by PD 98059 (not shown)

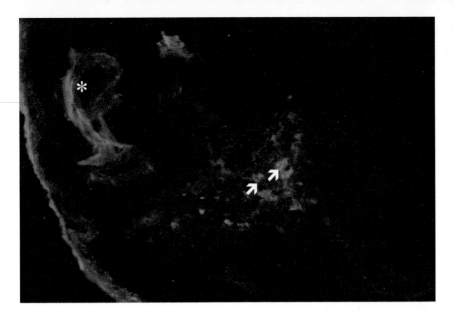

Fig. 3 Frozen section of retina from a Tie2-GFP transgenic mouse in which CNV has been induced by laser photocoagulation one week previously. A large choroidal vessel shows constitutive expression of Tie 2 (*). There is prominant Tie2 expression in the neovascular channels within the CNV (arrows). The normal adjacent choriocapillaris is only weakly positive at this exposure. The sclera at the left lower corner of the figure shows autofluorescence and does not signify Tie2 expression. Fluorescence image (X400).

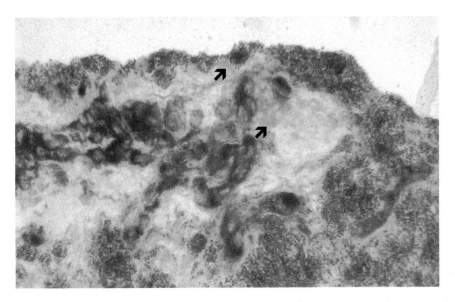

Fig. 4 Frozen section of human CNV membrane showing expression of TNF (blue, arrow) and CD31 (endothelial cells; red) by immunoperoxidase staining. The TNF positive cells are adjacent to the neovascular channels however colocolization does not occur. Brown pigment is present in residual RPE. (X800).

Preliminary Data:
The following data are presented in support of our hypotheses. **Specific Aim #1** concerns the expression of Ang1, Ang2 and Tie2 in human and experimental CNV membranes and the mechanism by which they are upregulated. We show here that: (Fig. 1), Ang1, Ang2, and Tie2 are expressed in human CNV membranes; (Fig. 2) while Ang2 is present mainly in CEC, it also colocalizes with cytokeratin positive RPE; many of the same cells that express VEGF also express Ang1, (Fig. 3), Tie2 is constitutively expressed in CEC and is upregulated in the newly formed vessels in a murine laser model; (Fig 4), TNF is present in human CNV membranes adjacent to the neovascular channels; (Fig. 5), VEGF stimulates Ang1 and Ang2 mRNA expression in RPE, while TNF increases Ang2 and Tie2 expression in CEC. **Specific Aim # 2** concerns the mechanism by which Tie2 activation stimulates choroidal neovascularization. We show that; (Fig. 6), Ang1 is chemotactic for CEC and rapidly activates protein kinase C and that (Fig. 7), we have developed adeno-viral vector concurrently producing green fluorescent protein (GFP) and Ang1 for proposed experiments. **Specific Aim # 3** concerns the effects of inhibiting Tie2 activation on CNV in vitro and in vivo. We show that (Fig. 8), while CEC but not RPE express Tie2 on the cell surface, both RPE and CEC demonstrate positive bands on Northern blot and secrete soluble Tie2 in their supernatants. We also show that (Fig. 9), an adenoviral vector producing systemic Tie2 can inhibit CNV formation in vivo.

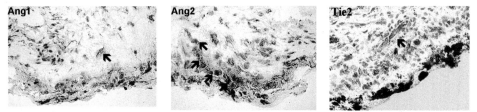

Fig.1 Frozen sections demonstrating Ang1, Ang2 and Tie2 expression (red reaction product, arrows) in active CNV membranes of AMD patients. Ang2 staining was always more prominent than Ang1 in active membranes. While Ang1 stains stromal cells, Ang2 mainly stains endothelial cells. Tie2 was predominantly expressed on endothelial cells. (X400)

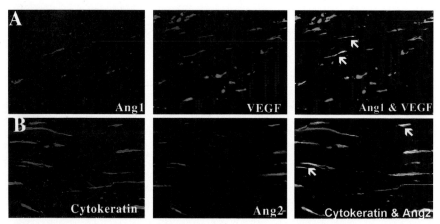

Fig. 2 Frozen section identification of cell types that express Ang1, Ang2, VEGF and cytokeratin by double staining with cell marker antibodies, (yellow color indicates colocalization, arrows). **(A)** Ang1 colocalizes with VEGF in a subset of stromal (RPE) cells. **(B)** While Ang2 was mainly expressed on endothelial cells coexpression with cytokeratin positive RPE was also seen. (X400)

Appendix D
Examples of Design Format

The following are examples of Experimental Design pages of several successful proposals.

Appendix D-1
Design Example

Specific Aim 2: Evaluate generation of cytotoxic agents (*cytokines and oxidants*) by the migrated microglia in the early phase of EAU.

Hypothesis: iNOS expression and peroxynitrite generation by migrated microglia occur early in the development of experimental EAU.

Experiment 3. Determine expression of iNOS by the migrated microglia and generation of peroxynitrite by these cells in the early phase of EAU.

Rationale: In the preliminary studies, we have demonstrated that at the early phase of EAU, the retinal microglia migrate to the outer retina/photoreceptor cell layer. We have also shown that microglia isolated from normal adult rats produce O_2^-, •NO, and peroxynitrite on stimulation in vitro, and in vivo microglia isolated from axotomized/EAU rats generate peroxynitrite. In this study, we further define these experiments to confirm the oxidant species peroxynitrite by determining iNOS expression, peroxynitrite being the combination product of O_2^- and •NO. Localization of iNOS and peroxynitrite in the migrated microglia will be also attempted.

Design:

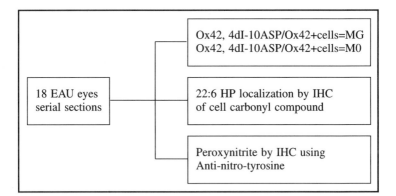

1. Induce EAU in 18 chimeric rats with optic nerve axotomy.
2. Sacrifice 6 animals each on days 8, 9, and 10.
3. Detect intracellularly generated peroxynitrite by nonfluorescent dihydrorhodamine, which in the presence of peroxynitrite forms a fluorescent rhodamine (Preliminary Studies, Experiment IX).
4. Counterstain with Ox42 and rhodamine to further confirm the identity of microglia. Similarly a different section of the retina will be processed to localize iNOS.

328

Data analysis/Significance: Examination of the sections with appropriate excitation/ emission filters should localize the intracellular presence of peroxynitrite. The presence of fluorescent rhodamine in Ox42-positive cells in the outer retina will suggest the generation of peroxynitrite by either microglia or macrophages. However, using the adjacent section, the co-localization of 4Di-10ASP axotomy dye and rhodamine will indicate the 4Di-10ASP-positive cells to be microglia and the dye-negative cells to be macrophages. The PCR study will reveal the presence or absence of any circulation-derived cells (macrophages) in the EAU retina.

Appendix D-2
Design Example

Experiment 9 (Specific Aim 2). Effects of Ang1 and Ang2 over-expression in RPE and CEC co-culture.

Hypothesis: When Ang2>Ang1, VEGF-induced 3D networks continue to grow and are sensitive to growth factor withdrawal. When Ang2<Ang1, VEGF-induced 3D networks show slower growth and are less sensitive to growth factor withdrawal.

Rationale. RPE and CEC can each be transduced using retroviruses to over-express genes of interest and can be selected to provide pure over-expressing cultures. Cells over-expressing Ang1 or Ang2 will be used in 3D co-cultures to show effects on CEC tubular networks. Over-expression of Ang1, relative to Ang2, in CEC and possibly RPE, should destabilize the RPE and, in the presence of VEGF, promote angiogenesis. The vessels should remain immature and will be sensitive to growth factor withdrawal. Over-expression of Ang1, relative to Ang2, in RPE and possibly CEC, should mature vascular networks and provide resistance against the effects of growth factor withdrawal.

Design.

1. Culture bovine CEC and human RPE; use early passages.
2. Develop retroviral vectors for Ang1 and Ang2.
3. Transduce cells with vectors, select with G418, collect high titer viral supernatants.
4. Co-culture CEC and RPE.
5. Treat co-cultures with varying concentrations of Ang1 and Ang2.
6. Measure volume of tubular formations.

Analysis and potential problems. Vector production and concentration are routine in this lab (see Preliminary Data). Cells will be examined for toxicity, although none is expected. Control experiments will employ "empty vector" retrovirus and B-gal retrovirus. Our system is sufficiently sensitive to detect a 25% difference in vascular tube volume.

Appendix D-3
Design Example

Table 1 *Experimental Design for Specific Aims 1 and 2*

Gp	Rabbits[1]	P. acnes Inoculum[2]	Serum[3]	Aqueous[4]	Vitreous[5]	IOL[6]	PLC[7]
Natural History Studies (Experiment 1)							
A	32 pseudo-phakic	Live	224	64	32	16 BC 16 FITC	16 BC 16 FITC
B	32 aphakic	Live	224	64	32		16 BC 16 FITC
C	16 pseudo-phakic	Saline (control)	112	32	16	8 BC 8 FITC	8 BC 8 FITC
D	16 aphakic	Saline (control)	112	32	16		8 BC 8 FITC
Nonviable P. acnes Studies (Experiment 2)							
E	16 pseudo-phakic	Heat killed	112	32	16	8 BC 8 FITC	8 BC 8 FITC
F	16 pseudo-phakic	Lysed	112	32	16	8 BC 8 FITC	8 BC 8 FITC

[1]Number of rabbits receiving unilateral ECCE surgery with (pseudophakic) or without (aphakic) IOL implantation, and followed clinically for 6 months (Specific Aim 1).

[2]Inoculum preparation injected into anterior chambers post-ECCE surgery (Specific Aim 1).

[3]Number of serum samples (7/rabbit) collected during 6-month follow-up period for the ELISA determination of antibody user to P. acnes and/or lens protein (Specific Aim 2).

[4]Number of aqueous specimens, collected at time of surgery and enucleation, for bacterial culture (Specific Aim 1) and ELISA determination of antibody liters to P. acnes and/or lens protein (Specific Aim 2).

[5]Number of vitreous specimens, collected at time of enucleation, for bacterial culture (Specific Aim 1) and ELISA determination of antibody titers to P. acnes and/or lens protein (Specific Aim 2).

[6]Number of IOLs collected at the time of enucleation for bacterial culture (BC) and immunofluorescent (FITC) identification of P. acnes (Specific Aim 1).

[7]Number of posterior lens capsules (PLC) collected at the time of enucleation for bacterial culture (BC) and immunofluorescent (FITC) identification of P. acnes (Specific Aim 1). The remainder of the enucleated eye will be submitted for histopathologic studies.

Timetable for Specific Aim 1: Experiment 1 will be performed over the first 17 months of the proposal period. We will complete the Group A and B animals in a series of four trials using 16 rabbits at a time (8 each, pseudophakic and aphakic). The Group C and D animals will be completed similarly in two trials. Experiment 2 will be performed over months 13 through 21 of the proposal period. We will complete Group E and F animals in two consecutive trials beginning at 2-month intervals as described for Groups A–D. There will be some overlap of time with the viable P. acnes long-term natural history studies described above. We will begin a trial every 2 months to provide for the appropriate use of space in the animal housing facilities and to optimize the scheduling and completion of the research week.

Appendix D-4
Design Example

AIM 1: Establish the cellular and molecular mechanisms by which HGF stimulates the formation of multilayered groups of RPE from the monolayer.

Overall Aim 1 Rationale: We hypothesize that HGF, produced by activated RPE cells, is a major mediator of phenotypic change in adjacent RPE; a relatively immotile monolayer of adherent RPE sitting on Bruch's membrane is changed into a motile population of relatively discohesive cells within a provisional ECM. Consistent with this hypothesis is the expectation that cells of the monolayer will respond differently to HGF than cells in culture. It is likely that effects on junctional proteins will be prominent in monolayer explants, while effects on ECM production, integrins and proteases may be more prominent in cultured cells.

Experiment 1: Define and compare temporal patterns of gene expression in cultured human RPE and human RPE monolayer explants after HGF treatment.

Hypothesis: RPE cultures and monolayer explants will each show distinct patterns of modulated gene expression after HGF treatment.

Rationale: Data mining and knowledge generation from expression array profiles will characterize differential HGF responses of the RPE monolayer from those of RPE cultures. Thus expression arrays will independently test the basic hypotheses of this grant and will be useful guides for subsequent experiments. Critical analysis of this data, followed by biologic validation, will reveal novel targets of HGF action.

Design:

1. Passage 2–4 human fetal RPE cultures and human RPE explant cultures

2. Expose to recombinant human HGF (20 ng/ml) for 0, 3, 6, 24 or 48 hours. Control cultures; vehicle alone.

3. Explant cultures will be dissected from fresh donor eyes (pg. 47).

4. Isolate total RNA using the Microarray core facility for generation and labeling of cDNA, and hybridization on Affymetrix U95A oligonucleotide arrays (representing over 12,000 human genes). All tests will be repeated three times from different donors.

Analysis:

1. Compare patterns of gene expression between samples at any one time point and then over time (3, 6, 24, and 48 hours) for the treated and untreated samples using weighted-linear regression t-tests.

2. "Treatment group" will be a predictor variable, coded as 1 if treated and 0 otherwise. We will stratify on replicates (1, 2 or 3) to account for the matching.

3. Measures in the untreated samples will be compared across all time points using repeated measures ANOVA.

4. Test whether average expression is constant over time, or whether a change is detected using the F-test. To compare treatment effects over time, we will perform a

general heterogeneity test followed by a test for differences in trends (slopes). A significant effect for the Treatment variable but not for the slopes will show an initial treatment effect that is maintained (constant) over all time points. A significant difference in slopes will show a treatment effect that changes over time.

5. The data from the RPE cultures will also be compared to the data from the RPE explant monolayers at each time point and over time using a linear regression model. Building on the model described for cell cultures, we can test for differences between RPE culture with RPE monolayer by introducing an indicator variable for the monolayer.

Expectations and Alternatives:

1. Both cultured RPE and monolayer explants will show significant alterations of gene expression after HGF treatment although the cultured cells and the explants will show different patterns of altered gene expression.

2. Differences may change over time as the RPE in the monolayer become dissociated and start to separate from the monolayer.

3. Variability in gene expression based on the retinal site is reduced by varying the site for each time point between experiments. We do not anticipate this to be a major problem since we have not previously seen significant differences between superior and inferior retina.

4. Through use of stringent statistical criteria only a small proportion of the genes on the chip will be identified as being of interest. The subset of genes to be studied in detail with biologic validation will be decided after temporal analysis of multiple time points with focus placed on genes that can be directly related to PVR pathogenesis.

Appendix D-5

Design Example

Experiment 7: Document photoreceptor damage by electron microscopy (E.M.) at the site of microglial infiltration.

Rationale: Damage to photoreceptors by the oxidants includes condensation and disruption of the outer segment discs of photoreceptors. This is the earliest morphologic change that can be documented by E.M. In recently reported methods, the axotomy dye 4Di-10ASP was photoconverted aerobically, and dye positive microglia were then readily identifiable in the E.M. by the inclusion of photoconverted dense granular 4Di-10ASP. Any morphologic damage of outer segments at the sites adjacent to microglia can then also be recognized.

Design: Eighteen chimeric/axotomized/EAU (days 8, 9 and 10) eyes (procedures on p. 37) will be processed for ultrastructural identification of 4Di-10ASP-positive microglia, using the oxygen-enriched photoconversion method. One half of the retina from the enucleated eye will be photoconverted following appropriate fixation for the E.M. visualization. The remaining half of the unfixed retina will be processed for DNA extraction and PCR amplification to detect the Y-chromosome, as described in our preliminary experiments (p. 25).

Data analysis/Significance: Based on our preliminary experiments (p. 27), we do not anticipate the infiltration of blood-derived macrophages in this early phase of EAU. This will be confirmed by PCR for Y-negativity, and only Y-negative retinas will be used for the study. Therefore, the photoreceptor damage adjacent to the microglia, which contain dense 4Di-10ASP deposits detectable by E.M., will indicate a pathogenic role for these cells.

Appendix E

Instructions to Reviewers Concerning Human Subjects

Yes, the world is different than 5 years ago in many ways. In the prior editions, this appendix contained two pages with the PHS Human Subjects regulations. The May 2001 revision of the PHS 398 Grant Application packet now contains more than 10 pages with instructions that pertain to human subjects. The prior edition, in April 1998, contained half as many. The many new topics and requirements are covered in Chapter 11. Study Section members must also be vigilant on these issues as they review each proposal. Incomplete detail on any of these topics requires a note in the Summary Statement as a flag to NIH staff. Severe irregularity can result in, "Not Recommended for Further Consideration."

Below is a copy of the NIH instructions to the reviewers.

NIH INSTRUCTIONS TO REVIEWERS FOR EVALUATING RESEARCH INVOLVING <u>HUMAN SUBJECTS</u> IN GRANT AND COOPERATIVE AGREEMENT APPLICATIONS
April 25, 2001

Please read the instructions contained in this document, whether this is your first time as a reviewer or you have reviewed previously. **NIH has revised the reviewer responsibilities and applicant requirements with respect to the <u>human subjects</u> elements identified below.** Each assigned application and project within an application involving human subjects must be evaluated with respect to elements listed below.

Note: The first two pages of this document summarize the reviewer responsibilities, and the subsequent pages of the document provide additional details, explanations and guidance.

REVIEWER CRITIQUE HEADINGS AND EVALUATION CODING OPTIONS

1. <u>PROTECTION OF HUMAN SUBJECTS FROM RESEARCH RISK: (page 3)</u>
  Absent (no information provided in the application – Call the Scientific Review Administrator.) or
  No Concern (acceptable risks and/or adequate protections) or
  Concerns (unacceptable risks and/or inadequate protections) or
  Exempt (See Glossary for Exemption Categories)

2. <u>DATA AND SAFETY MONITORING PLAN:</u>
(required only for clinical trials - page 4)
  Absent (no information provided in the application – Call the Scientific Review Administrator.) or
  Acceptable or
  Unacceptable

3. <u>INCLUSION OF WOMEN PLAN: (required for clinical research - page 5)</u>
  Not an NIH-defined Phase III Clinical Trial:
  Absent (no information provided in the application – Call the Scientific Review Administrator.) or
  Acceptable (representation coded 1-4, see instructions) or
  Unacceptable (representation coded 1-4 see instructions) or
  NIH-defined Phase III Clinical Trial: (see <u>special analyses requirements</u>)
  Absent (no information provided in the application – Call the Scientific Review Administrator.) or
  Acceptable (representation coded 1-4, see instructions) or
  Unacceptable (representation coded 1-4)

4. <u>INCLUSION OF MINORITIES PLAN: (page 6)</u>
  Not an NIH-defined Phase III Clinical Trial:

  Absent (no information provided in the application – Call the Scientific Review Administrator.) or
  Acceptable (representation coded 1-5, see instructions) or
  Unacceptable (representation coded 1-5) or
  NIH-defined Phase III Clinical Trial: (see <u>special analyses requirements</u>):
  Absent (no information provided in the application – Call the Scientific Review Administrator.) or
  Acceptable (representation coded 1-5, see instructions) or
  Unacceptable (representation coded 1-5)

5. <u>INCLUSION OF CHILDREN PLAN: (page 9)</u>
  Absent (no information provided in the application – Call the Scientific Review Administrator.) or
  Acceptable or
  Unacceptable

APPLICANT REQUIREMENTS (Page 2)

GLOSSARY OF TERMS (page 10)

ADDITIONAL GUIDANCE

Please refer to the Decision Trees on the NIH Peer Review Policy web page:

(http://grants.nih.gov/grants/peer/peer.htm)

Protection of Humans

Women in Clinical Research

Women in NIH-Defined Phase III Clinical Trials

Minorities in Clinical Research

Minorities in NIH-Defined Phase III Clinical Trials

Children in Human Subjects Research

Data and Safety Monitoring Plans in Clinical Trials

APPLICANT REQUIREMENTS:

1. <u>PROTECTION OF HUMAN SUBJECTS FROM RESEARCH RISK</u> (page 3)

In the <u>Human Subjects</u> Research section, applicants must (1) address the involvement of <u>human subjects</u> and protections from research risk relating to their participation in the proposed research plan, or (2) provide sufficient information on the research subjects to allow a determination by peer reviewers and NIH staff that a designated <u>exemption</u> is appropriate.

Note: NIH policy no longer requires documentation of Institutional Review Board (IRB) approval at the time of the initial peer review. <u>http://grants.nih.gov/grants/guide/notice-files/NOTOD-00-031.html</u>.

2. <u>DATA AND SAFETY MONITORING PLAN</u> (page 5)

As of the October 2000 receipt date (<u>http://grants.nih.gov/grants/guide/notice-files/NOTOD-00-038.html</u>) applicants must supply a general description of the Data and Safety Monitoring Plan for all <u>clinical trials</u> (see glossary definition) as part of the research application. The principles of data and safety monitoring require that all biomedical and behavioral clinical trials be monitored to ensure the safe and effective conduct of human subjects research, and to recommend conclusion of the trial when significant benefits or risks are identified or if it is unlikely that the trial can be concluded successfully. Risks associated with participation in research must be minimized to the extent practical and the method and degree of monitoring should be commensurate with risk.

3. <u>WOMEN AND MINORITY INCLUSION</u> (page 5)

The NIH Revitalization Act of 1993 (Public Law 103-43) requires that women and minorities must be included in all NIH-supported biomedical and behavioral <u>clinical research</u> projects involving <u>human subjects</u>, unless a clear and compelling rationale and justification establishes that inclusion is inappropriate with respect to the health of the subjects or the purpose of the research.

The most recent "NIH Guidelines on the Inclusion of Women and Minorities as Subjects in Clinical Research" (<u>http://grants.nih.gov/grants/guide/noticefiles/NOT-OD-00-048.html</u>) were published in the NIH Guide on August 2, 2000. All human clinical research (see glossary definition)

is covered by this NIH policy. Each project of a multi-project application must be individually evaluated for compliance with the policy.

Since a primary aim of <u>clinical research</u> is to provide scientific evidence leading to a change in health policy or a standard of care, it is imperative to determine whether the intervention or therapy being studied affects women or men or members of minority groups and their subpopulations differently.

Applicants must include a description of plans to conduct <u>valid analyses</u> (see glossary definition) to detect <u>significant differences</u> (see glossary definition) in intervention effect for an <u>NIH-defined Phase III Clinical Trial</u> (see glossary definition).

4. <u>INCLUSION OF CHILDREN</u> (page 9)

NIH requires that <u>children</u> (i.e., individuals under the age of 21) must be included in all <u>human subjects</u> research, conducted or supported by the NIH, unless there are scientific and ethical reasons not to include them.

This policy (<u>http://grants.nih.gov/grants/guide/noticefiles/not98-024.html</u>) applies to all NIH conducted or supported research involving <u>human subjects</u>, including research that is otherwise "exempt" in accord with Sections 101(b) and 401(b) of <u>45 CFR 46</u> - Federal Policy for the Protection of Human Subjects. The inclusion of children as subjects in research must be in compliance with all applicable subparts of 45 CFR 46 as well as with other pertinent federal laws and regulations. Therefore, applications for research involving human subjects must include a description of plan for including children. If children will be excluded from the research, the application must present an acceptable justification for the exclusion. This policy applies to all initial applications (Type 1) proposals and intramural projects submitted for receipt dates after October 1, 1998.

PROTECTION OF HUMAN SUBJECTS FROM RESEARCH RISK

REVIEWER RESPONSIBILITIES: Create a "Protection Of Human Subjects From Research Risk" heading in your written critique (using upper and lower case letters as shown).

Federal regulations (45 CFR 46.120) require that the information provided in the application (Human Subjects section e or other sections of the application) must be evaluated with reference to the following criteria:

Risk To Subjects; Adequacy Of Protection Against Risks; Potential Benefits Of The Proposed Research To The Subjects And Others; Importance Of The Knowledge To Be Gained.

Evaluate the information provided in the application, and indicate that the information is **"Absent"** or there are **"No Concerns"** or that there are **"Concerns"** or that the proposed research is **"Exempt"**.

Scoring Considerations:

If concerns are identified, they should be reflected in the priority score for scientific and technical merit assigned to the application. The negative impact on the score should reflect the seriousness of the human subjects concerns. Reviewers may also recommend limitations on the scope of the work proposed, imposition of restrictions, or elimination of objectionable (risky) procedures involving human subjects.

If the research risks are sufficiently serious and protections against the risks are so inadequate as to consider the proposed research unacceptable on ethical grounds, reviewers may recommend that no further consideration be given to the application and score the application as **NRFC** (Not Recommended for Further Consideration - An NRFC).

Your evaluation is independent of any other group who will review the research. (NIH policy no longer requires documentation of Institutional Review Board (IRB) approval at the time of the initial peer review http://grants.nih.gov/grants/guide/noticefiles/NOT-OD-00-031.html).

Absent If the applicant does not address any of the Human Subjects elements that are specifically required in the PHS 398 instructions, begin your comments in the Human Subjects section with the words **"Human Subjects Information Absent" and** call the Scientific Review Administrator.

No Concerns (acceptable risks and/or adequate protections): If the applicant has adequately and appropriately addressed the Human subjects criteria and there are no concerns as defined in the glossary of terms, then, enter the words "No Concerns (acceptable risks and/or adequate protections)".

Other issues related to the inclusion of human subjects, which are not concerns, may be communicated to the applicant or NIH staff in this section of your critique.

Concerns (actual or potentially unacceptable risk, or inadequate protection against risk, to human subjects): If the applicant has not adequately and appropriately addressed the four criteria in the application and/or you identify human subjects concerns, (defined below), then, begin your comments with the words **"Concerns (unacceptable risks and/or inadequate protections)."** Document and specify the actual or potential issues that constitute the unacceptable risks or inadequate protections against risks.

Concerns should be described in your reviews, whether or not you recommend that the application be scored.

Exempt: If the application indicates that the Human Subjects research is exempt from coverage by the regulations, then determine whether the information provided conforms to one of the categories of exempt research and whether the information justifies the exemption claimed. If it is exempt, state **"Exempt"** and specify which exemption or exemptions apply (see Glossary for list of Exemption categories).

If an exemption is claimed and you determine that the information provided does not justify the exemption, then, indicate that there is a "Concern" and indicate why you have determined that the information provided does not justify the exemption. Where is the human subjects information located in an application?

The PHS form 398 grant application requires that applicants provide information about human subjects involvement and protections from research risk in the RESEARCH PLAN and the Appendices (if applicable).

See decision tree for **Protection of Humans**

http://grants.nih.gov/grants/peer/tree_protection_hs.pdf

DATA AND SAFETY MONITORING PLAN

REVIEWER RESPONSIBILITIES: If the application contains clinical trials research, create a **"Data and Safety Monitoring Plan"** heading in your written critique (using upper and lower case letters as shown). **Required only if the application is clinical trials (see Glossary).**

Evaluate the acceptability of the proposed Data and Safety Monitoring Plan provided in the application's research plan. Data and Safety Monitoring Plan are required (http://grants. nih.gov/grants/guide/noticefiles/NOT-OD-00-038.html) of all applications that involve a clinical trial.

On the basis of the information provided in the application, document the extent to which you judge the plan is **"Absent"**, **"Acceptable,"** or **"Unacceptable."**

Scoring Considerations: If the Data And Safety Monitoring Plan is unacceptable, then, the unacceptability must be reflected in the priority score that you assign to the application.

The Data and Safety Monitoring Plan must be appropriate with respect to the potential risks to human participants, and complexity of study design.

Absent: If the applicant does not provide information about a Data and Safety Monitoring Plan, indicate **"Absent"** in the Data and Safety Monitoring section of the critique and call the Scientific Review Administrator.

Acceptable: If the general description of the Data and Safety Monitoring Plan is adequate, (e.g. defines the general structure of the monitoring entity and mechanisms for reporting Adverse Events to the NIH, the IRB, etc.), begin your comments with the word, **"Acceptable"** in the Data and Safety Monitoring section.

Unacceptable: If the information provided about Data and Safety Monitoring is inadequate, begin your comments with the word, **"Unacceptable"** and subsequently specify what is unacceptable about the plan and/or what information is missing.

Components of a Monitoring Plan

NIH requires the establishment of Data and Safety Monitoring Boards (DSMBs) for multi-site clinical trials involving interventions that entail potential risk to the participants.

(http://grants.nih.gov/grants/guide/notice-files/not98-084.html).

Generally, NIH-defined Phase III Clinical Trials require DSMBs. Smaller and earlier phase clinical trials may not require this level of oversight, and alternate monitoring plans may be more appropriate.

Applicants must submit a general description of the Data and Safety Monitoring Plan for all clinical trials. Monitoring plans are also required as part of the PHS 398 section "e. Human Subjects".

The general description of the Data and Safety Monitoring Plan should describe the entity that will be responsible for monitoring, and the policies and procedures for adverse event reporting. All monitoring plans must include a description of how Adverse Events (AEs) will be reported to the Institutional Review Board (IRB), the NIH, the Office of Biotechnology Activities (OBA) (if required), and the Food and Drug Administration (FDA) in accordance with IND or IDE regulations.

Monitoring entities may include, but are not limited to:

Principal Investigator
Independent individual/Safety Officer
Designated medical monitor
Internal Committee or Board with explicit guidelines
DSMB (required for multi-site NIH-defined Phase III Clinical Trials)
IRB (required)

A detailed Data and Safety Monitoring plan will be submitted to the applicant's IRB and subsequently to the funding IC for approval prior to award. The detailed monitoring plan must be approved by the funding IC prior to the accrual of human participants.

(http://grants.nih.gov/grants/guide/notice-files/NOTOD-00-038.html)

In addition applications involving human gene transfer research must comply with NIH Guidelines for Research Involving Recombinant DNA Molecules be and must submit protocols to the NIH Office of Biotechnology Activities (OBA), for review by the Recombinant DNA Advisory Committee(RAC) prior to final approval by the Institutional Biosafety Committee. OBA recommends that RAC review also occur prior to IRB review and submission to FDA for regulatory permission to proceed with the study.

See decision tree for **Data and Safety Monitoring Plans in Clinical Trials**

http://grants.nih.gov/grants/peer/tree_dsm_plans.pdf

WOMEN AND MINORITY INCLUSION

Reviewer Responsibilities:

Create two headings: **"Inclusion of Women"** and **"Inclusion of Minorities"** in your written critique (using upper and lower case letters as shown). Evaluate the assigned applications and each individual project within multicomponent applications to assess the plan for the inclusion of Women and Minorities or the acceptability of the justifications for exclusion provided in the application's research plan.

On the basis of the information provided in the application, designate that the information is **"Absent," "Acceptable"** or **"Unacceptable."**

Scoring Considerations: If the Inclusion Plan is unacceptable, then, the unacceptability must be reflected in the priority score that you assign to the application.

Provide a brief narrative text to answer each of the following questions separately for women and for minorities:

Inclusion Plan - Does the applicant propose a plan for the inclusion of minorities and both genders for appropriate representation? How does the applicant address the inclusion of women and members of minority groups and their subpopulations in the development of a research design that is appropriate to the scientific objectives of the study? Does the research plan describe the composition of the proposed study population in terms of sex/gender and racial/ethnic group, and does it provide a rationale for selection of such subjects.

Exclusion - Does the applicant propose justification when representation is limited or absent? Does the applicant propose exclusion of minorities and women on the basis that a requirement for inclusion is inappropriate with respect to the health of the subjects and/or with respect to the purpose of the research? Reviewers shall evaluate the justifications and assess whether they are acceptable.

Analysis Plans - Does the applicant propose an NIH-defined Phase III Clinical Trial (see Glossary for definition)? If yes, does the research plan include either (a) an adequate description of plans to conduct analyses to detect significant differences of clinical or public health importance in intervention effect by sex/gender and/or racial/ethnic subgroups when the intervention effect(s) is expected in the primary analyses, or (b) an adequate description of plans to conduct valid analyses (see Glossary) of the intervention effect in subgroups when the intervention effect(s) is not expected in the primary analyses.

Evaluation And Coding: For single project applications, assign an overall code as described below. For multi-project applications, a code should be assigned to each individual project or subproject in an application containing multiple projects or involving distinct populations or specimen collections. If only one project in a multiproject application involves clinical research, the codes assigned to that project will apply to the overall document; if there is more than one project covered by the policy, ALSO assign an overall code to the entire application as follows:

Absent: If no information is provided about the Inclusion of Women, indicate **"Absent"** in the appropriate heading section. In the absence of information or proposed plans for inclusion, reviewers should call the Scientific Review Administrator.

Representation Proposed in Project. Coding should reflect the total representation proposed for all projects or subprojects, even if some are singlegender.

Gender Codes

Format. Each code is a three digit alphanumeric string:

1st character **G** (indicates gender code)
2nd character **1, 2, 3, or 4** (representation proposed in project – see below)
3rd character **A or U** (acceptable or unacceptable – see guidance below)

Representation Proposed in Project
(2nd character)
1 = both genders
2 = only women
3 = only men
4 = gender unknown

GENDER CODES		
Gender Representation	Scientifically . . . Acceptable	Unacceptable
both included	G1A	G1U
women only	G2A	G2U
men only	G3A	G3U
unknown	G4A	G4U

Gender Inclusion In Clinical Research (Not A NIH-Defined Phase III Clinical Trial)

Acceptable: One or more of the following may apply:

Both genders are included in the study in scientifically appropriate numbers.

One gender is excluded from the study because: inclusion of these individuals would be inappropriate with respect to their health; <u>or</u> the research question addressed is relevant to only one gender; <u>or</u> evidence from prior research strongly demonstrates no difference between genders; <u>or</u> sufficient data already exist with regard to the outcome of comparable studies in the excluded gender, and duplication is not needed in this study.

One gender is excluded or severely limited because the purpose of the research constrains the applicant's selection of study subjects by gender (e.g., uniquely valuable stored specimens or existing datasets are single gender; very small numbers of subjects are involved; or overriding factors dictate selection of subjects, such as matching of transplant recipients, or availability of rare surgical specimens).

Gender representation of specimens or existing datasets cannot be accurately determined (e.g., pooled blood samples, stored specimens, or datasets with incomplete gender documentation are used), <u>and</u> this does not compromise the scientific objectives of the research.

Unacceptable: Representation fails to conform to NIH policy guidelines summarized in this document and the NIH Guidelines pertinent to the scientific purpose and type of study; or the application provides insufficient information, or does not adequately justify limited representation of one gender.

Gender Requirements for <u>NIH-defined Phase III Clinical Trials</u>:

Acceptable: One or more of the following may apply based on review of prior evidence:

Available evidence strongly indicates significant gender differences of clinical or public health importance in intervention effect, and the study design is appropriate to answer two separate primary questions — one for males and one for females — with adequate sample size for each gender. **The research plan must include a description of plans to conduct analyses to detect <u>significant differences</u> in intervention effect.**

Available evidence strongly indicates there is no significant difference of clinical or public health importance between males and females in relation to the study variables. (Representation of both genders is not required; however, inclusion of both genders is encouraged.)

There is no clear-cut scientific evidence to rule out <u>significant differences</u> of clinical or public health importance between males and females in relation to study variables, and study design includes sufficient and appropriate representation of both genders to permit <u>valid analyses</u> of a differential intervention effect. **The research plan must include a description of plans to conduct the <u>valid analyses</u> (see glossary definition) of the intervention effect.**

One gender is excluded from the study because:

inclusion of these individuals would be inappropriate with respect to their health; <u>or</u>

Inclusion of these individuals would be inappropriate with respect to the purposes of the research (e.g., the research question addressed is only relevant to one gender).

Unacceptable: Representation fails to conform to NIH policy guidelines summarized in this document and the NIH Guidelines pertinent to the scientific purpose and type of study; or the application fails to provide an appropriate analysis plan.

MINORITY CODING

A minority group is defined as "... a readily identifiable subset of the US population which is distinguished by either racial, ethnic and/or cultural heritage." In accordance with OMB Directive No.15, the basic racial and ethnic categories are: <u>American Indian or Alaska Native</u>; <u>Asian</u>; <u>Black or African American</u>, <u>Hispanic or Latino</u>; <u>Native Hawaiian or Other Pacific Islander</u> and <u>White</u>. It is not anticipated that every study will include all minority groups and subgroups. The inclusion of minority groups should be determined by the scientific questions under examination and their relevance to racial or ethnic groups. Applications should describe the subgroups that will be included in the research.

In foreign research projects involving human subjects, the definition of minority groups may be different than in the US; if there are scientific reasons for examining minority group or subgroup differences in such settings, studies should be designed to accommodate such differences.

Minority Codes

Format. Each code is a three digit alphanumeric string:

1st character **M** (indicated minority code)
2nd character **1, 2, 3, 4, or 5** (representation proposed in project – see below)
3rd character **A or U** (scientifically acceptable or unacceptable – see below)

Representation Proposed in Project (2nd character)

1 = minority and nonminority
2 = only minority
3 = only nonminority
4 = minority representation unknown
5 = only foreign subjects in study population (no U.S. subjects). If the study population includes both foreign and U.S. study subjects then use codes 1 thru 4 to describe the U.S. component (do not use code 5).

Acceptability/Unacceptability of Representation of Minorities (3rd character)

A = Representation is scientifically <u>acceptable</u> and recruitment/retention has been realistically addressed, or an acceptable justification for exclusion has been provided.

U = Representation is <u>unacceptable</u>. Application fails to conform to NIH policy guidelines in relation to the scientific purpose of the study; or fails to provide sufficient information; or does not adequately justify exclusion of minority consideration in subjects; or does not realistically address recruitment/retention.

MINORITY CODES		
Minority Representation	Scientifically . . . Acceptable	Unacceptable
minorities and non-minorities included	M1A	M1U
minorities only	M2A	M2U
non-minorities only	M3A	M3U
Unknown	M4A	M4U
Foreign	M5A	M5U

Minority Inclusion in Clinical Research; Not a NIH defined <u>NIH-defined Phase III Clinical Trial</u>.

Acceptable: One or more of the following may apply:

Minority individuals are included in scientifically appropriate numbers.

Some or all minority groups or subgroups are excluded from the study because:

Inclusion of these individuals would be inappropriate with respect to their health; <u>or</u>

The research question addressed is relevant to only one racial or ethnic group; <u>or</u>

Evidence from prior research strongly demonstrates no differences between racial or ethnic groups on the outcome variables; or a single minority group study is proposed to fill a research gap; <u>or</u>

Sufficient data already exists with regard to the outcome of comparable studies in the excluded racial or ethnic groups and duplication is not needed in this study; <u>or</u>

3. Some minority groups or subgroups are excluded or poorly represented because the geographical location of the study has only limited numbers of these minority groups who would be eligible for the study, <u>and</u> the investigator has satisfactorily addressed this issue in terms of the size of the study, the relevant characteristics of the disease, disorder or condition, or the feasibility of making a collaboration or consortium or other arrangements to include representation.

4. Some minority groups or subgroups are excluded or poorly represented because the purpose of the research constrains the applicant's selection of study subjects by race or ethnicity (e.g., uniquely valuable cohorts, stored specimens or existing datasets are of limited minority representation, very small numbers of subjects are involved, or overriding factors dictate selection of subjects, such as matching of transplant recipients or availability of rare surgical specimens).

5. Racial or ethnic origin of specimens or existing datasets cannot be accurately determined (e.g., pooled blood samples, stored specimens or data sets with incomplete racial or ethnic documentation are used) <u>and</u> this does not compromise the scientific objectives of the research.

Unacceptable: Minority representation fails to conform to NIH policy guidelines summarized in this document and in the NIH Guidelines pertinent to the scientific purpose and type of study, insufficient information is provided; or the application does not adequately justify limited representation of minority groups or subgroups.

Minority Requirements for NIH-defined Phase III Clinical Trials

Acceptable: One or more may apply:

Available evidence strongly indicates significant racial or ethnic differences in intervention effects, and the study design is appropriate to answer separate primary questions for each of the relevant racial or ethnic subgroups, with adequate sample size for each. **The research plan must include a description of plans to conduct analyses to detect** significant differences **in intervention effect.**

Available evidence strongly indicates that there are no significant differences of clinical or public health importance among racial or ethnic groups or subgroups in relation to the effects of study variables. (Minority representation is not required as a subject selection criterion; however, inclusion of minority group or subgroup members is encouraged.)

There is no clear-cut scientific evidence to rule out significant differences of clinical or public health importance among racial or ethnic groups or subgroups in relation to the effects of study variables, and the study design includes sufficient and appropriate representation of minority groups to permit valid analyses (see note below) of a differential intervention effect. **The Research Plan in the application or proposal must include a description of plans to conduct the** valid analyses **(see Glossary definition) of the intervention effect in subgroups.**

Some minority groups or subgroups are excluded from the study because:

Inclusion of these individuals would be inappropriate with respect to their health; or

Inclusion of these individuals would be inappropriate with respect to the purposes of the research (e.g., the research question addressed is not relevant to all subgroups).

Unacceptable: Minority representation fails to conform to NIH policy guidelines summarized in this document and in the NIH Guidelines pertinent to the scientific purpose and type of study, insufficient information is provided; or the application does not adequately justify limited representation of minority groups or subgroups, or the application fails to provide an appropriate analysis plan.

See decision trees for:

Women in Clinical Research

http://grants.nih.gov/grants/peer/tree_women_clinical_research.pdf

Women in NIH-Defined Phase III Clinical Trials

http://grants.nih.gov/grants/peer/tree_women_clinical_trials.pdf

Minorities in Clinical Research

http://grants.nih.gov/grants/peer/tree_minorities_clinical_research.pdf

Minorities in NIH-Defined Phase III Clinical Trials

http://grants.nih.gov/grants/peer/tree_minorities_clinical_trials.pdf

INCLUSION OF CHILDREN IN HUMAN SUBJECTS RESEARCH

REVIEWER RESPONSIBILITIES: Create an "Inclusion of Children Plan" heading in your written critique (using upper and lower case letters as shown)

Evaluate the acceptability of the proposed plan for the inclusion of children or the acceptability of the justifications for exclusion provided in the application's research plan.

On the basis of the information provided in the application document the extent to which you judge the plan is **"Absent"**, **"Acceptable,"** or **"Unacceptable."**

> **Scoring Considerations:** If the Inclusion Plan is unacceptable, then, the unacceptability must be reflected in the priority score that you assign to the application.

Reviewers are asked to evaluate the appropriateness of the population studied in terms of the aims of the research and ethical standards, the expertise of the investigative team in dealing with children at the ages included, and the appropriateness of the facilities. Evaluate and code (see instructions below) each project and subproject separately for inclusion of children.

The PI must describe in the application, under a section "Participation of Children," the plans to include children and a rationale for selecting or excluding a specific age range of child, or an explanation of the reason(s) for excluding children. Additional information is provided in the Human Subjects section.

Absent: If no information is provided about the Inclusion of Children, indicate **"Absent"** in the heading section.

In the absence of information on the proposed plans for inclusion, reviewers should call the Scientific Review Administrator.

An **Acceptable** plan is one in which the representation of children is scientifically appropriate and recruitment/retention has been realistically addressed, or an appropriate justification for exclusion has been provided.

For those plans, which are **"Acceptable"** provide one of the following codes:

C1A Both children and adults are included (e.g. inclusion is scientifically acceptable).

C2A Only children are represented in the study (e.g. inclusion is scientifically acceptable).

C3A No children included (e.g. acceptable justification for exclusion is provided).

C4A Representation of children is not known (e.g. The information on age of individuals providing specimens or in existing datasets cannot be accurately determined (e.g., pooled blood samples, stored specimens), and this does not compromise the scientific objectives of the research).

An **Unacceptable** plan is one, which fails to conform to NIH policy guidelines in relation to the scientific purpose of the study; or fails to provide sufficient information; or does not adequately justify that children are not included; or does not realistically address recruitment/retention

For those plans that are **Unacceptable** provide one of the following codes:

C1U Both children and adults are included; (e.g. no rationale is provided for selecting or excluding a specific age range of children).

C2U Only children are represented in the study (e.g. but age range is too restricted to be scientifically acceptable, such as including only children of ages 18-21).

C3U No children included (e.g. acceptable justification for exclusion is not provided).

C4U Representation of children is not known (e.g. the application does not provide sufficient information about the age distribution of the study population. the application does not comply with requirements and is unacceptable).

In all cases explain the basis for your judgment.

GLOSSARY OF TERMS

AMERICAN INDIAN OR ALASKA NATIVE:

A person having origins in any of the original peoples of North, Central, or South America and maintains tribal affiliation or community

ASIAN:

A person having origins in any of the original peoples of the Far East, Southeast Asia, or the Indian subcontinent including, for example, Cambodia, China, India, Japan, Korea, Malaysia, Pakistan, the Philippine Islands, Thailand, and Vietnam

BLACK OR AFRICAN AMERICAN:

A person having origins in any of the black racial groups of Africa. Terms such as "Haitian" or "Negro" can be used in addition to "Black or African American."

CHILD:

For purposes of this policy, a child is an individual under the age of 21 years. This policy and definition do not affect the human subject protection regulations for research on children 45 CFR 46) and their provisions for assent which remain unchanged.

It should be noted that the definition of child described above will pertain notwithstanding the FDA definition of a child as an individual from infancy to 16 years of age, and varying definitions employed by some states. Generally, state laws define what constitutes a "child," and such definitions dictate whether or not a person can legally consent to participate in a research study. However, state laws vary, and many do not address when a child can consent to participate in research. Federal Regulations (45 CFR 46, subpart D, Sec.401-409) address DHHS protections for children who participate in research, and rely on state definitions of "child" for consent purposes. Consequently, the children included in this policy (persons under the age of 21) may differ in the age at which their own consent is required and sufficient to participate in research under state law. For example, some states consider a person age 18 to be an adult and, therefore, one who can provide consent without parental permission (see also http://grants. nih.gov/grants/guide/notice-files/not98-024.html).

CLINICAL RESEARCH:

The NIH definition of clinical research is based on the 1997 Report of the NIH Director's Panel on Clinical Research that defines clinical research in the following three parts:

(1) Patient-oriented research. Research conducted with human subjects (or on material of human origin such as tissues, specimens and cognitive phenomena) for which an investigator (or colleague) directly interacts with human subjects. Excluded from this definition are in vitro studies that utilize human tissues that cannot be linked to a living individual. Patient-oriented research includes: (a) mechanisms of human disease, (b) therapeutic interventions, (c) clinical trials, or (d) development of new technologies.

(2) Epidemiologic and behavioral studies,

(3) Outcomes research and health services research.

Note: Autopsy material is not covered by the policy. When the research under review is essentially a service (e.g., statistical center or analysis laboratory) in support of another activity already found to be in compliance with this policy, a second review is not necessary.

Training grants (T32, T34, T35) are exempt from coding requirements but a term or condition of award will specify that all projects to which trainees are assigned must already be in compliance with the NIH policy on inclusion of women and minorities in clinical research.

CLINICAL TRIAL:

For purposes of reviewing applications submitted to the NIH, a clinical trial is operationally defined as a prospective biomedical or behavioral research study of human subjects that is designed to answer specific questions about biomedical or behavioral interventions (drugs, treatments, devices, or new ways of using known drugs, treatments, or devices).

Clinical trials are used to determine whether new biomedical or behavioral interventions are safe, efficacious and effective. Clinical trials of experimental drug, treatment, device or behavioral intervention may proceed through four phases:

Phase I clinical trials are done to test a new biomedical or behavioral intervention in a small group of people (e.g. 20-80) for the first time to evaluate safety (e.g. determine a safe dosage range, and identify side effects).

Phase II clinical trials are done to study the biomedical or behavioral intervention in a larger group of people (several hundred) to determine efficacy and to further evaluate its safety.

Phase III studies are done to study the efficacy of the biomedical or behavioral intervention in large groups of human subjects (from several hundred to several thousand) by comparing the intervention to other standard or experimental interventions as well as to monitor adverse effects, and to collect information that will allow the intervention to be used safely.

Phase IV studies are done after the intervention has been marketed. These studies are designed to monitor effectiveness of the approved intervention in the general population and to collect information about any adverse effects associated with widespread use.

NIH-Defined Phase III Clinical Trial:

For the purpose of the Guidelines on the Inclusion of Women and Minorities, an NIH-defined Phase III clinical trial is a broadly based prospective NIHdefined Phase III clinical investigation, usually involving several hundred or more human subjects, for the purpose of evaluating an experimental intervention in comparison with a standard or control intervention or comparing two or more existing treatments. Often the aim of such investigation is to provide evidence leading to a scientific basis for consideration of a change in health policy or standard of care. The definition includes pharmacologic, non-pharmacologic, and behavioral interventions given for disease prevention, prophylaxis, diagnosis, or therapy. Community trials and other population-based intervention trials are also included.

EXEMPTION CATEGORIES:

The six categories of research that qualify for exemption from coverage by the regulations include activities in which the only involvement of human subjects will be in one or more of the following six categories:

The six categories of research that qualify for exemption from coverage by the regulations include one or more of the following six categories:

Exemption 1: Research conducted in established or commonly accepted educational settings, involving normal educational practices, such as (a) research on regular and special education instructional strategies, or (b) research on the effectiveness of or the comparison among instructional techniques, curricula, or classroom management methods.

Exemption 2: Research involving the use of educational tests (cognitive, diagnostic, aptitude, achievement), survey procedures, interview procedures, or observation of public behavior, unless: (a) information obtained is recorded in such a manner that human subjects can be identified, directly or through identifiers linked to the subjects; and (b) any disclosure of the human subjects' responses outside the research could reasonably place the subjects at risk of criminal or civil liability or be damaging to the subjects' financial standing, employability, or reputation.

Exemption 3: Research involving the use of educational tests (cognitive, diagnostic, aptitude, achievement), survey procedures, interview procedures, or observation of public behavior that is not exempt under paragraph (2)(b) of this section, if: (a) the human subjects are elected or appointed public officials or candidates for public office; or (b) Federal statute(s) require(s) without exception that the confidentiality of the personally identifiable information will be maintained throughout the research and thereafter.

Exemption 4: Research involving the collection or study of existing data, documents, records, pathological specimens, or diagnostic specimens, if these sources are publicly available or if the information is recorded by the investigator in such a manner that subjects cannot be identified, directly or through identifiers linked to the subjects.

Exemption 5: Research and demonstration projects which are conducted by or subject to the approval of department or agency heads, and which are designed to study, evaluate, or otherwise examine: (a) public benefit or service programs; (b) procedures for obtaining benefits or services under those programs; (c) possible changes in or alternatives to those programs or procedures; or (d) possible changes in methods or levels of payment for benefits or services under those programs.

Exemption 6: Taste and food quality evaluation and consumer acceptance studies, (a) if wholesome foods without additives are consumed or (b) if a food is consumed that contains a food ingredient at or below the level and use found to be safe, or agricultural chemical or environmental contaminant at or below the level found to be safe, by the Food and Drug Administration or approved by the Environmental Protection Agency or the Food Safety and Inspection Service of the U.S. Department of Agriculture.

GENDER:

Refers to the classification of research subjects into either or both of two categories: women and men. In some cases, representation is unknown, because gender composition cannot be accurately determined (e.g., pooled blood samples or stored specimens without gender designation).

HISPANIC OR LATI'NO:

A person of Cuban, Mexican, Puerto Rican, South or Central American, or other Spanish culture or origin, regardless of race. The term, "Spanish origin," can be used in addition to "Hispanic or Latino".

HUMAN SUBJECTS:

The CODE OF FEDERAL REGULATIONS, TITLE 45, PART 46, PROTECTION OF HUMAN SUBJECTS (45-CFR-46) defines human subjects as follows:

Human subject means a living individual about whom an investigator (whether professional or student) conducting research obtains (1) data through intervention or interaction with the individual, or (2) identifiable private information. Intervention includes both physical procedures by which data are gathered (for example, venipuncture) and manipulations of the subject or the subject's environment that are performed for research purposes. Interaction includes communication or interpersonal contact between investigator and subject. Private information includes information about behavior that occurs in a context in which an individual can reasonably expect that no observation or recording is taking place, and information which has been provided for specific purposes by an individual and which the individual can reasonably expect will not be made public (for example, a medical record). Private information must be individually identifiable (i.e., the identity of the subject is or may readily be ascertained by the investigator or associated with the information) in order for obtaining the information to constitute research involving human subjects (see also the decision charts provided by the Office of Human Research Protection)

Legal requirements to protect human subjects apply to a much broader range of research than many investigators realize, and researchers using human tissue specimens are often unsure about how regulations apply to their research. Legal obligations to protect human subjects apply, for example, to research that uses–

Bodily materials, such as cells, blood or urine, tissues, organs, hair or nail clippings, even if you did not collect these materials

Residual diagnostic specimens, including specimens obtained for routine patient care that would have been discarded if not used for research

Private information, such as medical information, that can be readily identified with individuals, even if the information was not specifically collected for the study in question.

Research on cell lines or DNA samples that can be associated with individuals falls into this category.

HUMAN SUBJECTS CONCERN:

A human subject concern is defined as any actual or potential unacceptable risk, or inadequate protection against risk, to human subjects as described in any portion of the application.

HUMAN SUBJECTS RISK AND PROTECTION ISSUES:

The PHS 398 application instructions require that applicants address the following items in the Research Plan – Section e of their applications:

1. Subjects Involvement and Characteristics. Provide a detailed description of the proposed involvement of human subjects in the work previously outlined in the Research Design and Methods section. Describe the characteristics of the subject population, including their anticipated number, age range, and health status. Identify the criteria for inclusion or exclusion of any subpopulation. Explain the rationale for the involvement of special classes of subjects, such as fetuses, pregnant women, children, prisoners, institutionalized individuals, or others who are likely to be vulnerable populations.

2. Sources of Materials. Identify the sources of research material obtained from individually identifiable living human subjects in the form of specimens, records, or data. Indicate whether the material or data will be obtained specifically for research purposes or whether use will be made of existing specimens, records, or data.

3. Recruitment and Informed Consent. Describe plans for the recruitment of subjects and the consent procedures to be followed. Include the circumstances under which consent will be sought and obtained, who will seek it, the nature of the information to be provided to prospective subjects, and the method of documenting consent. The informed consent document should be submitted to the PHS only if requested.

4. Potential Risks. Describe the potential risks to subjects (physical, psychological, social, legal, or other) and assess their likelihood and seriousness to the subjects. Describe the procedures for protecting against or minimizing potential risks, including risks to confidentiality, and assess their likely effectiveness. Where appropriate, discuss provisions for ensuring necessary medical or professional intervention in the event of adverse effects to the subjects. Also, where appropriate, describe the provisions for monitoring the data collection to ensure the safety of subjects.

5. Protection Against Risk. Describe the procedures for protecting against or minimizing potential risks, including risks to confidentiality, and assess their likely effectiveness. Where appropriate, discuss provisions for ensuring necessary medical or professional intervention in the event of adverse effects to the subjects. Also, where appropriate, describe the provisions for monitoring the data collected to ensure the safety of subjects.

6. Benefits. Discuss the potential benefits of the research to the subjects and others, and the importance of the knowledge gained or to be gained. Discuss why the risks to subjects are reasonable in relation to the anticipated benefits to subjects and in relation to the importance of the knowledge that may reasonably be expected to result. Where appropriate, describe alternative treatments and procedures that might be advantageous to the subjects.

MAJORITY GROUP:

White, not of Hispanic Origin: A person having origins in any of the original peoples of Europe, North Africa, or the Middle East.

NIH recognizes the diversity of the U.S. population and that changing demographics are reflected in the changing racial and ethnic composition of the population. The terms "minority groups" and "minority subpopulations" are meant to be inclusive, rather than exclusive, of differing racial and ethnic categories.

MINORITY GROUPS:

A minority group is a readily identifiable subset of the U.S. population, which is distinguished by racial, ethnic, and/or cultural heritage.

It is not anticipated that every study will include all minority groups and subgroups. The inclusion of minority groups should be determined by the scientific questions under examination and their relevance to racial or ethnic groups.

Applicants should describe the subgroups to be included in the research. In foreign research projects involving human subjects, the definition of minority groups may be different than in the US.

NATIVE HAWAIIAN OR OTHER PACIFIC ISLANDER:

A person having origins in any of the original peoples of Hawaii, Guam, Samoa, or other Pacific Islands.

NIH-DEFINED PHASE III CLINICAL TRIAL:

For the purpose of the Guidelines on the Inclusion of Women and Minorities, an <u>NIH-defined Phase III Clinical Trial</u> is a broadly based prospective NIHdefined Phase III clinical investigation, usually involving several hundred or more human subjects, for the purpose of evaluating an experimental intervention in comparison with a standard or control intervention or comparing two or more existing treatments. Often the aim of such investigation is to provide evidence leading to a scientific basis for consideration of a change in health policy or standard of care. The definition includes pharmacologic, non-pharmacologic, and behavioral interventions given for disease prevention, prophylaxis, diagnosis, or therapy. Community trials and other population-based intervention trials are also included.

OUTREACH STRATEGIES:

These are outreach efforts by investigators and their staff(s) to appropriately recruit and retain populations of interest into research studies. Such efforts should represent a thoughtful and culturally sensitive plan of outreach and generally include involvement of other individuals and organizations relevant to the populations and communities of interest, e.g., family, religious organizations, community leaders and informal gatekeepers, and public and private institutions and organizations. The objective is to establish appropriate lines of communication and cooperation to build mutual trust and cooperation such that both the study and the participants benefit from such collaboration.

RACIAL AND ETHNIC CATEGORIES:

The Office of Management and Budget (OMB) Directive No. 15 defines the minimum standard of basic racial and ethnic categories, which are used by NIH. These definitions are used because they allow comparisons to many national databases, especially national health databases.

Therefore, the racial and ethnic categories described in this document should be used as basic guidance, cognizant of the distinction based on cultural heritage.

RESEARCH PORTFOLIO:

Each Institute and Center at the NIH has its own research portfolio, i.e., its "holdings" in research grants, cooperative agreements, contracts and intramural studies. The Institute or Center evaluates the research awards in its portfolio to identify those areas where there are knowledge gaps or which need special attention to advance the science involved. NIH may consider funding projects to achieve a research portfolio reflecting diverse study populations. With the implementation of this new policy, there will be a need to ensure that sufficient resources are provided within a program to allow for data to be developed for a smooth transition from basic research to NIH-defined Phase III clinical trials that meet the policy requirements

SCIENTIFICALLY ACCEPTABLE OR UNACCEPTABLE:

A determination, based on whether or not the gender or minority representation proposed in the research protocol conforms with NIH policy guidelines pertinent to the scientific purpose and type of study. A determination of unacceptable is reflected in the priority score assigned to the application. In addition, the definition of what constitutes SCIENTIFICALLY ACCEPTABLE OR UNACCEPTABLE changes if the research being conducted is a clinical trial, as opposed to merely being clinical research.

SIGNIFICANT DIFFERENCE:

For purposes of the NIH policies, a "significant difference" is a difference that is of clinical or public health importance, based on substantial scientific data. This definition differs from the commonly used "statistically significant difference," which refers to the event that, for a given set of data, the statistical test for a difference between the effects in two groups achieves statistical significance. Statistical significance depends upon the amount of information in the data set. With a very large amount of information, one could find a statistically significant, but clinically small difference that is of very little clinical importance. Conversely, with less information one could find a large difference of potential importance that is not statistically significant.

SUBPOPULATIONS:

Each minority group contains subpopulations, which are delimited by geographic origins, national origins and/or cultural differences. It is recognized that there are different ways of defining and reporting racial and ethnic subpopulation data. The subpopulation to which an individual is assigned depends on selfreporting of specific racial and ethnic origin. Attention to subpopulations also applies to individuals of mixed racial and/or ethnic parentage. Researchers should be cognizant of the possibility that these racial/ethnic combinations may have biomedical and/or cultural implications related to the scientific question under study.

VALID ANALYSIS:

The term "valid analysis" means an unbiased assessment. Such an assessment will, on average, yield the correct estimate of the difference in outcomes between two groups of subjects. Valid analysis can and should be conducted for both small and large studies. A valid analysis does not need to have a high statistical power for detecting a stated effect. The principal requirements for ensuring a valid analysis of the question of interest are:

Allocation of study participants of both sexes/genders (males and females) and from different racial/ethnic groups to the intervention and control groups by an unbiased process such as randomization,

Unbiased evaluation of the outcome(s) of study participants, and

Use of unbiased statistical analyses and proper methods of inference to estimate and compare the intervention effects among the gender and racial/ethnic groups.

WHITE:

A person having origins in any of the original peoples of Europe, the Middle East, or North Africa.

Appendix F

Suggested Reading

SUGGESTED READING

There are a number of articles and books in print concerning scientific writing, and several devoted to grant proposals. We have found the following helpful.

Browner, W. S.: *Publishing and Presenting Clinical Research.* Baltimore: Lippincott, Williams and Wilkins, 1999. The focus of this book is the scientific paper, but the principles apply very well to proposal writing. The sections on designing an effective experiment are excellent. This should be required reading for all graduate students in the life sciences.

Gregory, M. W.: The infectiousness of pompous prose. *Nature* **360:** 11, 1992. This wonderful commentary precisely targets our most common failing: pomposity! (See below for article.)

Hulley, S. B., and Cummings, S. R.: *Designing Clinical Research.* Baltimore: Williams and Wilkins, 2001. This book should be required reading for every clinical scientist. Its focus is the many new requirements, particularly statistical, of a well-designed clinical study. The last chapter, "Writing and Funding a Research Proposal," provides a somewhat different perspective on grantsmanship applicable to clinical research.

Iverson, C. (Ed.): *American Medical Association Manual of Style,* 9th ed. Baltimore: Lippincott, Williams and Wilkins, 1998. This is probably the most convenient authority on questions of style, references, journal format, and avoidable errors. A must for the scientific writer's library.

King, S.: *On Writing: A Memoir of the Craft.* New York: Simon and Schuster, 2000. This seems an unlikely source of inspiration for the scientific writer, but trust us—it is a worthy read.

Schermer, M.: Colorful pebbles and Darwin's dictum. *Science,* April 2001, p.11. This two-page editorial is a perfect companion to the remarks of Martin Gregory. Short is best! (See below for this editorial.)

SHOULD ANIMALS BE ANESTHETIZED BEFORE DECAPITATION?

Some IACUC groups prohibit euthanasia of experimental animals by decapitation without anesthesia, except in those experiments that would be invalidated by the use of anesthesia. The IACUC may request literature citations to support the waiver of anesthesia. The following references may be used to support the claim that anesthesia is detrimental to research involving neuroendocrinology and/or stress.

Barnes, D. M.: Steroids may influence changes in mood. *Science* **232:** 1344, 1986.

Feldman, S.: Neural pathways mediating adrenocortical responses. *FED. Proc.,* **44:** 169, 1986.

Majewski, D., Harrison, N., Schwartz, R., Barker, J., and Paul, S.: Steroid hormone metabolites are barbiturate-like moderators of the GABA receptor. *Science* **232:** 1004, 1986.

Morgan, J. J., Cohen, D. R., Hempstead, J. L., and Curran, T.: Mapping patterns for c-fos expression in the central nervous system after seizures. *Science* **237:** 192, 1987.

Siegal, R. A., Chowers, I., Conforti, N., and Feldman, S.: The role of the medial forebrain bundle in the mediation of the hypothalamic-hypophyseal-adrenal responses to acute neurogenic stress. *Brain Res. Bull.* **6:** 113, 1981.

Colorful Pebbles
and Darwin's Dictum*
Science is an exquisite blend of data and theory
MICHAEL SHERMER

Writing to a friend on September 18, 1861, Charles Darwin reflected on how far the science of geology had come since he first took it up seriously during his five-year voyage on the HMS Beagle:

> *About thirty years ago there was much talk that geologists ought only to observe and not theorise; and I well remember some one saying that at this rate a man might as well go into a gravel-pit and count the pebbles and describe the colours. How odd it is that anyone should not see that all observation must be for or against some view if it is to be of any service!*

For my money, this is one of the deepest single statements ever made on the nature of science itself, particularly in the understated denouement. If scientific observations are to be of any use, they must be tested against a theory, hypothesis or model. The facts never just speak for themselves. They must be interpreted through the colored lenses of ideas: percepts need concepts.

When Louis and Mary Leakey went to Africa in search of our hominid ancestors, they did so not because of any existing data but because of Darwin's theory of human descent and his argument that we are obviously closely related to the great apes. Because the great apes live in Africa, it is there that the fossil remains of our forebears would most likely be found. In other words, the Leakeys went to Africa because of a concept, not a percept. The data followed and confirmed this theory, the very opposite of how we usually think science works. Science is an exquisite blend of data and theory, facts and hypotheses, observations and views. We can no more expunge ourselves of biases and preferences than we can find a truly objective, Archimedean perspective—a god's-eye view—of the human condition. We are, after all, humans, not gods.

In the first half of the 20th century, philosophers and historians of science (who were mostly scientists doing philosophy and history on the side) presented science as a progressive march toward a complete understanding of Reality—an asymptotic curve to Truth. It was only a matter of time before physics (and eventually even the social sciences) would round out their equations to the sixth decimal place. Later, professional philosophers and historians took over and, in a paroxysm of postmodern deconstruction, proffered a view of science as a relativistic game played by European white males who, in a reductionistic frenzy of hermeneutical hegemony, were hell-bent on suppressing the masses beneath the thumb of dialectical scientism and technocracy. (Yes, some of them actually talk like that, and one really did call Newton's Principia a "rape manual.")

Thankfully, intellectual trends, like social movements, have a tendency to push both ends to the middle, and these two extremist views of science are now largely passé. Physics is nowhere near explaining everything to six decimal places, and as for the social sciences, in the words of a friend from New Jersey, "fuhgeddaboudit." Yet science does progress, and some views really are superior to others, regardless of the color, gender or country of origin of the scientist holding that view. Although scientific data are "theory laden," as philosophers like to say, science is truly different from art, music, religion and other forms of human expression in that it has a self-correcting mechanism built into it. If you don't catch the flaws in your theory, the slant in your bias or the distortion in your preferences, someone else will. The history of science is littered with the debris of downed theories.

Future columns will explore these borderlands of science where theory and data intersect. Let us continue to bear in mind Darwin's dictum: all observation must be for or against some view to be of any service.

The Infectiousness
of Pompous Prose*

MARTIN W. GREGORY

For centuries, scientists have been bombarded with pleas for plain language. Why have these pleas had no effect, when the problem of unreadable prose could be solved at a stroke?

There are two kinds of scientific writing: that which is intended to be read, and that which is intended merely to be cited. The latter tends to be infected by an overblown and pompous style. The disease is ubiquitous, but often undiagnosed, with the result that infection spreads to writing of the first type. I would like to present a few examples of the problem, and to offer a solution.

In 1667, Bishop Thomas Sprat implored[1] the newly formed Royal Society of London for the Improving of Natural Knowledge to "reject all the amplifications, digressions, and swellings of style; to return back to the primitive purity, and shortness, when men delivered so many *things,* almost in as many *words.*" I have quoted only one sentence, but the bishop, evidently used to a captive audience, took two pages to extol brevity.

The most common problems that occur in scientific writing are (1) too many words, and (2) the adoption of a supposed 'literary' style in the mistaken belief that the written language is different from the spoken.

A typical example of the first problem is shown in a figure (not reproduced here). The following is another: "The *main* purpose of any scientific article is to convey in the fewest *number of* words the ideas, procedures, and conclusions of an investigator *to the scientific community.* Whether *or not* this *admirable* aim is accomplished depends *to a large extent* on how skillful the author is in *assembling the words of* the *English* language."

That is the opening sentence of an editorial[2] entitled "Use, misuse and abuse of language in scientific writing". The italics are mine: all these words can be omitted without loss of meaning. The last sentence can be reduced from twenty-seven words to eight: "Whether he succeeds depends on his writing skill." Thus the problem is so insidious that it appears even in works devoted to its eradication.

Distorted prose

In the second type of problem, prose is perverted and distorted to make it difficult to understand. It is like a neoplastic transformation, rendering the original tissue (the spoken word) unidentifiable. To illustrate this point, I shall present a case, and ask you to imagine yourself using it to explain your work to a colleague in the bar. Try opening the conversation with: "The availability of culture methods to measure either the formation of antibody in mixtures of T and B cells or the antigen-driven proliferation of T cells has allowed a more precise evaluation of the phenomenon involved in induction of the immune response[3]." If I have understood the authority correctly, he means: "Some culture

---

*Reprinted by permission from *Nature* Vol. 360, pp. 11. Copyright © 1992 Macmillan Magazines Ltd.

methods have helped us to understand the immune response better. Using cell culture we can measure antibody formation in a mixture of T and B cells—or we can measure the proliferation of T cells driven by antigen."

This may not be much shorter, but it is more likely to get you a drink. Try this one: "That the sense of smell was used by these cattle was established because of the marked audible variation in inhalation intensity as the animals grazed[4]." Presumably, "marked audible variation in inhalation intensity" means loud sniffing.

Here is a severe case: "As the practical relevance of intestinal immunity in diarrhoeal disease relates to the possibility of developing effective immunisation programmes for the control of gut infections, this review will focus on insights into the functioning of the immune system particularly relevant to this goal[5]." In other words: "This review will focus on aspects relevant to vaccine development."

Aaronson wrote an article[6] called *On Style in Scientific Writing*. He cited C. D. Graham, who compiled a glossary of pompous phrases, of which Aaronson gave some examples. Rather than cite any of these examples, I quote Aaronson's comment on them: "Although Graham is pressing the point for the sake of humor, working scientists will recognise the essential veracity of his translations." Had Aaronson been talking, he would have said "he's funny but he's right".

If you wish to be unintelligible, start your sentences in the middle so that the reader doesn't know what you're talking about until half-way through: "Similar to figurative language in function, humor is another way by which we come to know the world." That quotation has taken from the book *Breathing Life into Medical Writing*[7], in which this abominable style is actively encouraged. With skill, the technique can be refined to the point where the reader has to go back to the beginning to find out how it all started: "No avicide myself and, indeed, not much of a wide-ranging aviphage, I had always assumed that the so-called glorious twelfth occurred only in August when the aristocratic victim of your matched pair of Churchills or Boss' or Purdies (or what have you at £12,000 a throw) is, of course, our only and uniquely indigenous bird, and red grouse[8]."

That sentence deserves a prize. Read enough times, it becomes apparent that the author is not talking about avicides, or about himself, or about wide-ranging aviphages, or about aristocratic victims or about throwing matched pairs of Churchills, Bosses or Purdies (whatever they are), or even about the red grouse. He's talking about *the so-called glorious twelfth*. What would a non-British reader make of all that?

When a paper of this type is read aloud, the effect is stunning. In 1880, T. H. Huxley is said to have opened his speech to the Zoological Society with this sentence: "There is evidence, the value of which has not been disputed, and which, in my judgement, amounts to proof, that between the commencement of the tertiary epoch and the present time the group of the equidae has been represented by a series of forms, of which the oldest is that which departs least from the general type of structure of the higher mammalia, while the latest is that which most widely differs from that type[9]."

The titles of some scientific journals are admirably brief. Not so the contents. Here is an example from *Gut:* "All of these measurements have wide ranges of values in both control (Doniach and Shiner, 1957; Butterworth and Perez-Santiago, 1958; Rubin *et al.,* 1960a and b; Shiner and Doniach, 1960; Chacko, Job, Johnson, and Baker, 1961; Cameron *et al.,* 1962; Jos, 1963; Yardley, Bayless, Norton, and Hendrix, 1962; Astaldi, Conrad, Ratto, and Costa, 1965; Madanagopalan *et al.,* 1965; Swanson and Thomassen, 1965; Stewart, Pollock, Hoffbrand, Mollin, and Booth, 1967; Pollock, Nagle, Jeejeebhoy, and Coghill, 1970) and coeliac (Rubin *et al.,* 1960a; Shiner and Doniach, 1960; Chacko, *et al.,* 1961; Cameron *et al.,* 1962; Jos, 1962; Yardley *et al.,* 1962; Bolt, Parrish, French, and Pollard, 1964; Madanagopalan *et al.,* 1965; Stewart *et al.,* 1967; Hamilton, Lynch, and

Reilly, 1969; Pollock *et al.,* 1970) mucosae and the differences between the means are small (Rubin *et al.,* 1960a; Shiner and Doniach, 1960; Jos, 1962; Madanagopalan *et al.,* 1965; Stewart *et al.,* 1967)[10]."

That is not verbosity. It is simply the unspeakable Harvard system, to which so many journals are needlessly committed. The 149 words can be reduced to 22 at a stroke: "All these measurements have wide ranges of values in both control[1–12] and coeliac[3–7,9,11–14] mucosae and the differences between the means are small[3,4,6,9,13–15]". The original passage is unspeakable and unreadable, but neither the author nor the editor is interested in whether anyone *reads* this article. Indeed, they prefer that no one reads beyond the summary, or better still, beyond the authors' names.

Treatment

The first of these stylistic problems is easy to treat. Authors need to reduce their articles to the fewest possible words. William Strunk dealt with the subject well in his classic *The Elements of Style*[11]. Strunk was an enthusiast. One of his students described his zeal in a later edition[12] of Strunk's book: "Omit needless words!" cries the author on page 23, and into that imperative Will Strunk really put his heart and soul. In the days when I was sitting in his class, he omitted so many needless words, and omitted them so forcibly and with such eagerness . . . that he often seemed in the position of having shortchanged himself—a man left with nothing more to say yet with time to fill . . . Will Strunk got out of this predicament by a simple trick: he uttered every sentence three times. When he delivered his oration on brevity to the class, he leaned forward over the desk, grasped his coat lapels in his hands, and, in a husky, conspiratorial voice said, 'Rule Seventeen. Omit needless words! Omit needless words! Omit needless words!' " This advice is easy to follow: all you need is a blue pencil and practice.

Treatment of the pseudo-literary style problem is difficult, and rarely attempted, even though editorial boards of journals could solve it at a stroke by rejecting incomprehensible manuscripts. The best advice to authors is to throw the draft away and start again. How can a plain, clear text emerge by this process? The scientific literature itself will provide little guidance. Some of it may be good, but in my view the best advice is to be found elsewhere. John Whale, for instance, wrote a series of articles for the *Sunday Times* which has been gathered into one volume[13] which I found particularly readable. In chapters 5 and 6 he urges us to write as we would speak. If this rule is followed, the problem virtually disappears. The solution may be simple, but that doesn't mean it is always easy to apply. You will no doubt find signs of the problem in this paper: I am only a scientist, after all.

Discussion

Pleas for scientists to write readably have failed for at least 300 years. This is because the pleas have been aimed at the wrong people: the scientists. They should have been aimed at editors. The most important aspect of a scientific paper is its scientific value, but no matter how important it is, no one will read it if it is unreadable. Most scientists have no expertise in writing. We need help. The people who should be best qualified to help us are the editors through whom our efforts pass on the way to publication. But whom do we find as editors? More scientists!

Everyone can write, so it is assumed that writing is easy, or unimportant. Everyone can paint as well, but not everyone's paintings are worth hanging on walls. To expect scientists to produce readable work without any training, and without any reward for success or retribution for failure, is like expecting us to play violins without teachers or to observe speed limits without policemen. Some may do it, but most won't or can't.

With no guidance, scientists copy what they see, and we see things like this: "The author is of the opinion that it is appropriate to write scientific papers in the third person." This is ridiculous. *I* am the author, not a third person.

If there must be scientists on editorial boards of journals, their job must be only to reject bad science. The editor's job is to reject bad writing. The editor has the power to enforce standards of readability, and should be allowed to use this power.

In conclusion, my suggestion for the elimination of unreadable papers is first to omit needless words, and second, to write as you would speak. This magnificent advice will certainly have no measurable effect. For centuries, we scientists have been showered with advice on how to write readably, and still we all ignore it. Isn't it time we sought another solution?

In my opinion, editors should be writers, not scientists. Scientists should be judged according to how many times their work is *read,* not cited. (Audience research reveals how many people listen to or watch which programmes; readership research could in principle reveal how many read our articles.) Peer review will continue to uphold scientific standards, but badly written work should be rejected, whatever its scientific standard. Authors will be prepared to work (or pay) to get their paper re-written to have it published in the best journals if the only grounds for rejection by the journals are those of unreadability. An editor could offer to rewrite such articles (for an exorbitant fee). Thus, editors will get rich, journals will get read, readers will retain their hair, and real progress will be made.

Martin W. Gregory is in the British Veterinary Project, Republic of Yemen, and can be contacted at the Foreign and Commonwealth Office, King Charles St, London SW1A 2AH, UK.

1. Sprat, T. from *The History of the Royal Society of London for the Improving of Natural Knowledge (1667)* reprinted in Ryan, L. V. *A Science Reader* (Rinehart, New York, 1959).
2. Gaafar, S. M. *Vet Parasit.* **8,** 199–200 (1981).
3. Unanue, E. R. *New Engl. J. Med.* **303,** 977–985 (1980).
4. Arnold, G. W. & Dudzinski, M. L. *Ethology of Free-Ranging Domestic Animals* (Elsevier, Oxford, 1978).
5. Rowley, D. & La Brody, J. *J. Diarrhoeal. dis. Res.* **4,** 1–9 (1986).
6. Aaronson, S. *Curr. Cont. Life Sci.* No 2, 10 (1977).
7. Sheen, A. P. *Breathing Life into Medical Writing* (Mosby, St. Louis, 1987).
8. Hillaby, J. *New Scient.* (6 May 1976).
9. Huxley, T. H. *Science* **2** (1st series, 1881). (Cited in *Science* **207,** 750; 1980).
10. Chapman, B. L., Henry, K., Paice, F., Stewart, J. S. & C. Oghill, N. F. *Gut* **5,** 905–909 (1973).

Index

363